AF604799

Air Fryer

THE ULTIMATE COLLECTION

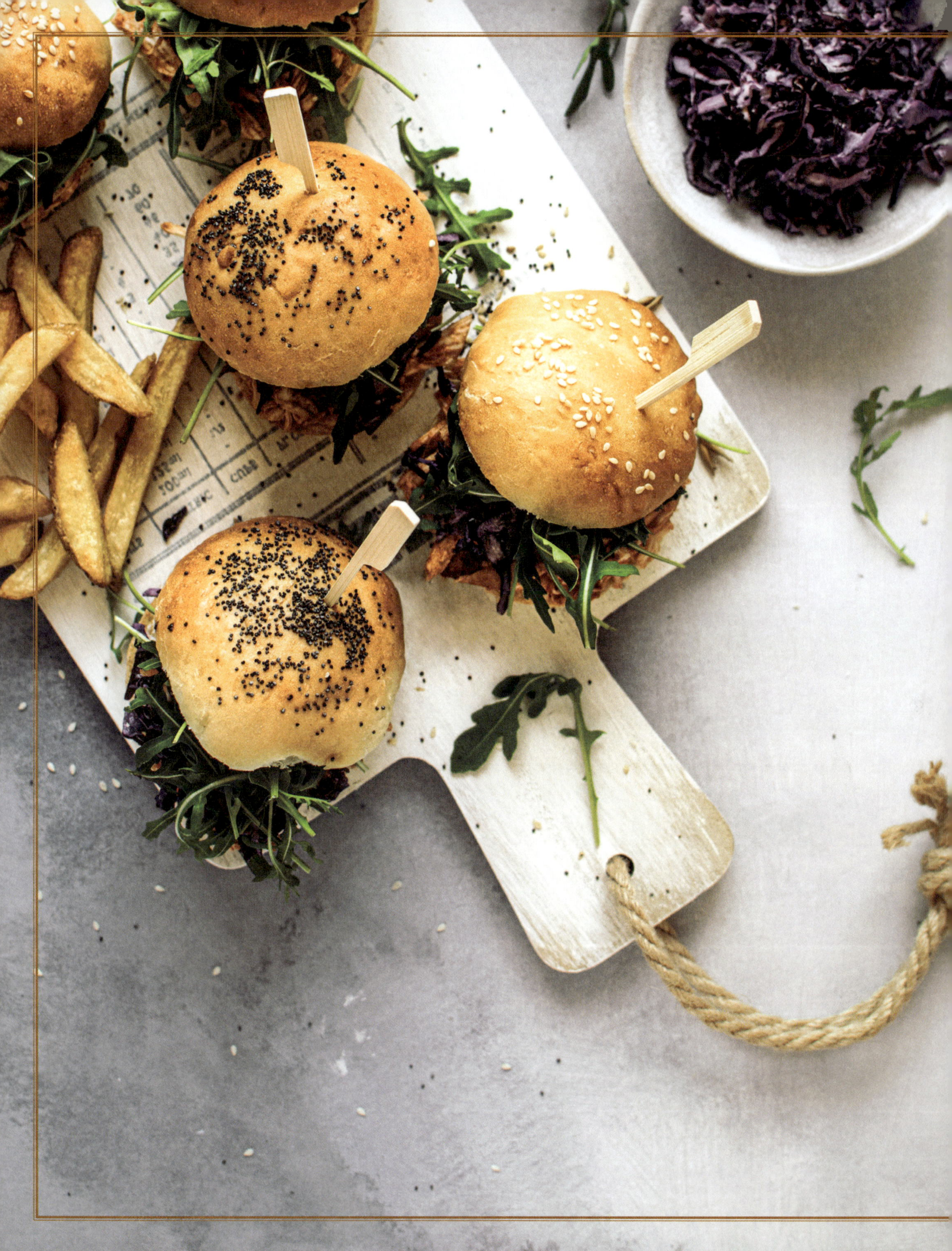

Air Fryer

THE ULTIMATE COLLECTION

The absolute best recipes, so you can make the most out of your appliance.

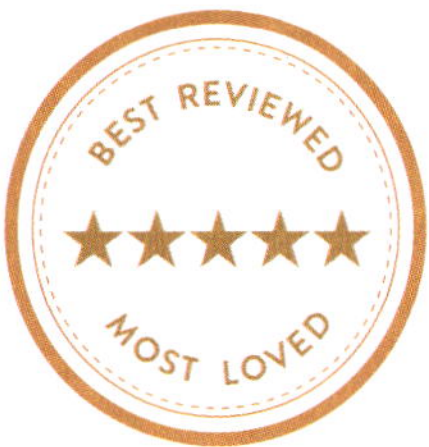

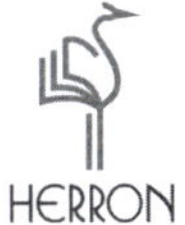

Contents

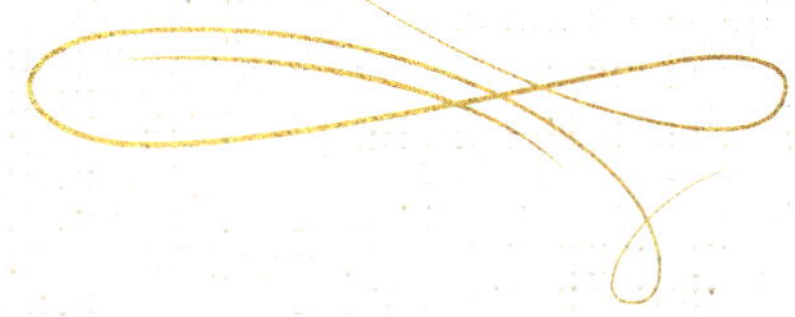

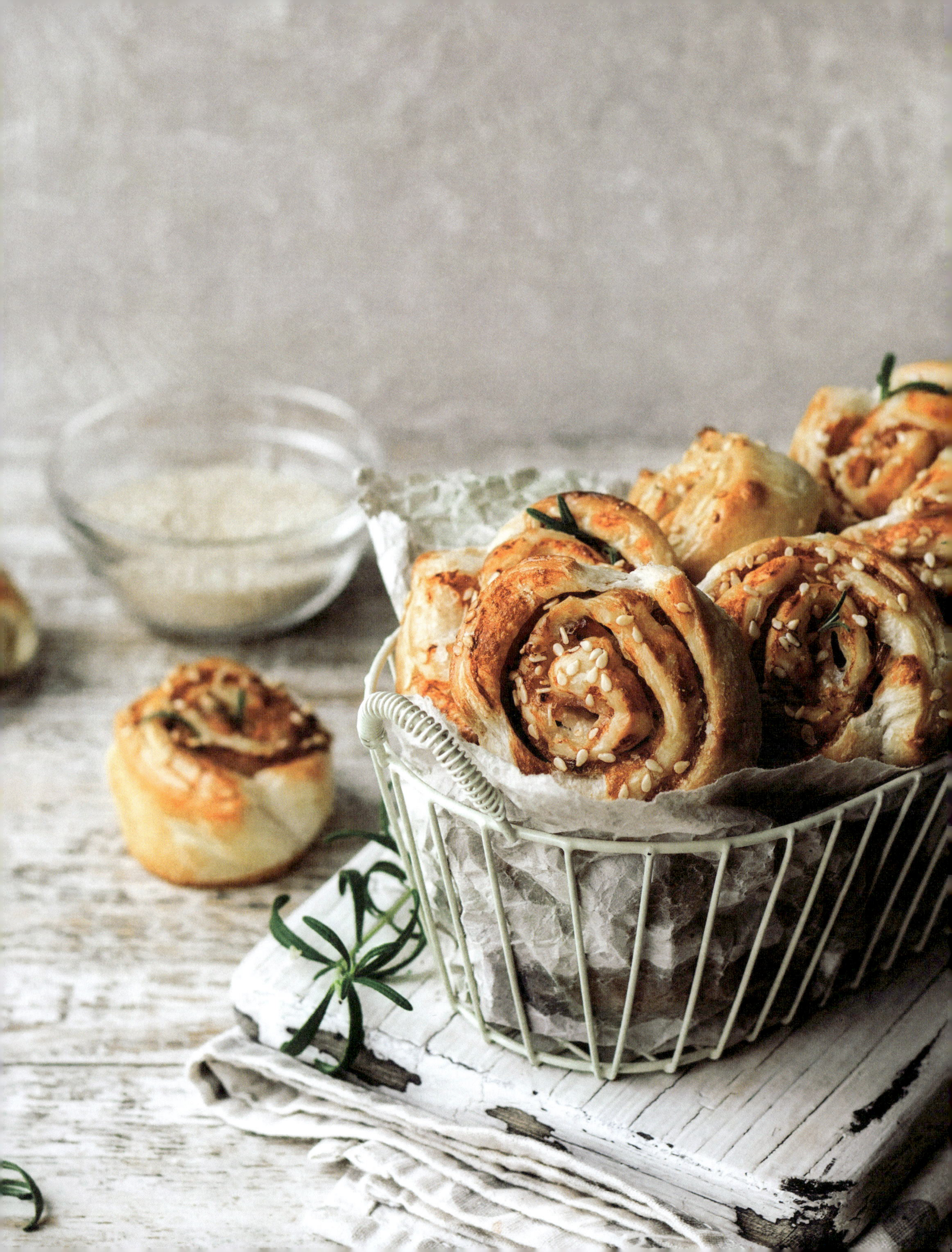

Welcome to the Ultimate Collection of Air Fryer Recipes.

The recipes in this book are the best of the best. They have been handpicked from a selection of Australia's bestselling air fryer cookbooks, so that you have the most useful, versatile and successful collection of recipes all in one place. Packed full of inspiration, ideas and practical tips, they will set you on track to air frying success.

If you are new to air fryers, you might be wondering what the fuss is about. Air fryers provide a healthier alternative to deep-frying food, but with similar (some say better) results. That's why they are such a hit with families who want to keep on eating their favourite crispy chips and nuggets but with little or no fat. The health benefit of an air fryer is number one for many, especially those looking to conserve calories or make the shift to a healthier diet, but there are other benefits too.

For busy people, the air fryer delivers when it comes to speed. Ready-made food can be cooked in about half the time a conventional oven would take. Food can be cooked from frozen too, so you save on defrosting time (and you don't have to remember to get it out of the freezer in advance).

It's called a 'fryer', but as you'll discover this machine can grill, bake and roast foods as well, so it's not limited to chicken nuggets and chips. It is extremely versatile and should be viewed like a conventional oven in terms of its capability to cook different foods. You can bake a cake in it, roast a chicken, poach an egg, cook a quiche or make sausage rolls.

Last but not least for busy people is the ease of clean up. Traditional fryers and even ovens tend to use a lot of oil and make a splashy mess around the place. The air fryer, by contrast, uses little oil and all 'mess' is contained within the appliance. Most have been designed to be very easy to clean, with removable nonstick parts that are dishwasher friendly.

Enjoy this selection of winning air fryer recipes, and embrace your appliance. It has the capacity to transform your cooking, making it easier and faster to get healthier food on the table.

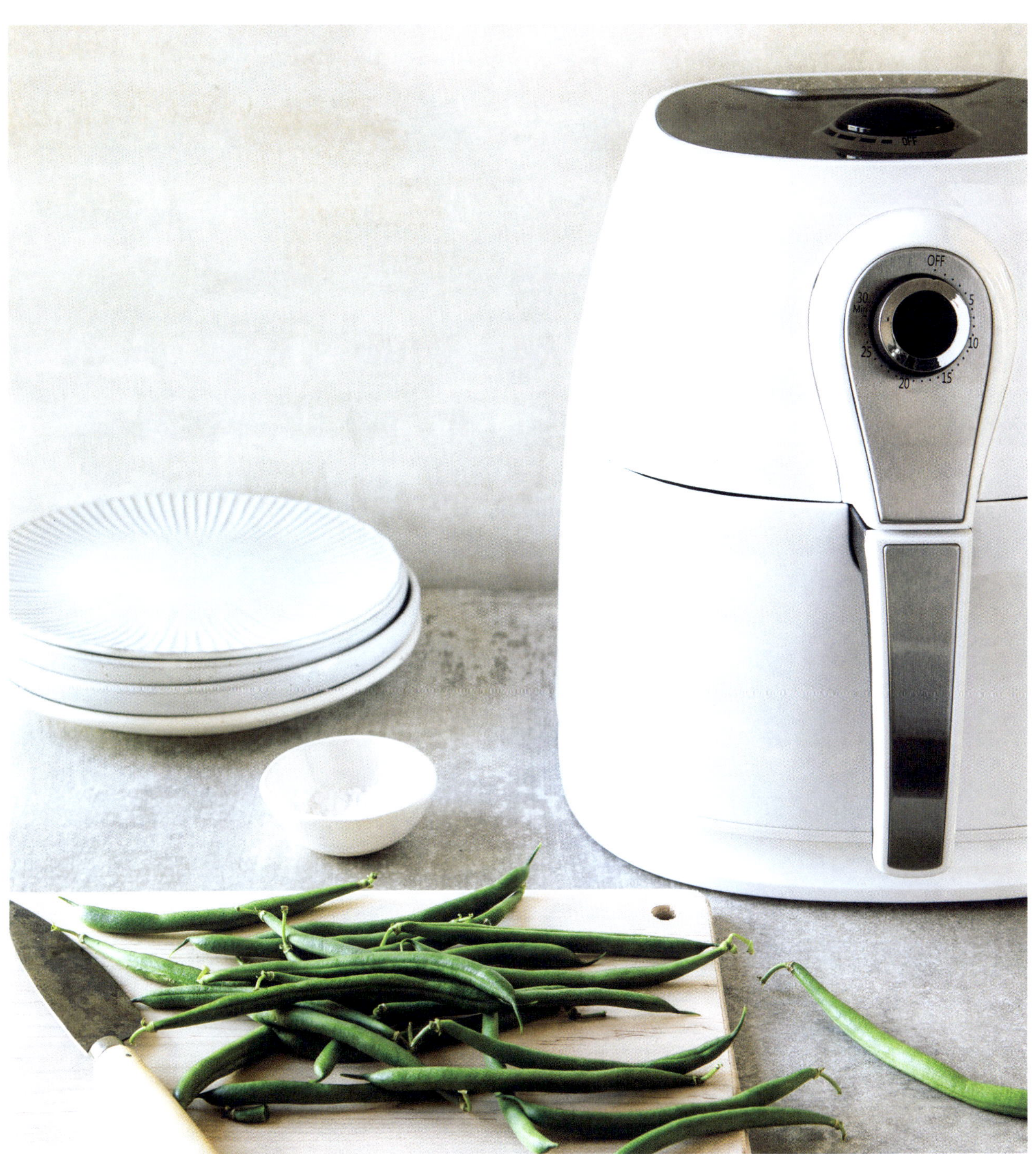
OFF
OFF
5
10
15
20
25
30 Min

Choosing an air fryer

The two factors to consider when choosing the best air fryer for you are size (capacity) and wattage (power).

Size is measured by litre capacity. Air fryers come in three main sizes - small, medium and large. The small sizes range between 3L and 3.5L, the medium between 4L and 5L, and large sizes range from 7L to 12L in capacity. These larger versions take up more bench space, but they often come with extra features such as a rotisserie or dehydrator.

If you have a large family to cook for, you will probably want to opt for a medium or large air fryer, or maybe even more than one. For couples or small families, a small air fryer may be enough. Do your homework and decide what's best for you.

Power is an important consideration during your research too. Power is measured by wattage. A higher wattage means greater power which means food will cook more quickly. If this is a priority, look for an air fryer with a high wattage.

Cooking times and temperatures

If you want to experiment with recipes beyond those in this book, you can find excellent tools online to assist with converting conventional oven temperatures to air fryer temperatures. Just google 'air fryer calculator'. A good rule of thumb to bear in mind though is the 20:20 rule: that you will generally reduce the temperature by approximately 20°C and reduce the cook time by 20%.

As with conventional cooking, the size of an ingredient, such as a potato, will influence the cooking time. Likewise, the extent to which you fill muffin trays or the size of your pies will influence cooking times. Check regularly until you are very familiar with your machine.

Accessories

The great news is that you don't have to make a big investment in air fryer accessories up front. You can use any existing dish, ramekin, cake tin, bowl or other utensil in your air fryer so long as it is made from an ovenproof material such as glass, ceramic, metal or silicone, and fits in your air fryer basket. Likewise you can use baking paper, patty pans (paper or silicone) and aluminium foil in your air fryer, just as long as this does not completely cover the bottom of the basket, which would disrupt air flow.

However, you might decide to invest in extras designed specifically for the air fryer that you feel would be helpful. Experiment with the recipes in this book and see what you most need. We have provided a list of the basics opposite. Or, if you are a complete beginner, you might prefer to purchase a starter pack, which will generally include a cake tin with a convenient handle, a double layer accessory (to expand your cooking surfaces), a pizza pan, a cooking rack with skewer holders, and a silicone mat to protect cooking surfaces. You can also buy accessory kits to suit your cooking interests, such as baking accessory kits or grilling accessory kits.

Note: One of the best things about appliances made specifically for the air fryer is their shape and size. They are designed to fit in the air fryer, whereas utensils designed for the oven tend to be bigger.

COMMON AIR FRYER ACCESSORIES

Baking pan
Cake tin
Pizza pan
Ramekins
Grill pan
Double layer accessory (or metal rack)
Bread rack
Silicone cupcake moulds
Silicone mat

The double layer accessory is especially useful because it doubles the space you have available to cook in. As the air fryer is small compared to the conventional oven, it will enable you to create food for the family without having to cook in batches.

Note: For the purposes of this book, we have assumed that you don't have any special air fryer accessories. Where a utensil is required, we have listed it in the ingredients. You will need to ensure that it fits in your air fryer and is ovenproof.

PANS AND TINS

When placing a pan or tin in the air fryer basket, leave a little space around it so that the air can circulate. For the same reason, always put the pan into the air fryer basket and never directly into the air fryer. Use oven mitts when removing pans and tins from the air fryer.

COOKING SPRAY

Not exactly an accessory, cooking oil spray is nonetheless an essential ingredient for cooking in an air fryer. Invest in a sprayer bottle (or two) that you can refill. Depending on how and what you cook, you might like to have one filled with a nonstick cooking oil and the other with olive oil (for flavour as well as its nonstick properties).

A pastry brush is also handy for applying oil to food and glaze or egg wash to pies and pastries.

Note: We have not included cooking spray in the ingredients lists for recipes, but have assumed it is a kitchen staple.

THERMOMETER

A great investment if you are serious about cooking in an air fryer is an instant-read kitchen thermometer. This will be particularly helpful for cooking meat, helping you achieve the best (and safest) results with the least fuss.

Sometimes meat and fish are simply cooked to preference, such as rare or well done (see below), but some meat, such as chicken, needs to reach a certain temperature to be safe. Chicken is cooked when the internal temperature reaches 74°C, but note that a thicker piece of meat might require a few more minutes' cooking.

Practice makes perfect, but a good rule of thumb for cooking red meat is:

For rare meat: 50°C
For medium meat: 55°C
For well-done meat: 60°C

Cooking tips

PREHEAT

If a recipe specifies preheating, you can use the preheat setting on your air fryer or, if it doesn't have one, simply set to the desired temperature and let it run for 3 minutes.

PAT DRY

Use paper towel to pat foods dry before cooking to avoid splattering and excess smoke.

SPRITZ

Lightly spritz foods with cooking spray or toss in a small amount of oil to minimise the chance of sticking to the basket and to maximise results.

SPRITZ AGAIN DURING COOKING

You don't need to do this on fatty foods, such as steak, but for anything that's coated in breadcrumbs give an extra spritz with oil during cooking, especially on any dry, floury areas, for a crispier result.

DON'T OVERCROWD THE BASKET

Give food plenty of space so that the air can circulate. This will deliver the best and crispiest results. Cook in batches or use a double layer accessory to maximise available space.

SHAKE THE BASKET

For best results, shake the basket and/or rotate food every 5-10 minutes. This will allow the air to circulate better and will result in more uniform cooking.

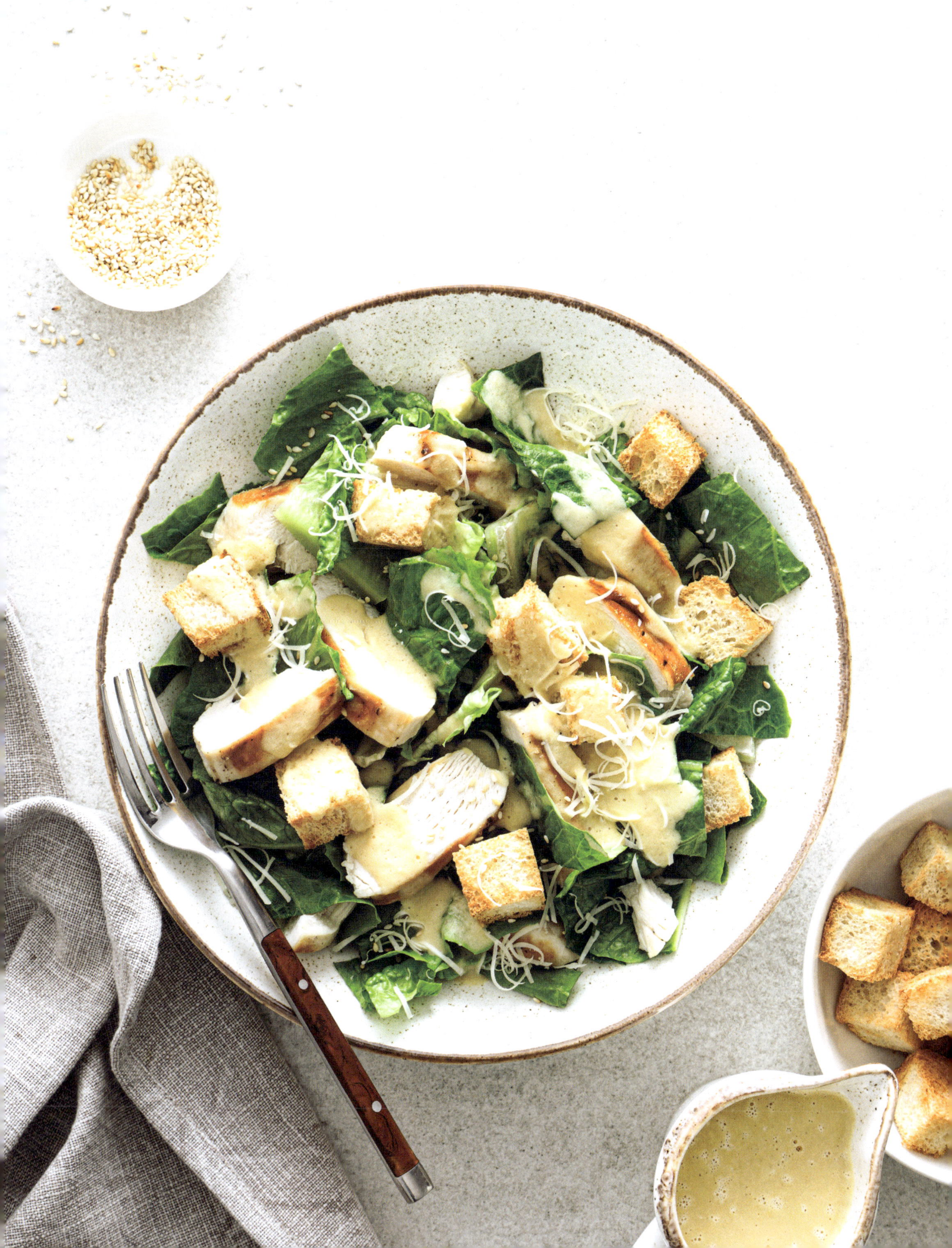

Chapter One

Hearty Breakfasts

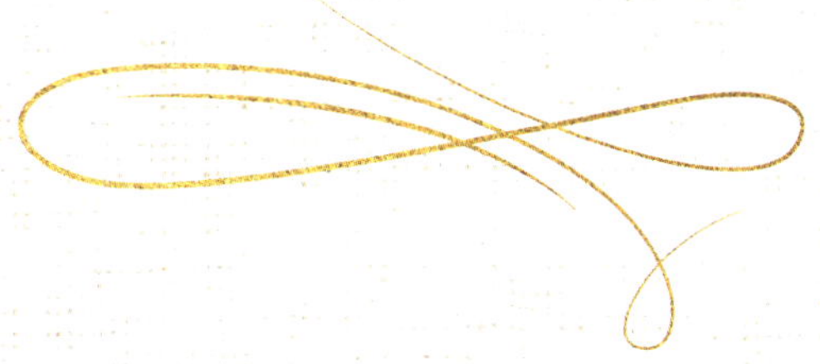

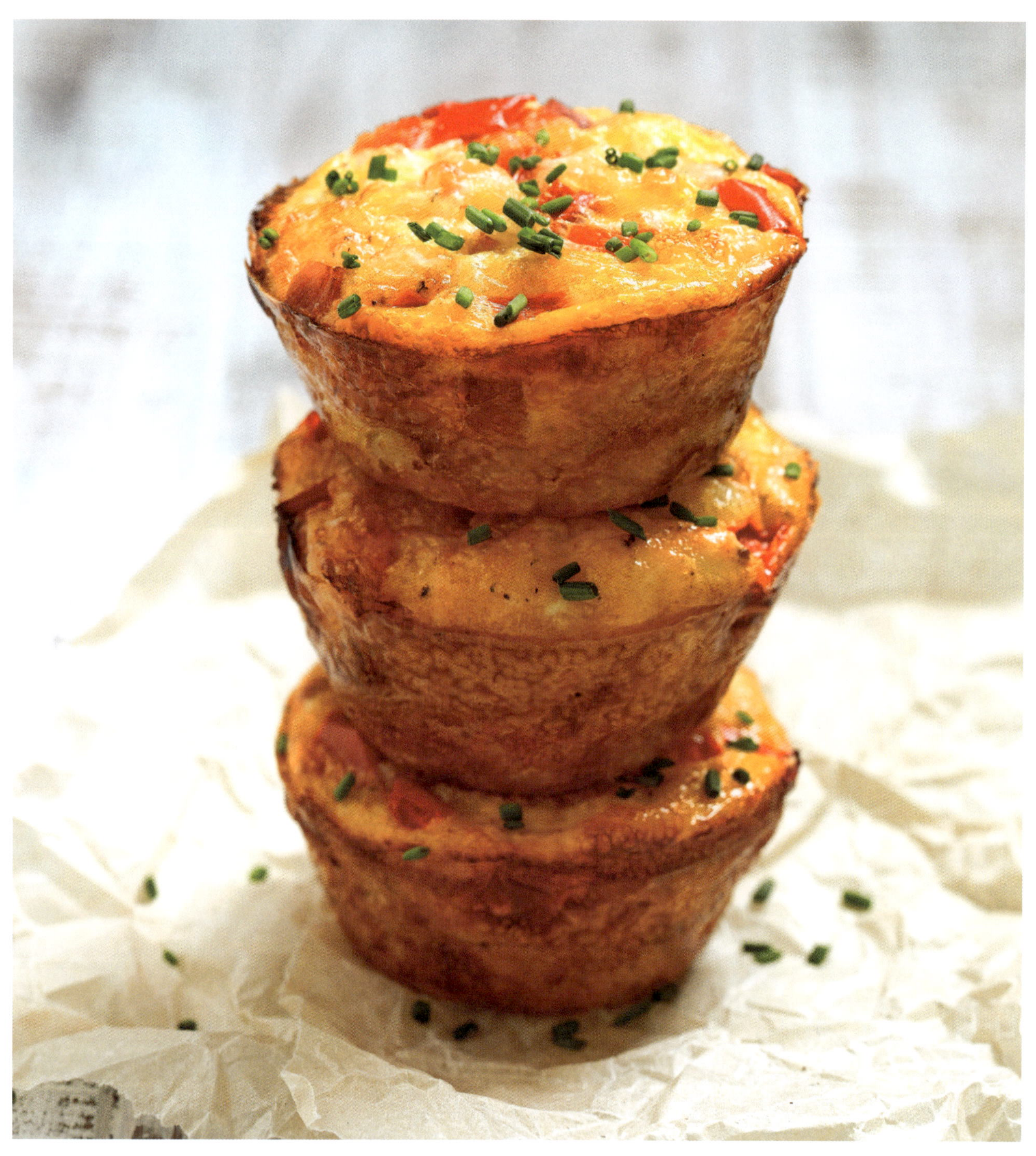

Bacon & Egg Cups

MAKES 6

PREP + COOK TIME: 25 MINS

GLUTEN FREE

BACON & EGG CUPS

6 large eggs

2 tbsps cream

Pinch of salt and pepper

½ red capsicum, diced

¼ small onion, diced

½ cup (60g) grated Cheddar cheese

3 rashers bacon, cooked and chopped

¼ cup (30g) grated mozzarella cheese

1 tbsp chopped fresh chives, to garnish

Muffin tray or silicone moulds

Lightly spray six silicone moulds with oil and transfer to the air fryer.

Place the eggs, cream, salt and pepper in a large mixing bowl and whisk to combine. Sprinkle in the capsicum, onion, Cheddar cheese and bacon and stir to combine.

Pour the egg mixture into the moulds. Sprinkle the mozzarella cheese over the top.

Cook for 15 minutes at 160°C. Garnish with chives, if desired.

Pesto, Tomato & Cheese Bruschetta

SERVES 4
PREP + COOK TIME: 30 MINS
VEG

PESTO

¼ cup (45g) pine nuts

1½ cups (20g) fresh basil leaves

2 small cloves garlic, halved

¾ cup (60g) grated Parmesan cheese

5 tbsps olive oil

BRUSCHETTA

8 x 2cm-thick slices of baguette, ciabatta or sourdough

2 cups (250g) grated mozzarella cheese

32 cherry tomatoes, halved

2 tbsps olive oil

Salt and pepper to taste

2 tbsps chopped fresh basil

Place pine nuts, basil, garlic and Parmesan in the bowl of a food processor and process until finely chopped. With the motor running, gradually add the oil in a thin steady stream until well combined.

Spread pesto generously over each slice of bread. Sprinkle with mozzarella and top with cherry tomato halves. Drizzle with olive oil and season with salt and pepper.

Cook in batches in air fryer for 4-5 minutes at 220°C.

Sprinkle with chopped basil to serve.

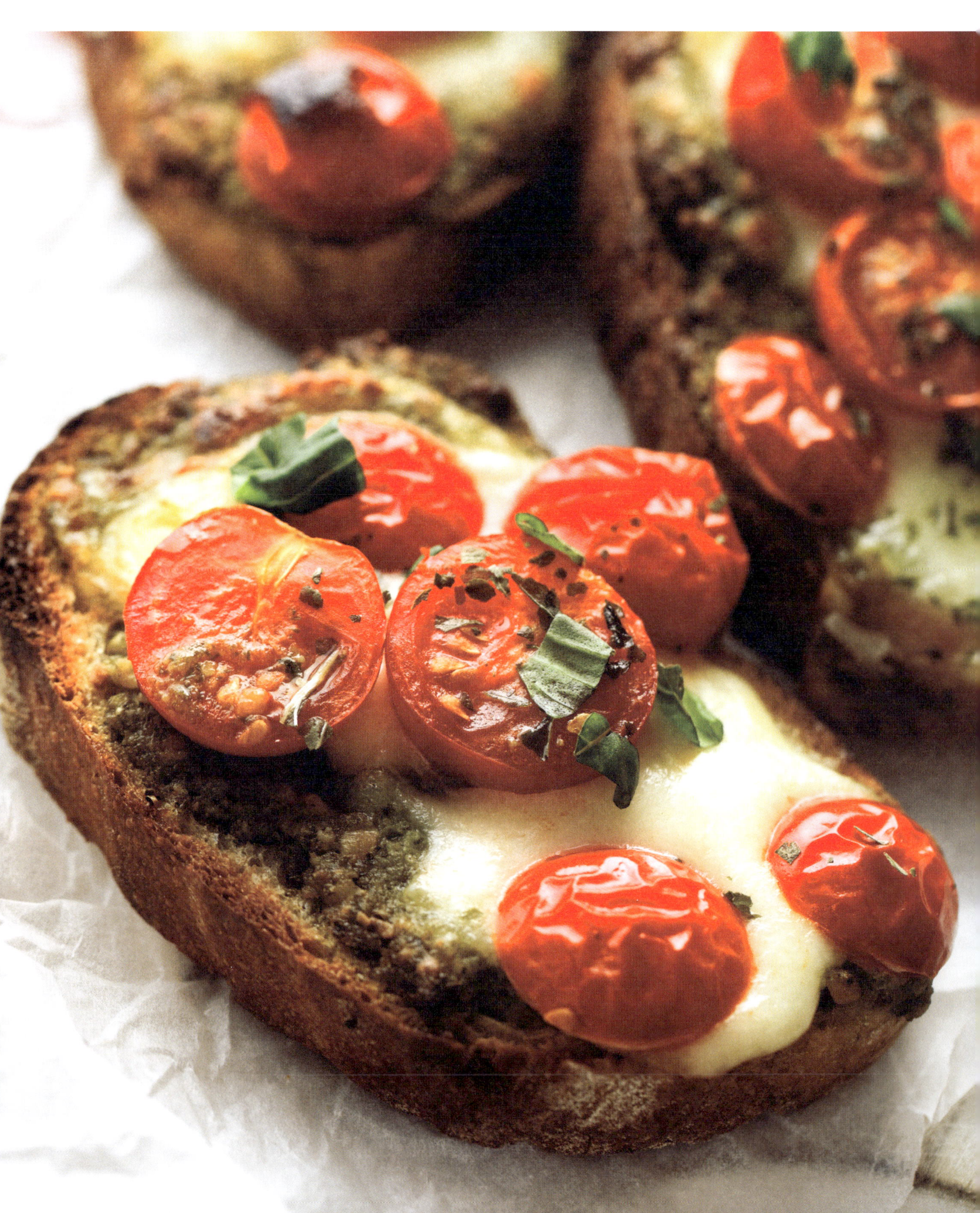

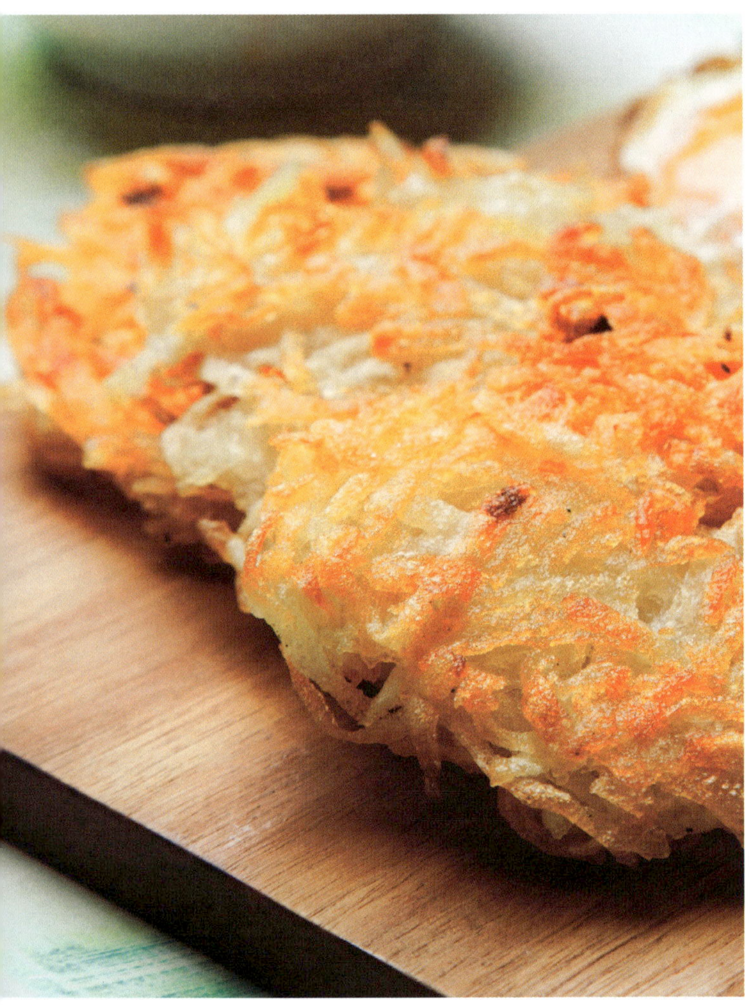

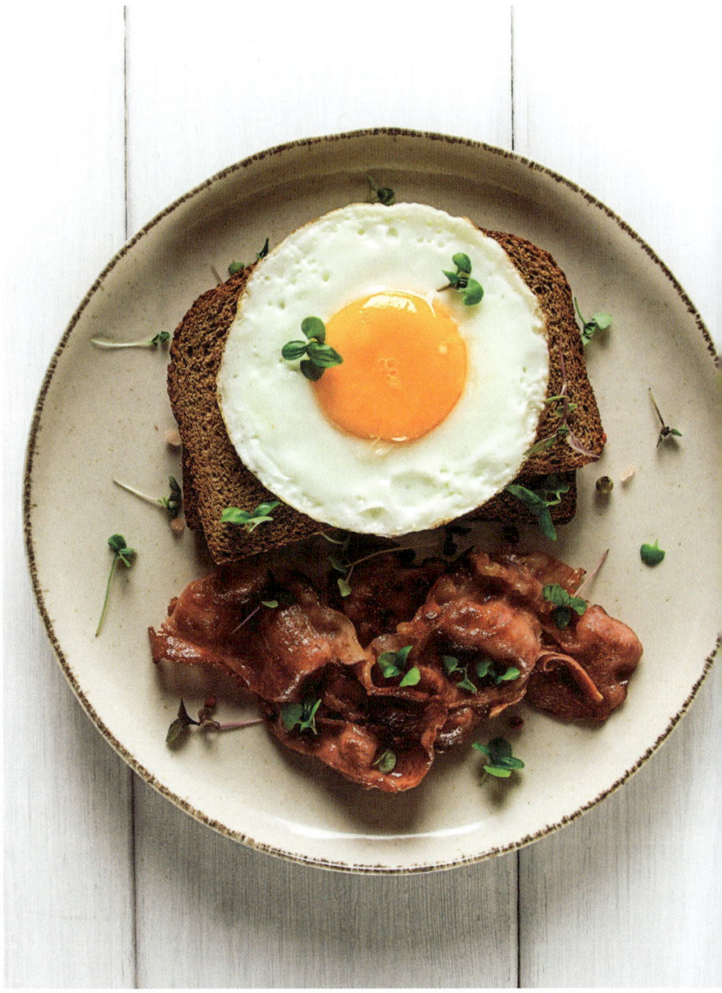

Homemade Hash Browns

SERVES 2

PREP + COOK TIME: 20 MINS + SOAKING AND CHILLING

VEG • DAIRY FREE

Bacon & Eggs

SERVES 2

PREP + COOK TIME: 20 MINS

HOMEMADE HASH BROWNS

4 large potatoes, peeled and finely grated

2 tbsps cornflour

½ tsp salt

2 tsps olive oil

Place the grated potatoes in a bowl of cold water and soak for 30 minutes. Drain and then pat dry with a paper towel. Transfer to a clean, dry bowl.

Add the cornflour, salt and oil and mix together. Form into small patties and transfer to the fridge for 10 minutes.

Preheat the air fryer to 200°C.

Lightly spray the air fryer basket. Place the patties in the basket and cook for 15 minutes, flipping halfway through cooking.

Note:

Don't skip the soaking stage as this will remove the starch from the potatoes, making the hash browns crispier.

BACON & EGGS

8 thin rashers bacon

2 tbsps butter

2 eggs

Salt and pepper to taste

4 slices toast

Preheat the air fryer to 200°C.

Place the bacon in the air fryer basket in a single layer (you may need to cook in two batches or use a double-layer accessory).

Cook for 5 minutes, checking halfway and rearranging with tongs as needed. For thicker bacon, cook for 10 minutes. Set aside and keep warm.

Place butter in a baking pan that will fit in your air fryer and insert the pan into the air fryer. Heat butter until just melted (approximately 1 minute).

Remove the pan and crack both eggs into it. Season with salt and pepper. Return to the air fryer and cook at 160°C. For soft yolks, cook for 4 minutes. For hard yolks, cook for 8 minutes. Check occasionally during cooking to ensure eggs are cooked to your preference.

Serve the bacon and eggs with toast.

Note:

Cook bacon for an extra minute or two if you'd like it extra crispy. If cooking in batches, drain the grease after each cook time to avoid the fat smoking.

Frittata

SERVES 2
PREP + COOK TIME: 25 MINS
GLUTEN FREE

4 eggs

3 tbsps double cream

½ cup (40g) mushrooms, sliced

1 cup (165g) lightly steamed broccoli florets

2 rashers bacon, cooked and chopped

¼ cup (60g) crumbled feta

¼ cup (30g) grated Cheddar cheese

Pinch of dried chilli flakes

Salt and pepper to taste

Handful of pea shoots, to garnish

Baking pan

Preheat the air fryer to 180°C.

Line a deep 19cm baking pan with greaseproof paper, spray with cooking spray and set aside.

In a bowl, whisk together the eggs and cream.

Add mushrooms, broccoli, bacon, feta, Cheddar and chilli flakes. Season with salt and pepper and stir to combine.

Pour mixture into the baking pan and place inside the air fryer basket.

Cook for 12-16 minutes, or until eggs are set. To check, insert a toothpick in the centre of the frittata. The eggs are set if it comes out clean.

Scatter with pea shoots to serve.

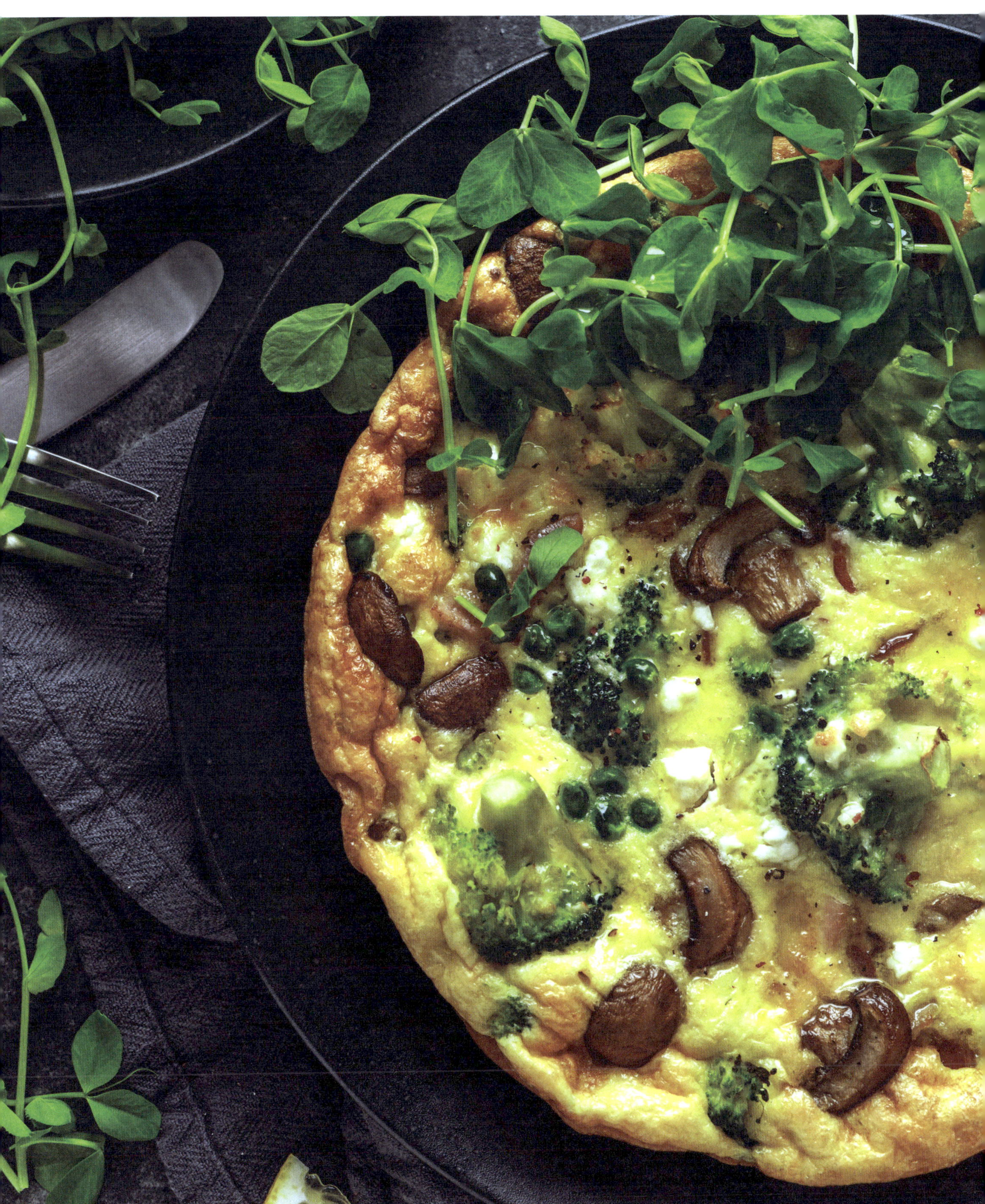

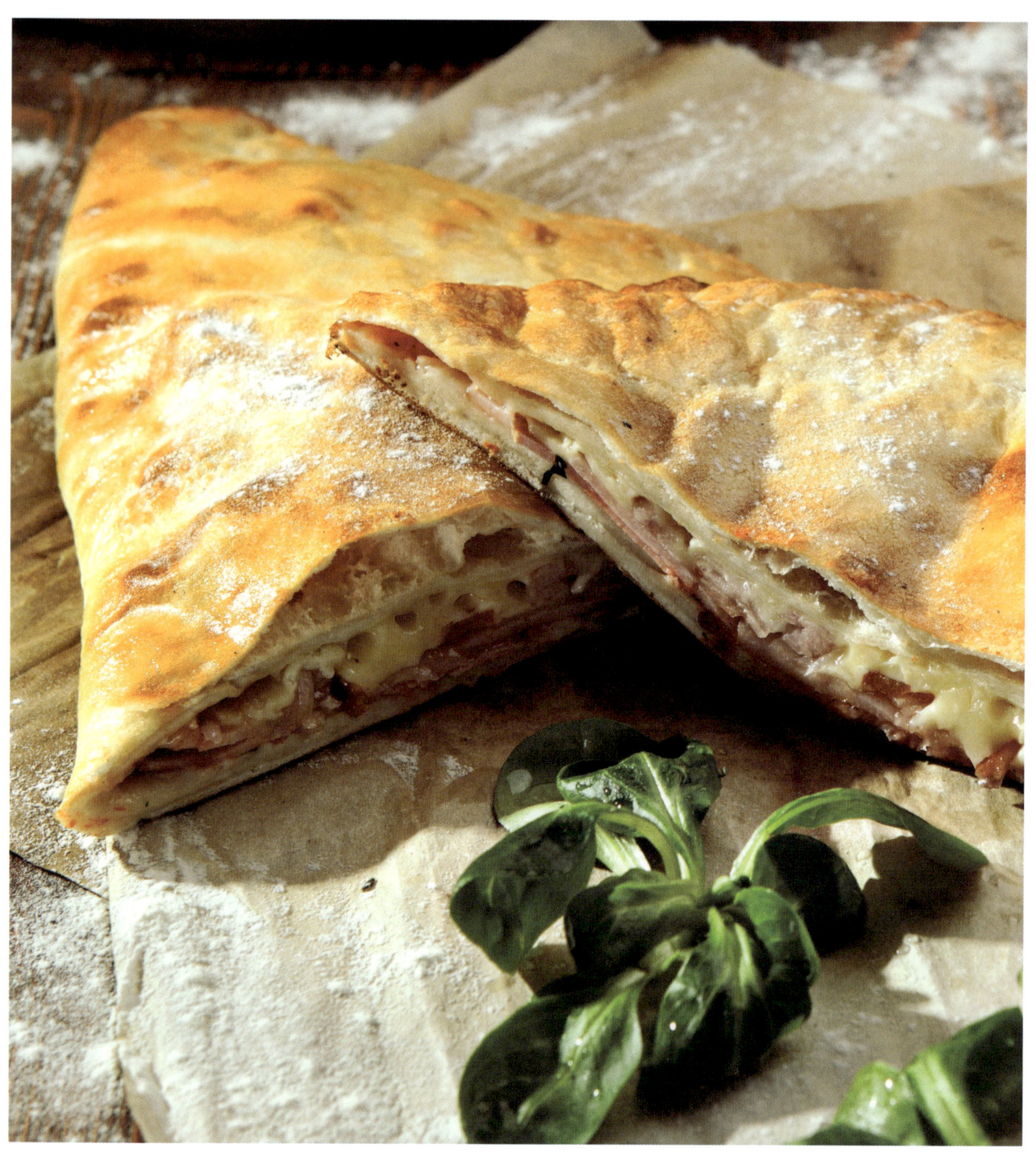

Ham & Mozzarella Calzone

SERVES 4

PREP + COOK TIME: 55 MINS

HAM & MOZZARELLA CALZONE

8g sachet instant dried yeast
¼ tsp salt
1 tsp caster sugar
¾ cup (185ml) warm water
2 cups (250g) plain flour
2 tbsps olive oil
150g thinly sliced ham
2 tomatoes, thinly sliced
250g mozzarella cheese, sliced

Combine yeast, salt, sugar and warm water in a jug. Stir with a fork. Cover with plastic wrap. Set aside in a warm place for 5 minutes or until bubbles form on the surface.

Sift flour into a large bowl. Add yeast mixture and olive oil. Mix to form a soft dough.

Turn dough onto a lightly floured surface. Knead for 8 minutes or until smooth and elastic. Place in a lightly greased bowl. Cover with plastic wrap. Set aside in a warm place for 15-20 minutes or until doubled in size.

Punch dough with your fist. Knead gently on a lightly floured surface. Cut dough into four pieces. Knead each piece into a ball. Roll each ball into a 15cm (diameter) round.

Arrange ham, tomato and cheese over half of each round, leaving a 2cm border around the edge. Brush edge with water. Fold dough over to enclose filling. Press edges together to seal. Spray lightly with cooking spray.

Preheat air fryer to 160°C.

Place calzones in air fryer basket and cook for 8 minutes. Turn calzones over and cook for a further 4 minutes until golden brown.

Spinach & Feta Muffins

SERVES 12

PREP + COOK TIME: 25 MINS

VEG

350g frozen chopped spinach, thawed and squeezed to remove moisture

2 large eggs

¼ cup (60ml) olive oil

1 cup (250ml) milk

¼ cup (60ml) Greek yoghurt

2 cups (250g) plain flour

2 tsps baking powder

150g feta cheese, diced

Muffin tray or silicone moulds

Place spinach, eggs, olive oil, milk and yoghurt in a large bowl. Mix well. Add flour, baking powder and cheese. Stir to combine.

Preheat air fryer to 175°C. Spoon mixture into silicone moulds or a muffin tray filled with paper liners.

Cook in batches or use a double layer accessory for 15-20 minutes, until an inserted skewer comes out clean.

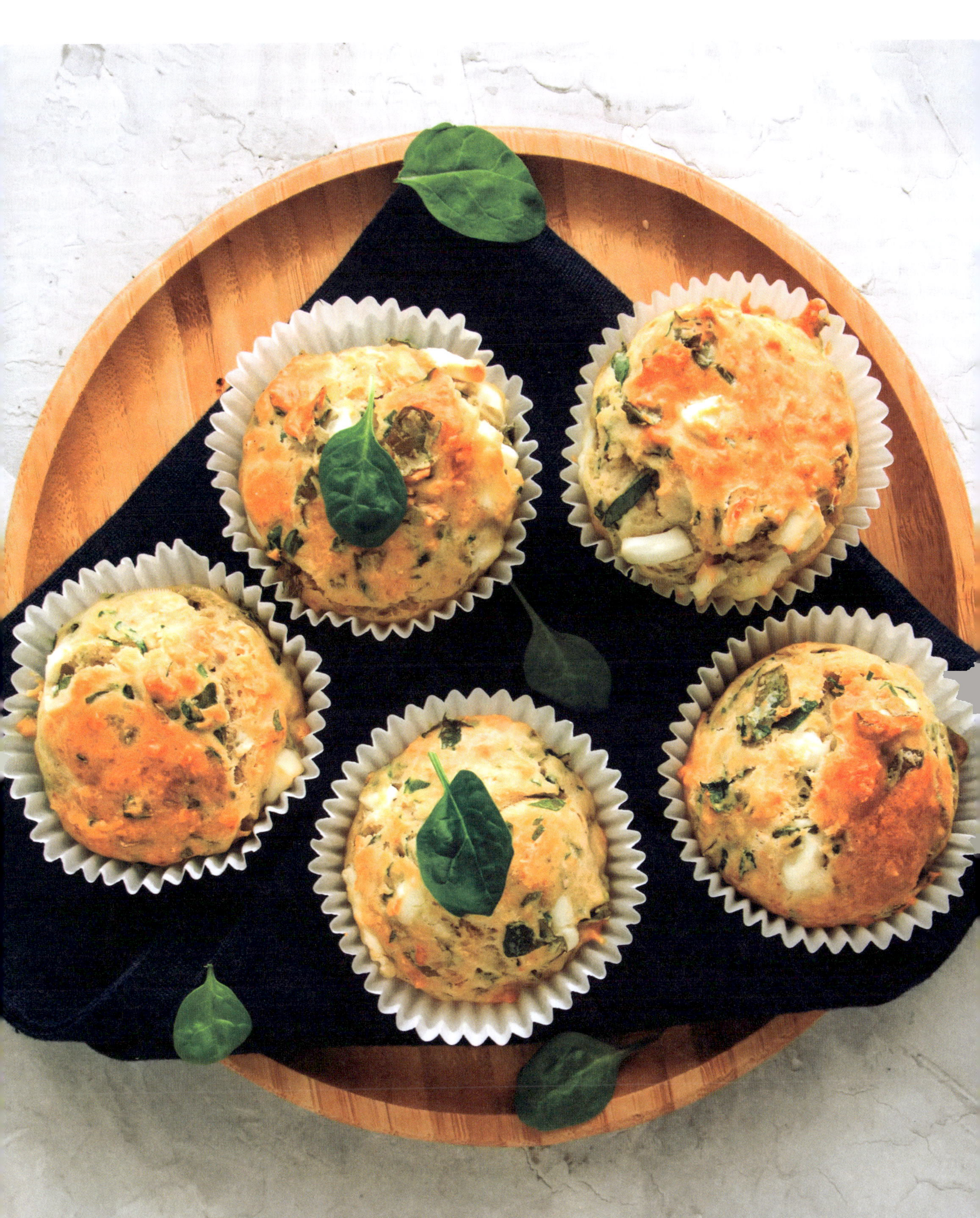

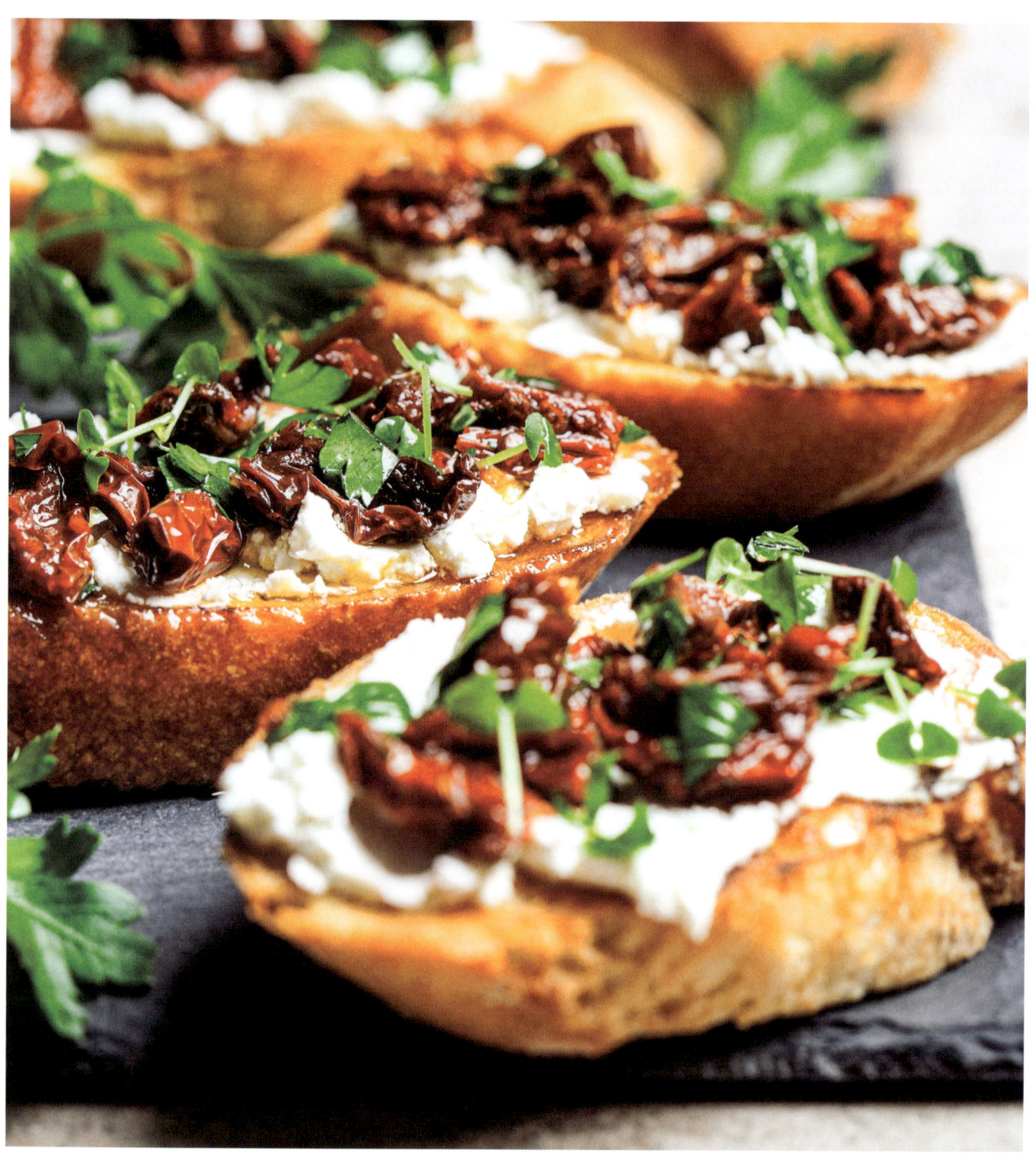

Sun-Dried Tomato Toast

SERVES 4

PREP + COOK TIME: 15 MINS

VEG

SUN-DRIED TOMATO TOAST

1 medium, crusty baguette

1 clove garlic

3-4 tbsps olive oil

150g cream cheese

1 cup (50g) sun-dried tomatoes, sliced

Salt and pepper to taste

¼ cup (5g) roughly chopped parsley leaves

Preheat air fryer at 190°C for 3 minutes.

Cut the baguette into slices. Slice garlic clove in half and generously rub the top of each bread slice with the garlic.

Brush each slice with olive oil.

Working in batches, place bread slices in one even layer in air fryer basket and cook for 3-4 minutes until golden brown. Repeat with remaining bread.

Spread each slice with cream cheese and top with sun-dried tomatoes. Drizzle with remaining olive oil and season with salt and pepper.

Scatter over parsley to serve.

POACHED EGGS

4 eggs
Baking pan

Place the baking pan in the air fryer basket.

Using a jug or the kettle, fill to halfway with boiling water.

Carefully crack the eggs and slide them into the water.

Cook the eggs at 200°C for 3½ minutes for soft yolks or longer to suit your preference.

Remove from the air fryer using a slotted spoon.

APPLE PANCAKES

60g butter, melted
1 egg
1 cup (250ml) milk
1¼ cups (150g) plain flour, sifted
1 tsp baking powder
Pinch of ground cinnamon
2 tbsps brown sugar
1 apple, grated
Baking pan, lightly greased

Preheat the air fryer to 180°C.

Whisk together the butter, egg and milk in a large bowl.

Combine the flour, baking powder, cinnamon and sugar in a separate bowl.

Pour the wet ingredients into the dry and stir until just combined. Gently stir in the apple.

Scrape 2 heaped tablespoons of batter into the pan. Cook for 7 minutes or until golden.

Repeat for remaining mixture.

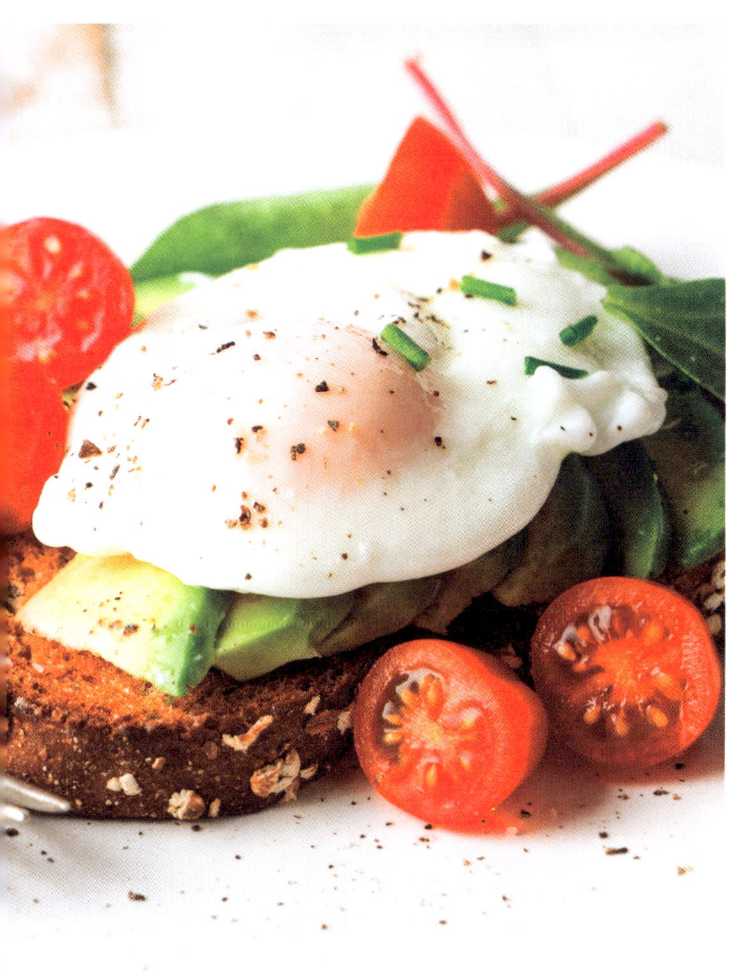

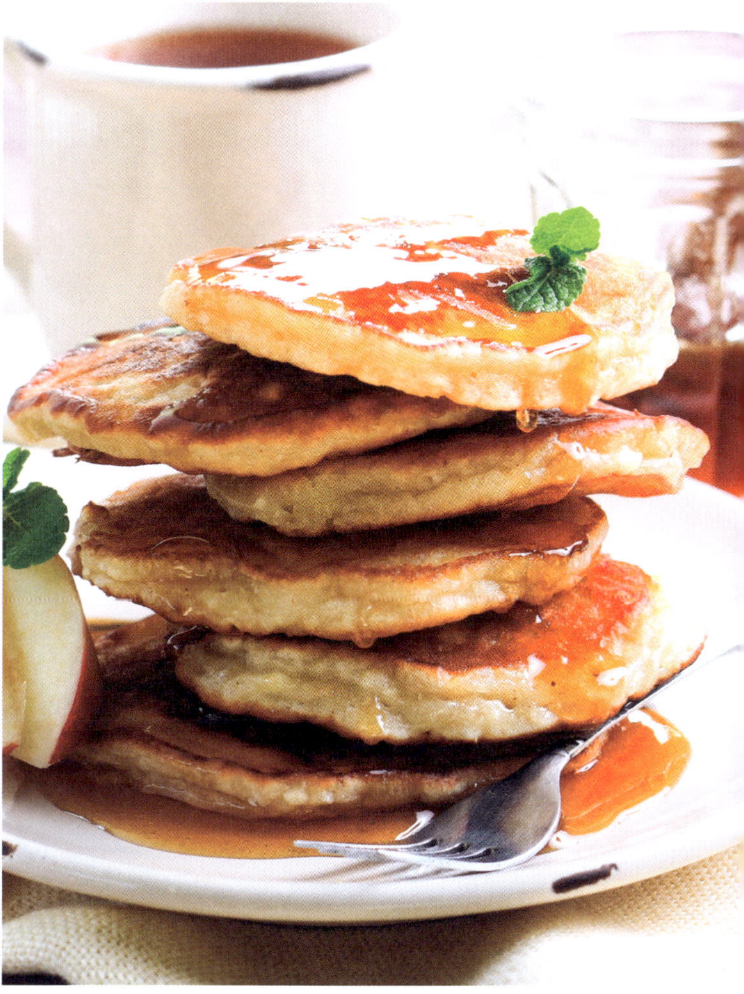

Poached Eggs

SERVES 4

PREP + COOK TIME: 4 MINS

VEG • GLUTEN FREE • DAIRY FREE

Apple Pancakes

SERVES 2

PREP + COOK TIME: 20 MINS

VEG

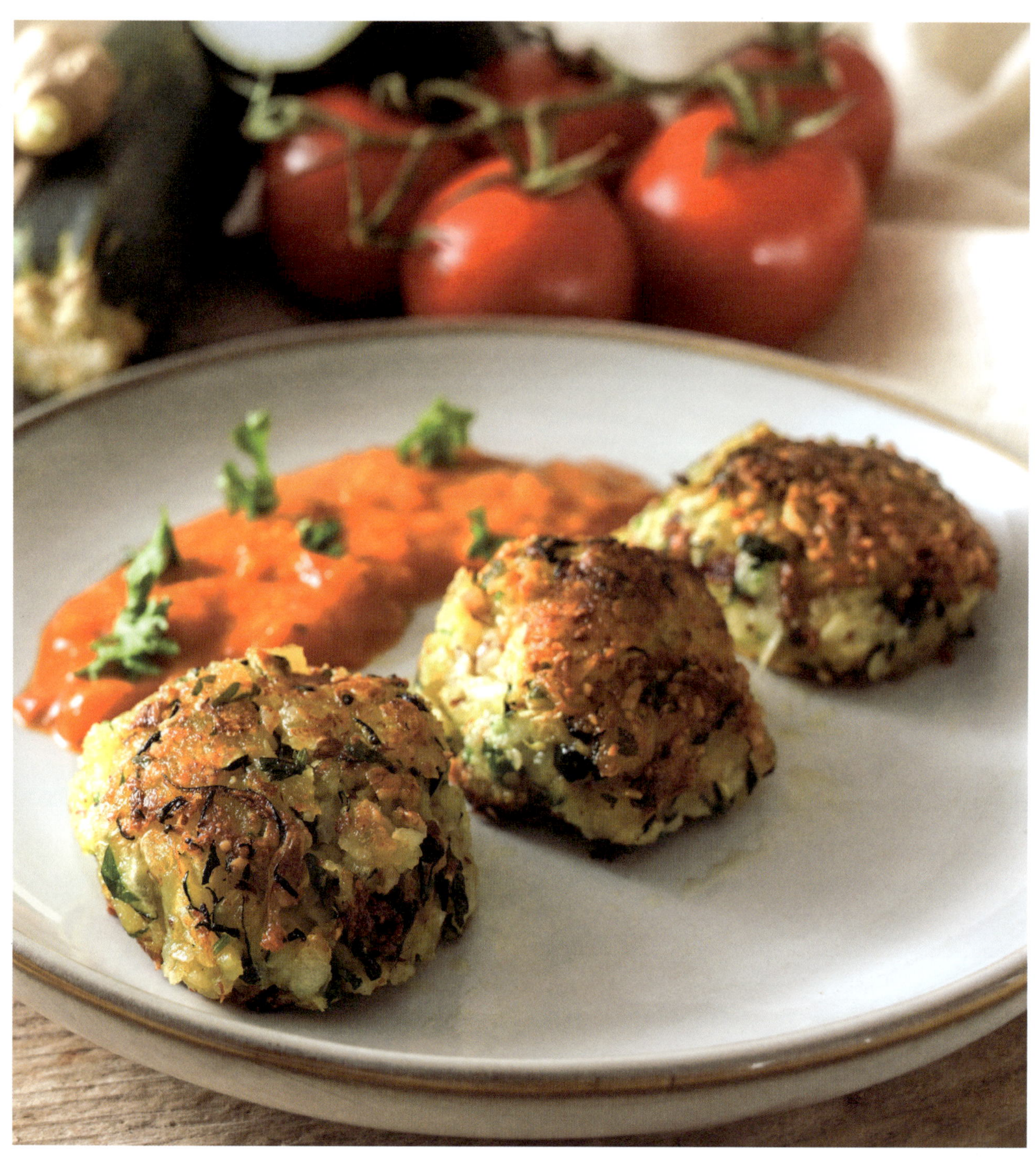

Zucchini Croquettes

SERVES 4

PREP + COOK TIME: 35 MINS

VEG • GLUTEN FREE

ZUCCHINI CROQUETTES

2 medium zucchinis, grated (to make 2 cups)
1 tsp salt
1 medium sweet potato, grated (to make 1 cup)
1 egg, beaten
⅓ cup (40g) almond meal + more if needed
⅓ cup (30g) grated Parmesan cheese
1 tsp olive oil
1 tsp Italian seasoning
½ tsp garlic powder
½ tsp baking powder
Tomato sauce or relish to serve (optional)

Place the grated zucchini in a sieve over a bowl. Mix in the salt and set aside for a 10 minutes. Transfer the zucchini to a clean tea towel and squeeze out the extra moisture.

Add the zucchini, sweet potato, egg, almond meal, Parmesan cheese, olive oil, Italian seasoning, garlic powder and baking powder to a medium bowl and mix well to combine into a chunky batter. Add a little more almond meal if the mixture is too wet.

Use a ¼ cup scoop to form into balls.

Preheat the air fryer to 190°C.

Spray the air fryer basket with cooking spray. Place the balls into the air fryer basket in a single layer and spray with cooking spray. Air fry for 10-11 minutes until golden and crispy. Serve with tomato sauce or relish, if desired.

Egg, Tomato & Thyme Tarts

MAKES 4

PREP + COOK TIME: 30 MINS

VEG

Plain flour, for dusting

1 sheet frozen puff pastry, just thawed

¾ cup (90g) grated Cheddar cheese

4 large eggs

8 cherry tomatoes, halved

1 tbsp fresh thyme leaves

Preheat the air fryer to 200°C.

Place the pastry sheet on a floured workbench and cut into four squares. Place one or two squares (depending on space) in the air fryer basket, spacing them apart so they do not touch. Cook for 10 minutes or until pastry is golden brown.

Remove the basket from the air fryer. Using a spoon, press down in the centre of the pastry to make an indentation. Sprinkle cheese into each indentation and then crack an egg into it. Dot the cherry tomato halves around the corners of each and sprinkle with thyme leaves.

Return to the air fryer and cook for a further 6-8 minutes or until cooked to your preference. Transfer to a wire rack and allow to cool for 5 minutes. Serve warm.

Repeat steps with the remaining ingredients until you have made four tarts.

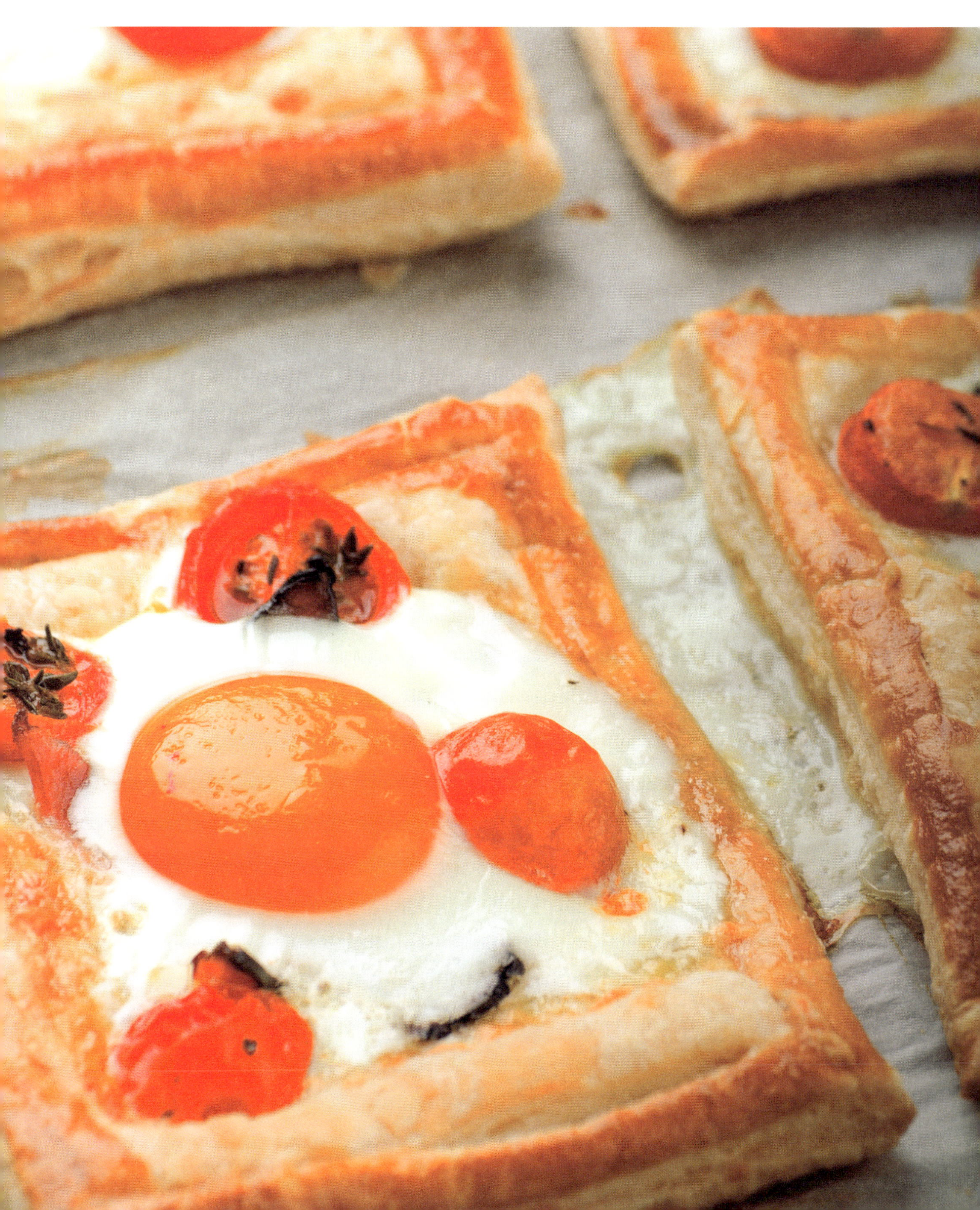

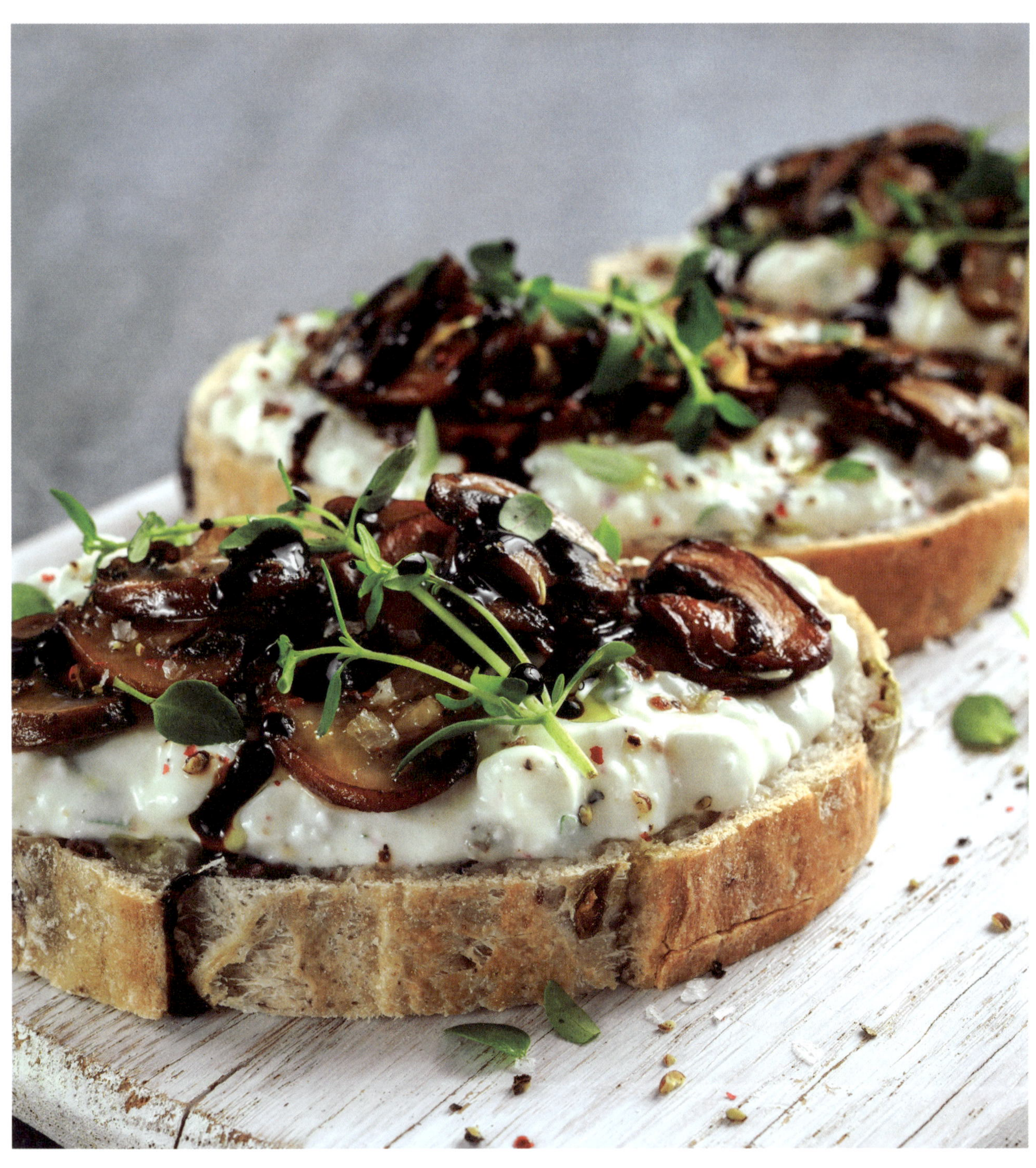

Garlic Mushrooms with Ricotta on Toast

SERVES 4

PREP + COOK TIME: 20 MINS

VEG

GARLIC MUSHROOMS WITH RICOTTA ON TOAST

8 slices wholegrain bread

1 tbsp olive oil + more for brushing and drizzling

300g button mushrooms, sliced

2 cloves garlic, minced (or ½ tsp garlic powder)

Salt and pepper to taste

½ cup (125g) ricotta cheese

½ cup (110g) cream cheese

⅓ cup (30g) grated Parmesan cheese

1 tbsp chopped chives

1 tbsp chopped parsley

1 tsp minced thyme leaves

Juice of ½ lemon

2 tbsps balsamic glaze

Pinch of dried chilli flakes (optional)

Fresh herbs, to serve

Brush bread slices lightly with olive oil. Place bread in air fryer basket in one even layer, working in batches if needed, and cook for 3 minutes at 190°C.

Place mushrooms in a bowl with 1 tablespoon olive oil and garlic. Season with salt and pepper. Toss to coat.

Cook for 10 minutes at 190°C, removing and shaking the basket halfway through cooking.

Meanwhile place ricotta, cream cheese, Parmesan, chives, parsley and thyme in a large bowl. Squeeze in lemon juice and mix well to combine.

Spoon ricotta mixture on top of toast slices.

Spoon over the mushrooms then drizzle with balsamic glaze and olive oil and scatter with dried chilli flakes, if using. Season with salt and pepper and top with fresh herbs.

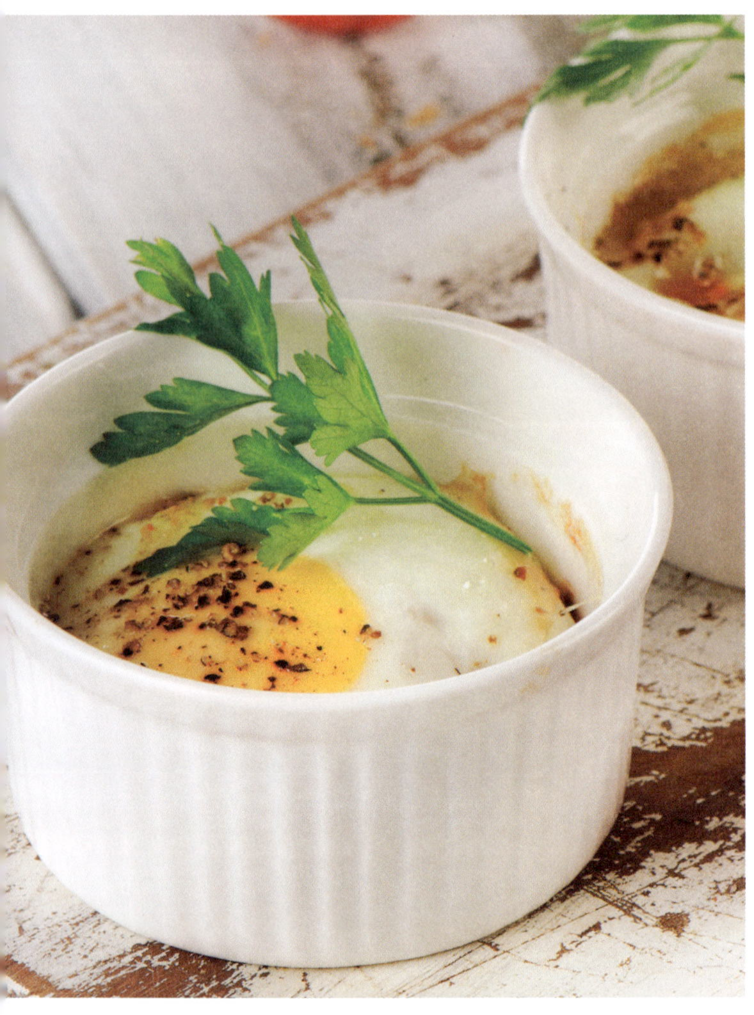

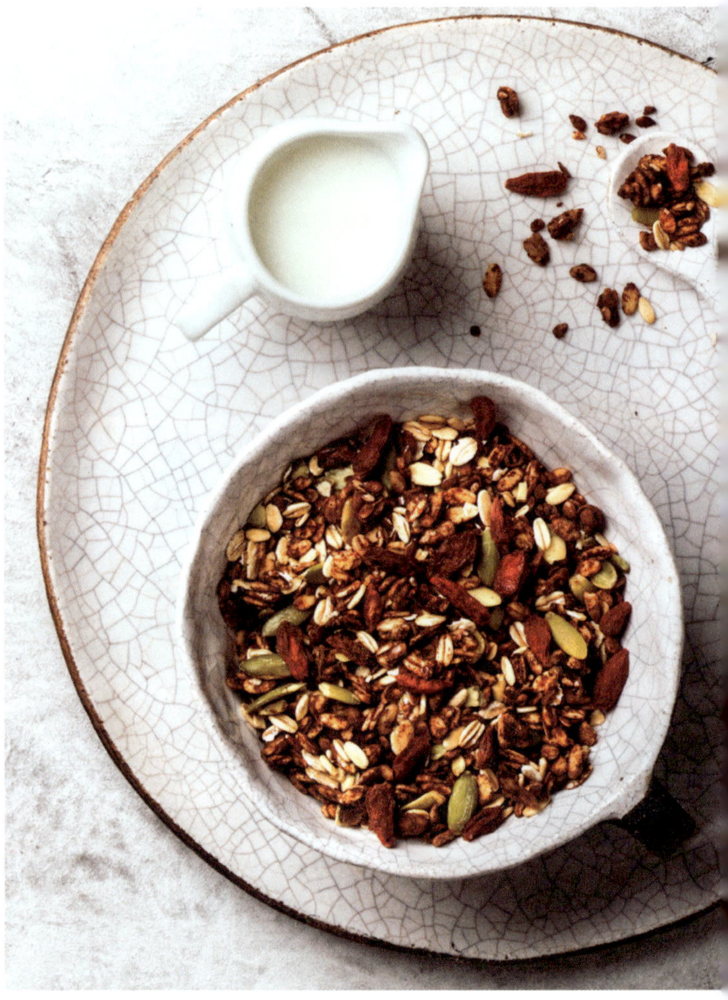

Baked Eggs

SERVES 2

PREP + COOK TIME: 10 MINS

VEG • GLUTEN FREE • DAIRY FREE

Cinnamon Granola

SERVES 12

PREP + COOK TIME: 40 MINS + COOLING

VEG • DAIRY FREE

BAKED EGGS

2 large eggs

⅛ tsp paprika

Salt and pepper to taste

2 ramekins

Preheat air fryer to 180°C. Spray the ramekins with nonstick spray.

Crack each egg into a small ramekin. Sprinkle with paprika, salt and pepper to taste.

Bake the eggs for 5-8 minutes or until the eggs have cooked to desired consistency.

CINNAMON GRANOLA

1½ cups (130g) rolled oats

½ cup (60g) walnuts, chopped

½ cup (60g) almonds, chopped

½ cup (60g) sunflower seeds

½ cup (60g) pepitas (pumpkin seeds)

¼ cup (80g) maple syrup or honey

1 tbsp coconut oil

2 tsps cinnamon

½ tsp salt

½ cup (50g) goji berries

Place all the ingredients except the goji berries in a large bowl and mix to combine.

Place the mixture in the air fryer basket and cook for 35 minutes at 120°C, stirring every 10 minutes.

Remove from the air fryer and spread out on a baking tray to cool for 30 minutes.

Pour into a large bowl, add goji berries and mix.

Corn Fritters

SERVES 4
PREP + COOK TIME: 45 MINS
VEG • GLUTEN FREE

2 medium zucchinis, grated
Salt and pepper to taste
½ cup (130g) cooked mashed potato
1 cup (175g) corn kernels
2 tbsps chickpea flour
3 cloves garlic, minced
2 tbsps olive oil

In a large bowl mix grated zucchini with ½ teaspoon salt and leave for 15 minutes. Then place on a clean tea towel and twist to squeeze out excess liquid.

Combine zucchini, potato, corn, chickpea flour, garlic, salt and pepper in a mixing bowl. Mix well.

Use your hands to shape the mixture into patties. Brush each fritter with olive oil.

Preheat air fryer to 180°C.

Arrange fritters in one layer in air fryer basket. Cook in batches or use a double-layer accessory if necessary.

Cook for 8 minutes then flip and cook for a further 3-4 minutes until brown.

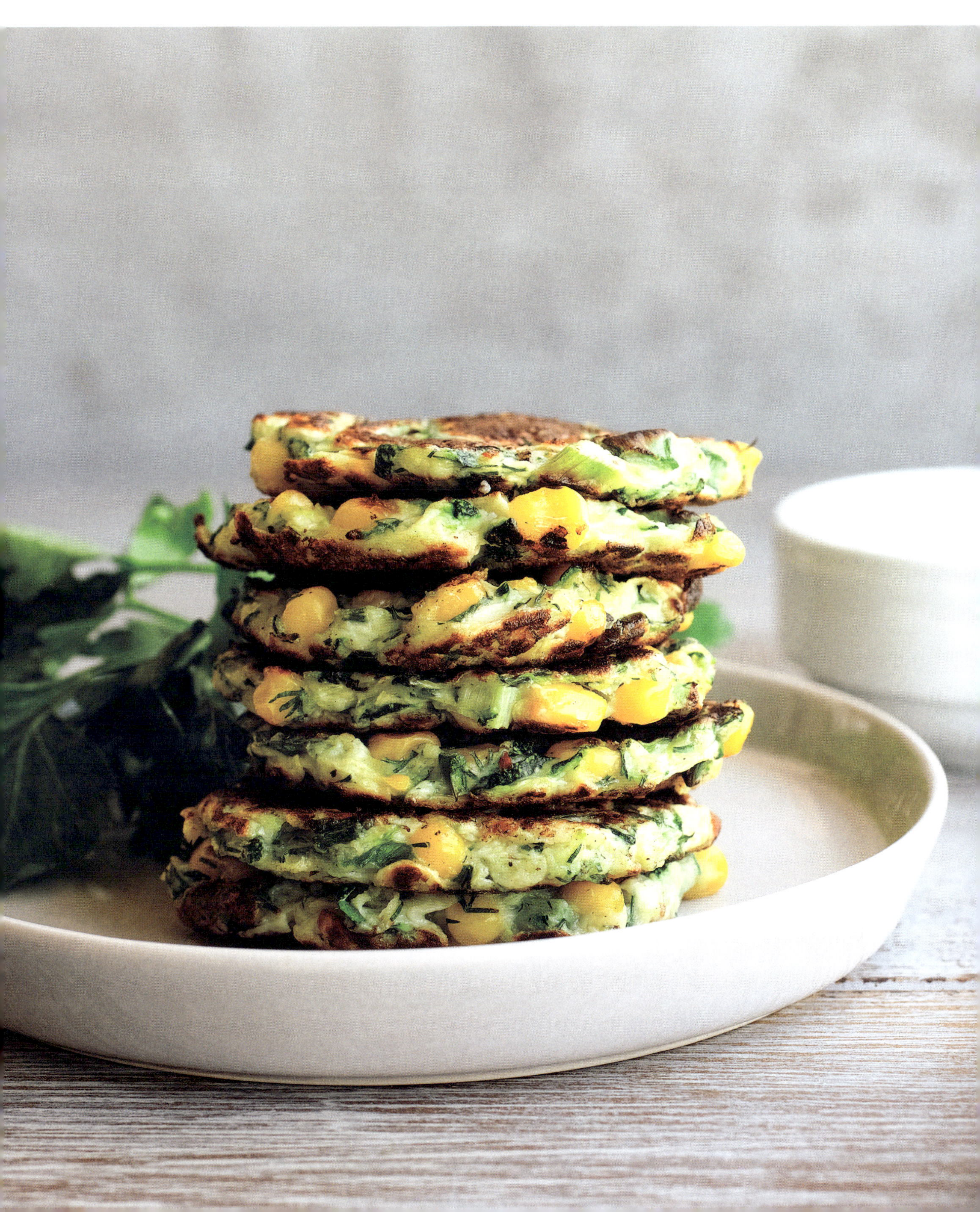

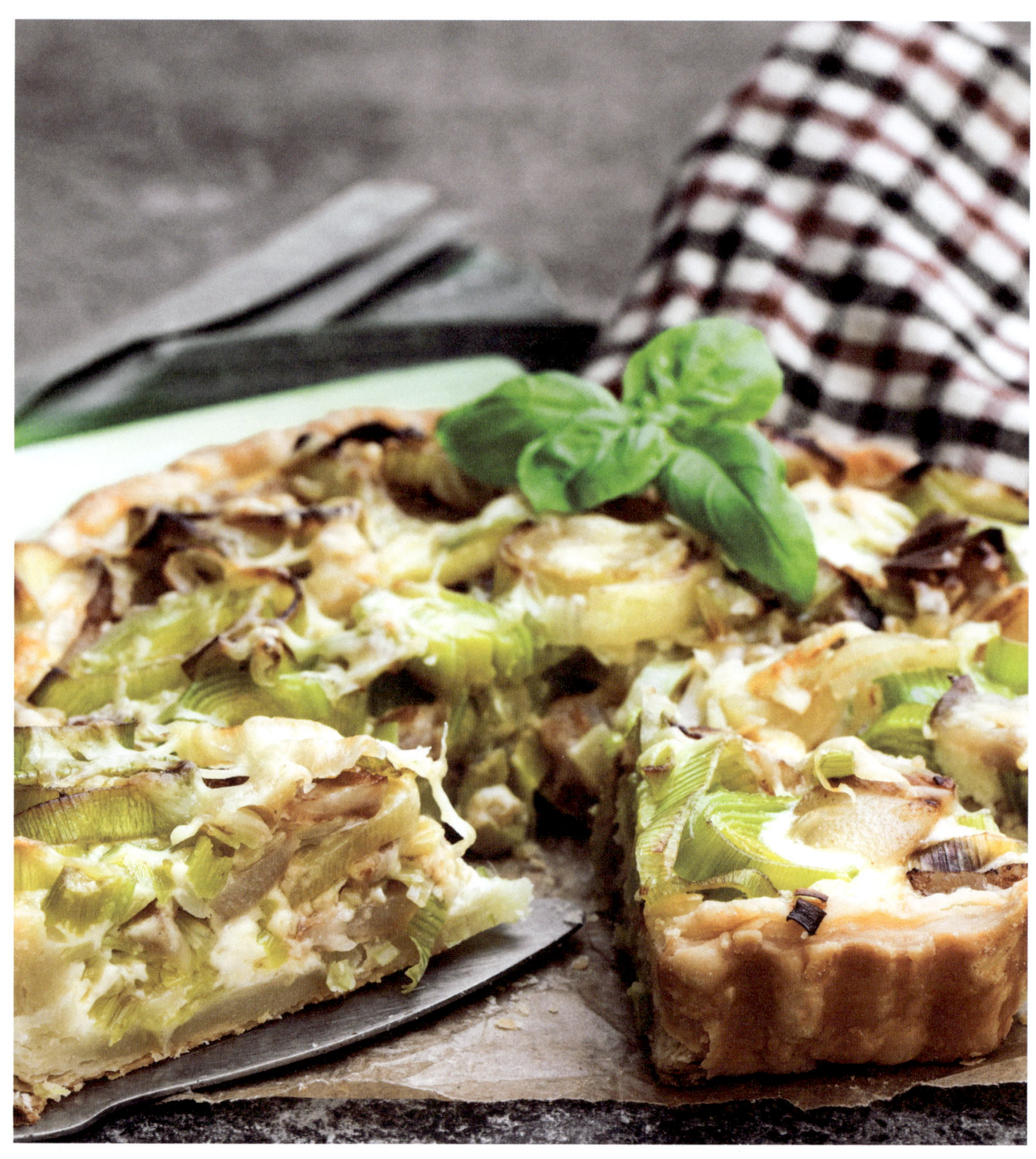

Leek & Mushroom Tart

SERVES 4

PREP + COOK TIME: 1 HOUR + 1 HOUR CHILLING

VEG

LEEK & MUSHROOM TART

25g butter

3 leeks, sliced and washed

150g chestnut mushrooms, sliced

1 egg

¾ cup (180ml) thickened cream

¾ cup (100g) coarsely grated Gruyere cheese

PASTRY

1½ cups (190g) plain flour

100g cold butter, diced

6 tbsps cold water

For the pastry, place flour and butter in a large bowl. Rub together with your fingertips until crumbly. Add water 1 tablespoon at a time, mixing with a knife. Bring pastry together, wrap in plastic wrap and chill for 1 hour.

Heat butter in a pan over medium heat. Add leeks and cook for 10 minutes, then add mushrooms and cook for a further 5 minutes until soft. Set aside.

In a large bowl mix together egg, cream and half of the cheese. Add leeks and mushrooms. Stir to combine.

Roll out pastry, transfer to a flan dish or cake tin that fits into your air fryer. Trim the edges and prick with a fork.

Place into air fryer and cook at 160°C for 10-15 minutes.

Pour filling into pastry, top with remaining cheese. Cook for 15-20 minutes at 160°C until set and golden brown.

SPINACH OMELETTE

2 eggs
¼ cup (60ml) milk
Pinch of salt
100g baby spinach
¼ cup (30g) grated Cheddar cheese
Baking pan

Whisk the eggs, milk and salt in a small bowl until well combined. Add the spinach and loosely combine.

Pour the mixture into a well-greased baking pan.

Place the pan into the air fryer basket and cook for 4 minutes at 180°C.

Sprinkle the cheese over the top and return to cook for a further 4 minutes.

Use a thin spatula to loosen the omelette from the sides of the pan and transfer to a plate.

Flip one half of the omelette over before serving.

ZUCCHINI CHICKPEA PATTIES

1 large zucchini, grated
1 x 400g can chickpeas, drained and rinsed
3 spring onions, chopped
1 tsp garlic powder
3 tbsps ground coriander
½ tsp chilli powder
1 tsp ground cumin
Salt and pepper to taste

Preheat air fryer to 200°C.

Place grated zucchini in a clean tea towel with chickpeas and squeeze to remove any excess liquid.

Place zucchini and chickpeas in a large bowl with spring onions, garlic powder, spices and seasoning. Use your hands to combine, then shape mixture into patties.

Arrange patties in air fryer. Spray with cooking spray.

Cook for 12 minutes, turning halfway, until golden brown.

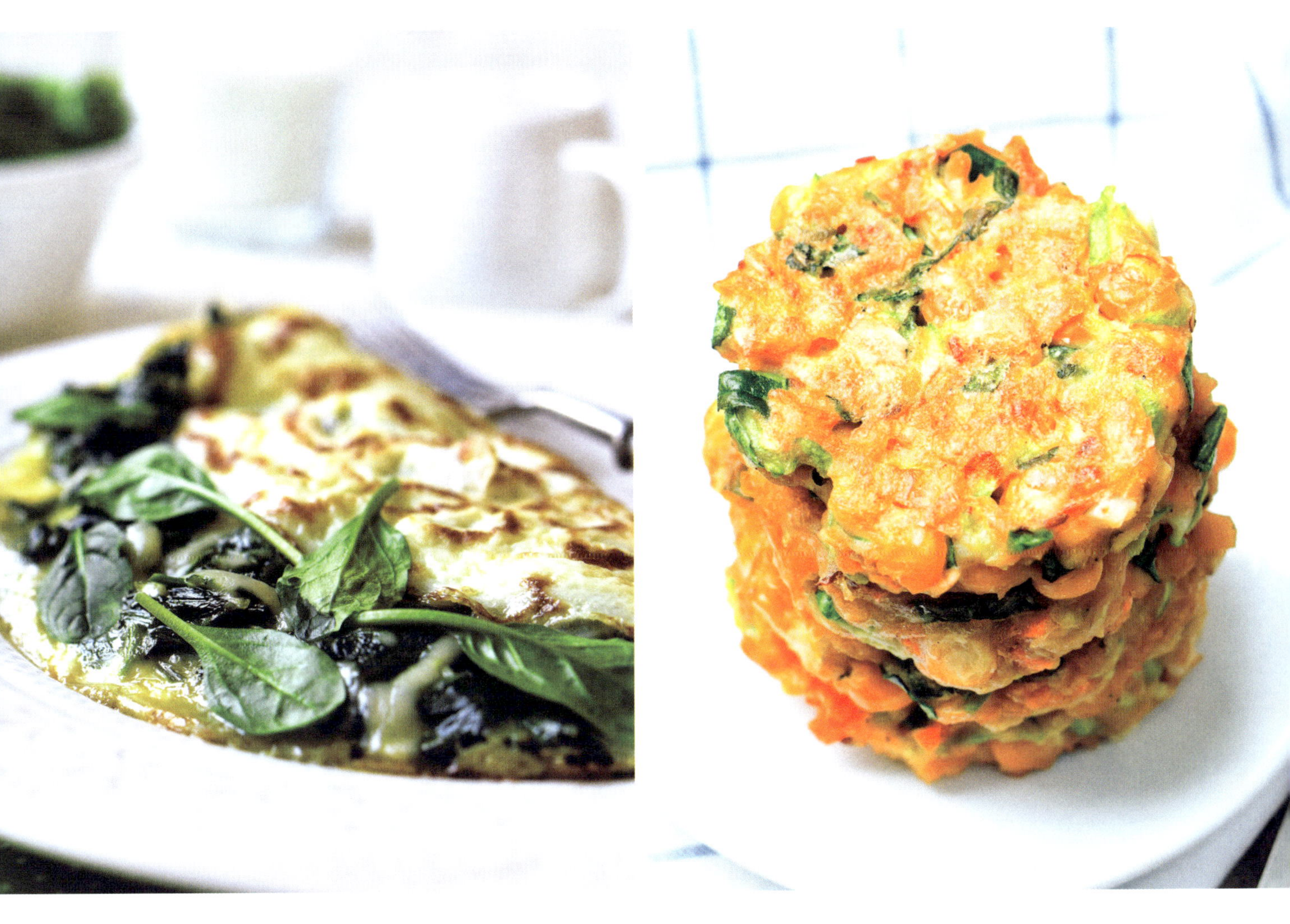

Spinach Omelette

SERVES 1

PREP + COOK TIME: 15 MINS

VEG • GLUTEN FREE

Zucchini Chickpea Patties

SERVES 2

PREP + COOK TIME: 25 MINS

VEG • GLUTEN FREE • DAIRY FREE

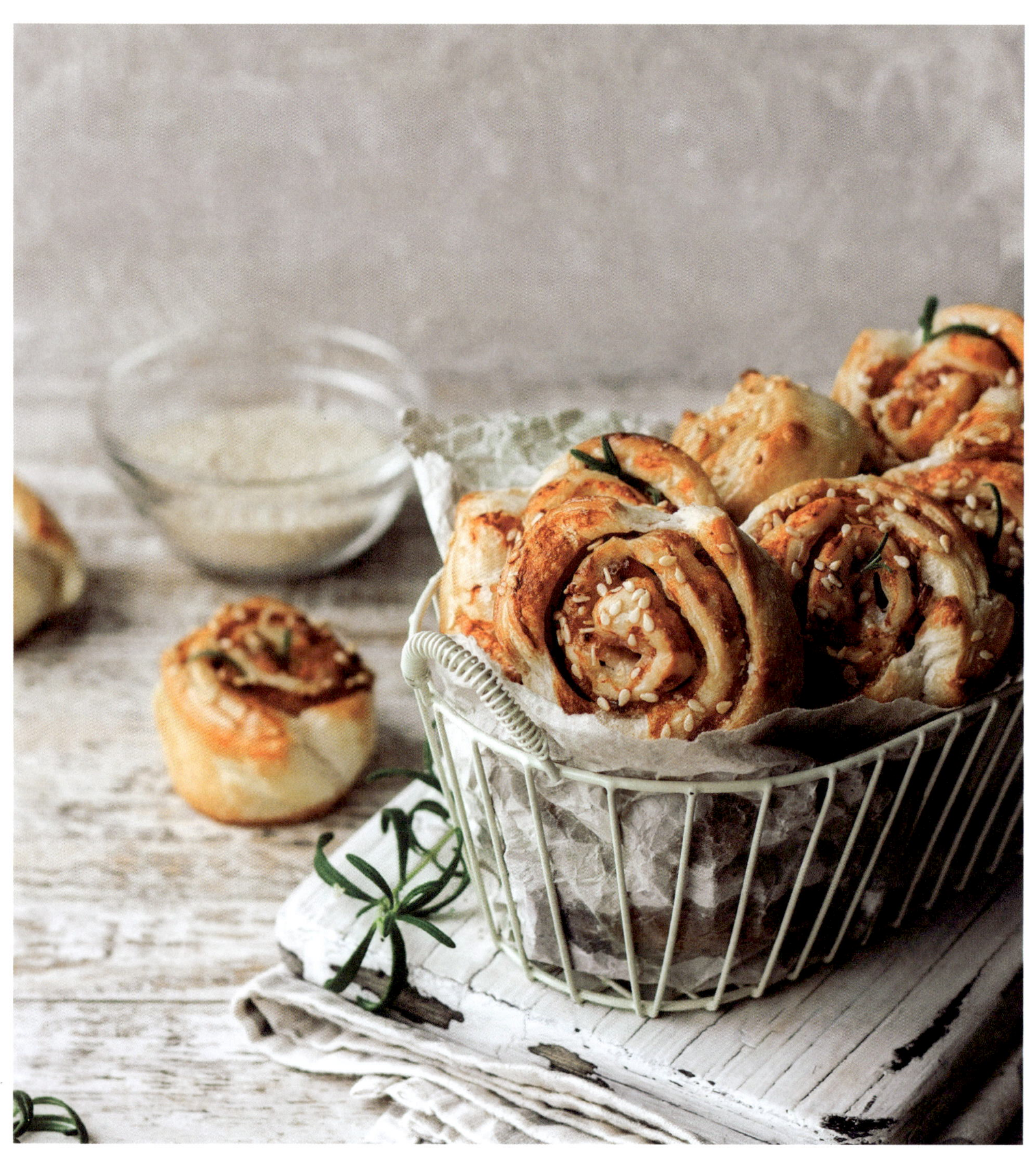

Cheese & Bacon Scrolls

MAKES 12-14

PREP + COOK TIME: 30 MINS

CHEESE & BACON SCROLLS

1 cup (250ml) Greek yoghurt

1½ cups (185g) self-raising flour + more as needed

2 tbsps tomato paste

1 cup (125g) shredded mozzarella cheese

225g bacon, diced

1 tbsp sesame seeds

Mix yoghurt and flour in a medium-sized bowl until well combined. Form into a ball and knead well until smooth. Add extra flour if dough is too sticky.

Sprinkle extra flour over a well-cleaned benchtop.

Use a rolling pin to roll dough into a thin rectangle, around 1cm thick. Spread with tomato paste and scatter with cheese and bacon.

Roll from the long side of the dough to form a sausage shape. Cut rolled dough into 2cm-wide sections. Place in the air fryer basket, leaving a little space in between each one. Sprinkle the tops with sesame seeds. Work in batches or use a double-layer accessory, if needed.

Air fry at 180°C for 12-15 minutes until golden.

TOFU SCRAMBLE

300g silken tofu
¼ tsp garlic powder
1 tbsp nutritional yeast flakes
1 tsp dried oregano
¼ tsp dried chilli flakes
⅛ tsp turmeric
Salt and pepper to taste
200g mushrooms, sliced
2 spring onions, sliced
Baking pan

Preheat air fryer to 180°C.

Spray baking pan with cooking spray.

Place the tofu in a bowl and mash with a fork, then stir through garlic powder, nutritional yeast, herbs and spices. Season with salt and pepper. Add the mushrooms and spring onions and stir to combine.

Transfer the mixture to a pan. Place pan in air fryer basket and cook for 15 minutes.

COTTAGE CHEESE PANCAKES

400g cottage cheese
4 eggs
2 tbsps melted butter
1 tsp vanilla extract
1 cup (125g) flour
1 tbsp baking powder
2 tbsps maple syrup

Combine cottage cheese, eggs, butter and vanilla extract in a large bowl. Mix well to combine. Add flour, baking powder and syrup and beat thoroughly.

Preheat air fryer to 160°C.

Line air fryer basket with greaseproof paper and spray with avocado oil. Cooking in batches, spoon half ladlefuls at a time of batter onto the paper.

Cook for 5-7 minutes without flipping until browned. Repeat with remaining batter, spraying each batch.

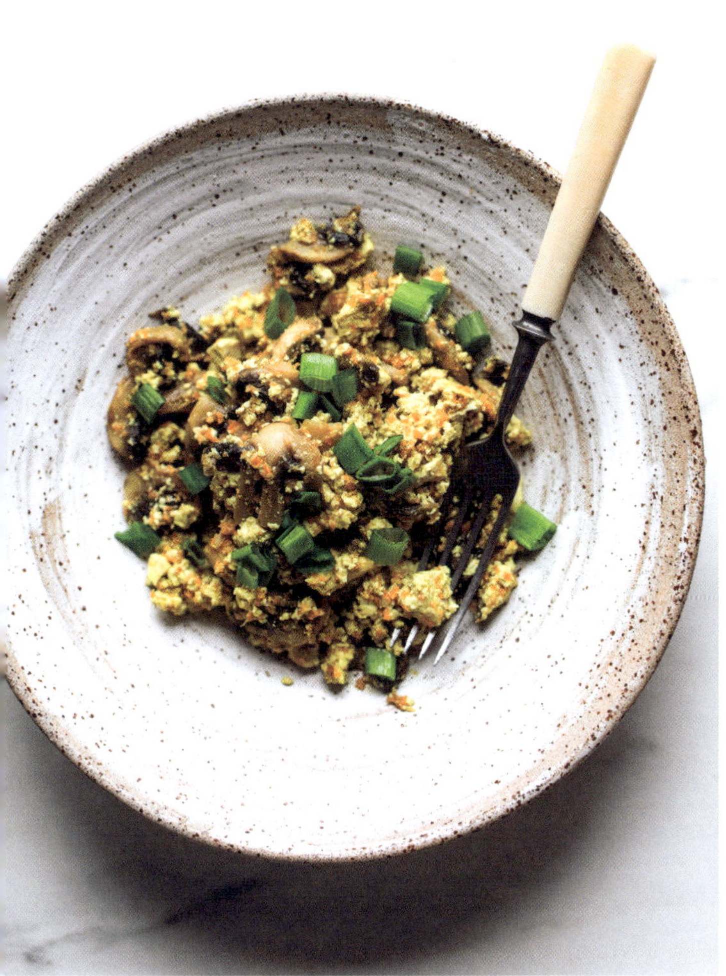

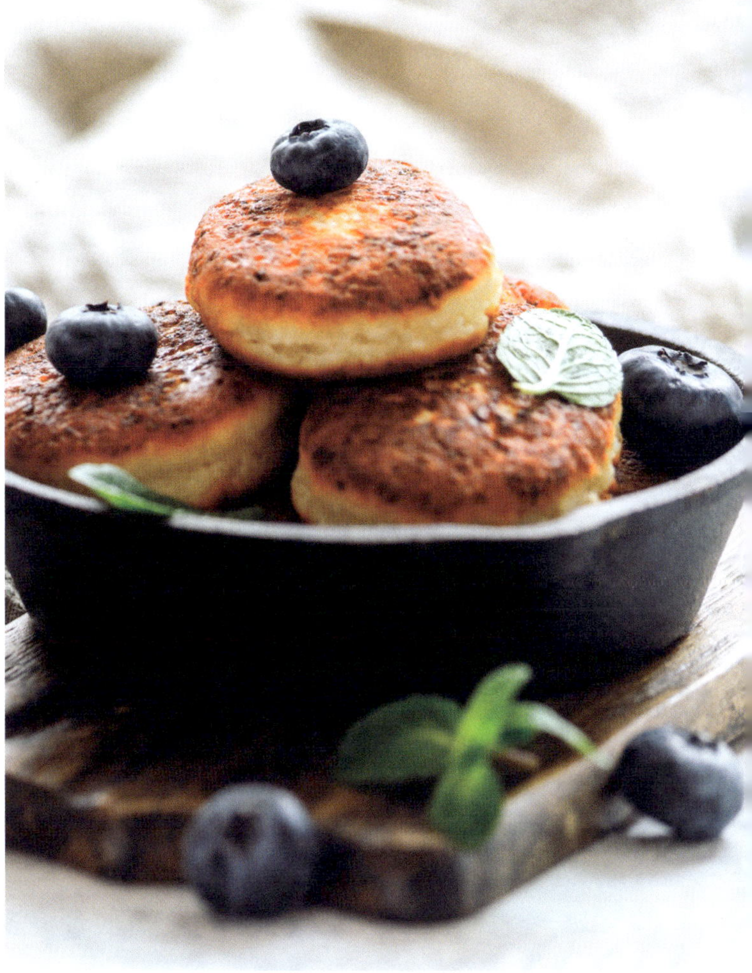

Tofu Scramble

SERVES 2

PREP + COOK TIME: 20 MINS

VEG • GLUTEN FREE • DAIRY FREE

Cottage Cheese Pancakes

SERVES 8

PREP + COOK TIME: 20 MINS

VEG

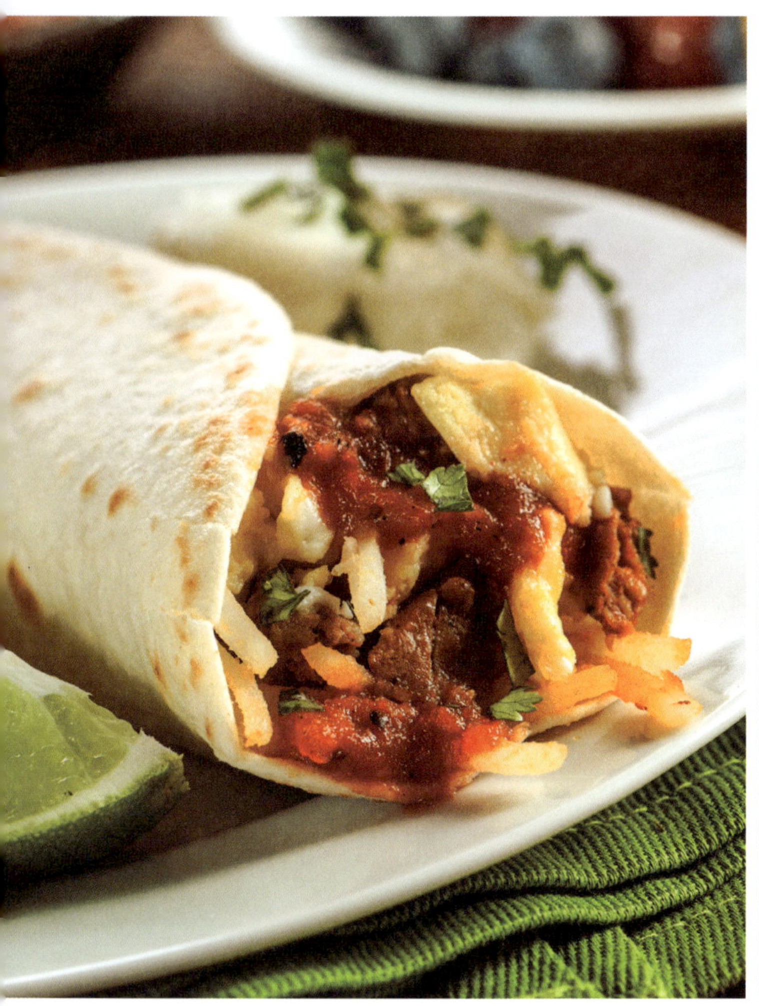

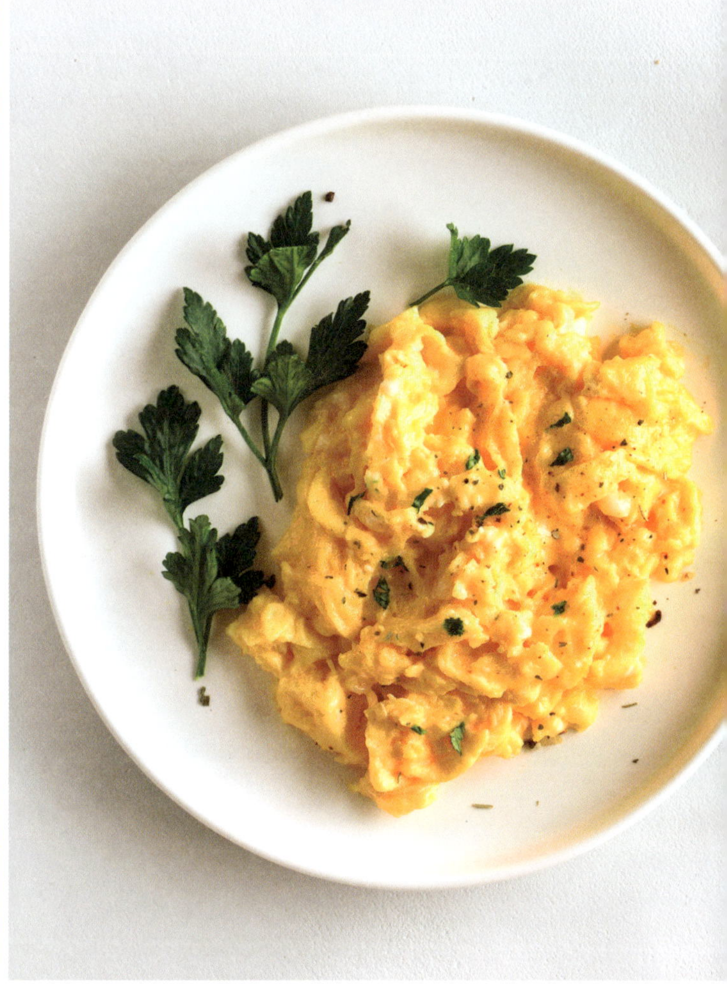

Breakfast Burritos

SERVES 3

PREP + COOK TIME: 15 MINS

Scrambled Eggs

SERVES 2

PREP + COOK TIME: 10 MINS

VEG • GLUTEN FREE

BREAKFAST BURRITOS

6 eggs, scrambled (see next recipe)

4 cooked sausages, chopped

½ cup (60g) grated Cheddar cheese

1 cup (270g) tomato salsa

6 flour tortillas

Fresh parsley, to serve

Preheat the air fryer to 180°C. Spray the air fryer basket with olive oil spray.

Combine the egg, sausage, cheese and salsa in a mixing bowl. Spoon ½ cup of the mixture into the centre of a flour tortilla. Fold in the sides and then roll to form a burrito.

Repeat with the remaining ingredients.

Place the burritos into the air fryer basket and cook for 5 minutes. Serve garnished with fresh parsley, if desired.

SCRAMBLED EGGS

4-5 eggs

Salt and pepper to taste

Knob of butter

Baking pan

Preheat the air fryer to 220°C.

Whisk the eggs until fully combined. Season to taste.

Place butter in the baking pan and insert the pan into the air fryer. Heat butter until just melted (approximately 1 minute).

Add the eggs and cook for 1 minute. Remove, stir and check the consistency. Repeat until the eggs are cooked to your liking.

Cauliflower Fritters

SERVES 4

PREP + COOK TIME: 25 MINS

VEG • GLUTEN FREE

1 head cauliflower, cut into florets

2 tbsps olive oil

½ onion, diced

Salt and pepper to taste

2 eggs

½ cup (50g) grated Parmesan cheese

5 tbsps blanched almond meal

1 tbsp chopped parsley

1 tsp garlic powder

Guacamole or favourite dipping sauce to serve

Place cauliflower florets into a food processor and pulse until it resembles rice. Transfer to a clean tea towel and squeeze out any excess water.

Heat olive oil in a large frying pan over medium-high heat. Add onion and cook for 3-5 minutes until soft and translucent. Add cauliflower and season with salt and pepper. Cook for 3-4 minutes until softened.

In a large bowl whisk together eggs, Parmesan, almond meal, parsley and garlic powder. Add cauliflower and stir to combine.

Preheat air fryer to 190°C.

Scoop up mixture into small balls and flatten into patties with your palms.

Spray air fryer basket with cooking spray and lay patties in a single layer. Spray tops with cooking spray. Work in batches or use a double-layer accessory, if needed. C

ook for 3 minutes, then flip over, spray the other side and cook for another 3 minutes until crispy. Serve hot with guacamole or your favourite dipping sauce.

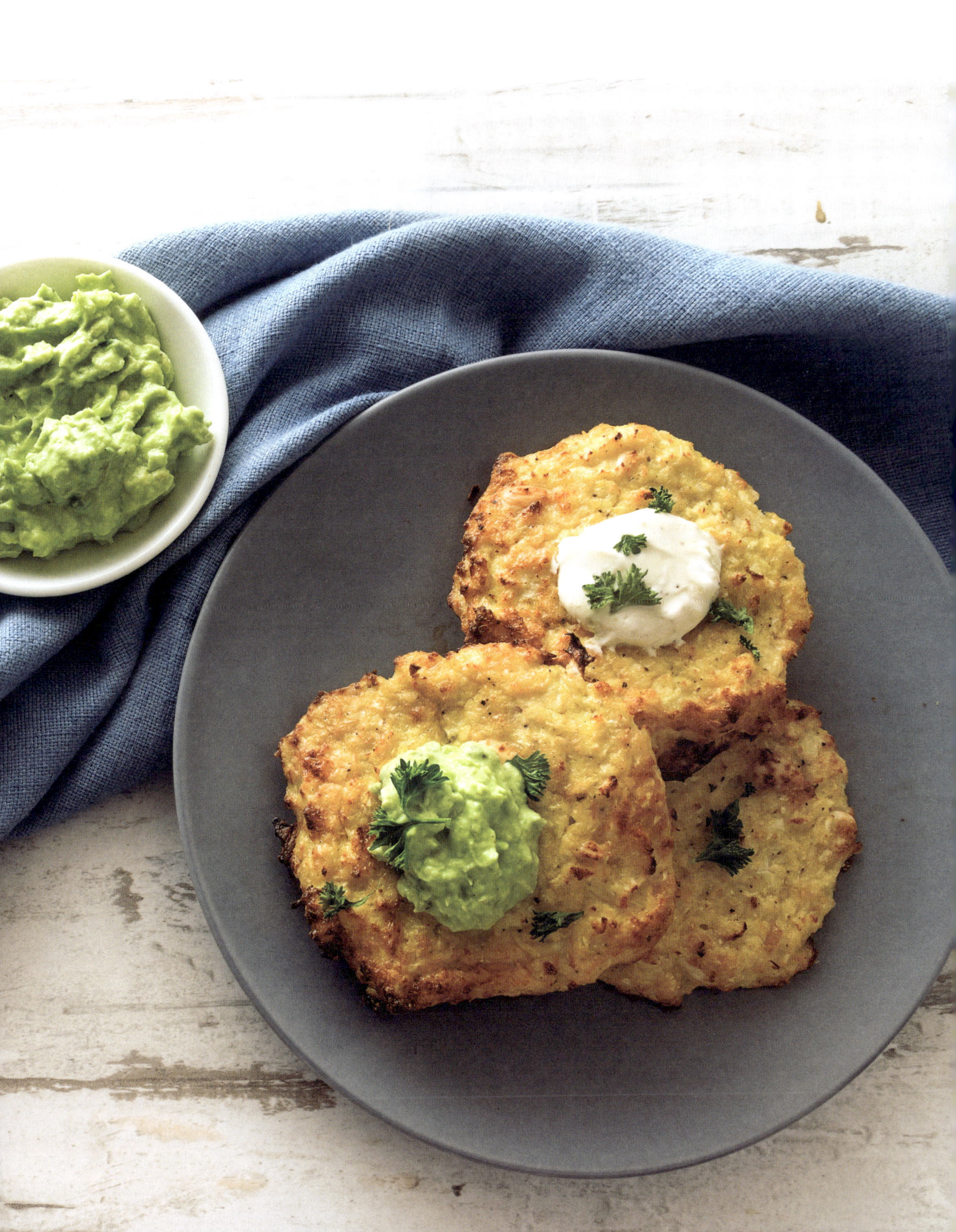

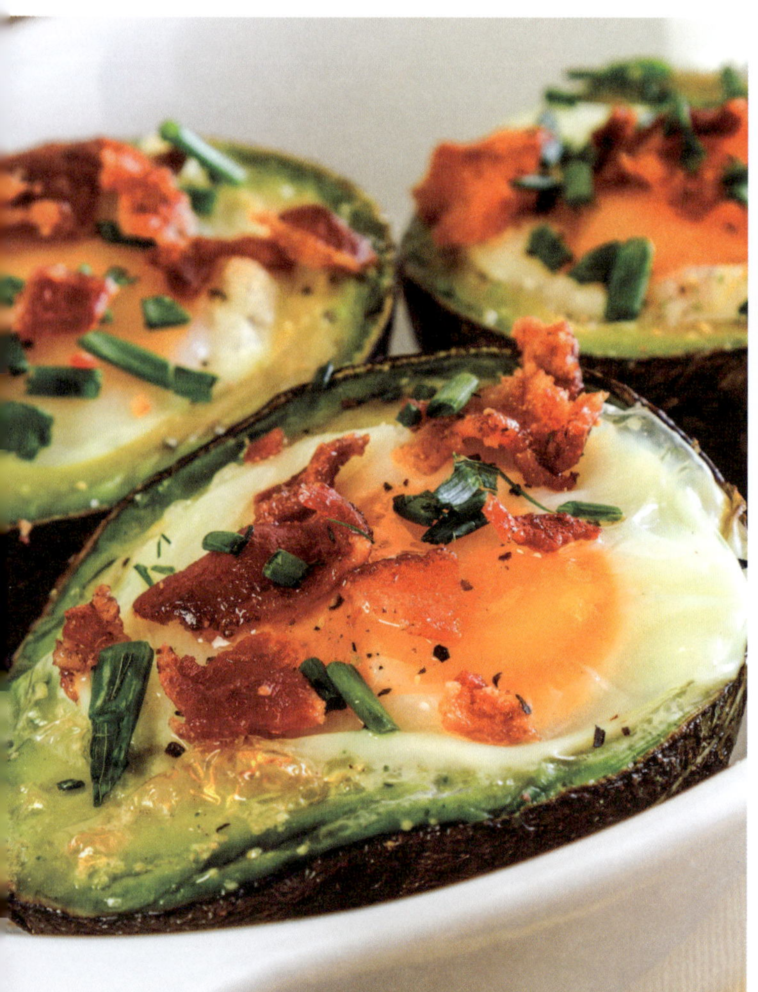

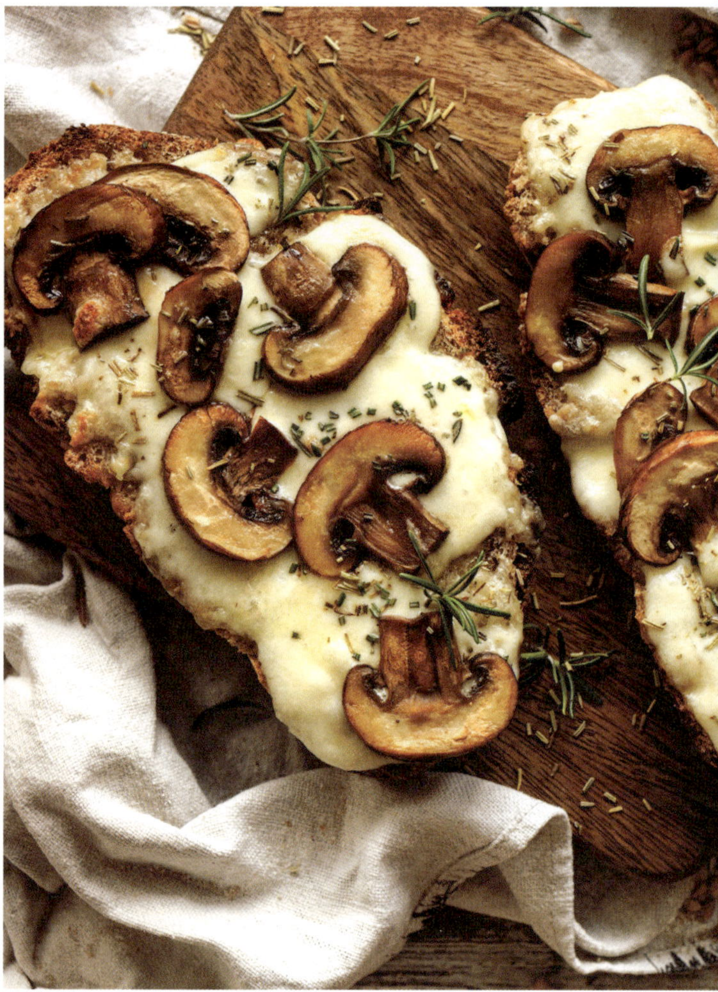

Avo Eggs with Bacon

SERVES 2

PREP + COOK TIME: 20 MINS

GLUTEN FREE • DAIRY FREE

Mushrooms & Cheese on Toast

SERVES 1

PREP + COOK TIME: 20 MINS

VEG

AVO EGGS WITH BACON

2 rashers bacon

2 avocados

4 eggs

Salt and pepper to taste

1 tbsp chives, chopped

Place bacon in air fryer. Cook for 4 minutes at 200°C, then turn with tongs and cook for a further 4 minutes. Set aside to cool.

When bacon is cool enough to handle snip it into small pieces. Set aside.

Cut avocados in half and remove the stone.

Place avocados in air fryer basket then crack an egg into each one, keeping the yolk intact.

Cook at 200°C for 9 minutes or until egg is done to your liking.

Season the eggs with salt and pepper. Sprinkle over bacon pieces and chives to serve.

MUSHROOMS & CHEESE ON TOAST

2 tsps olive oil

½ cup (40g) sliced mushrooms

1 clove garlic, minced

Salt and pepper to taste

2 slices of sourdough bread

Butter for spreading

1 cup (125g) grated mozzarella or Gruyere cheese

1 tsp chopped rosemary

Heat the olive oil in a small pan over medium heat. Add the mushrooms and garlic and cook, stirring regularly, for 5-8 minutes until the mushrooms are tender. Season with salt and pepper.

Toast the bread in a toaster.

Spread toast with butter. Top with grated cheese, followed by sliced mushrooms and chopped rosemary.

Place in the air fryer and cook at 200°C for 4-5 minutes until the cheese is melted and golden.

CAULIFLOWER HASH BROWNS

3½ cups (350g) grated cauliflower
1 onion, finely chopped
1 egg
½ cup (45g) chickpea flour (besan)
1 cup (125g) grated Cheddar cheese
½ tsp paprika
1 tsp salt
Pepper to taste

Place grated cauliflower in a clean tea towel and twist to squeeze out moisture.

Place the cauliflower in a large bowl and add onion, egg, flour, cheese, paprika, salt and pepper. Mix until well combined.

Shape the mixture into eight patties and freeze for at least 1 hour.

Preheat air fryer to 200°C.

Spray air fryer basket with oil. Arrange patties in one layer in air fryer basket, Cook in batches or use a double layer accessory if necessary.

Cook for 10 minutes, turning halfway through the cooking process.

BREAKFAST FRITTATA

4 eggs
3 tbsps double cream
¼ cup (30g) grated Cheddar cheese
3 cherry tomatoes, halved
1 spring onion, finely sliced
Pinch of salt
Baking pan

Preheat the air fryer to 180°C.

Lightly spray and line a baking pan with greaseproof paper and set aside.

Whisk the eggs and cream together in a mixing bowl.

Add the remaining ingredients to the bowl, and stir to combine.

Pour the mixture into the baking pan and place inside the air fryer basket.

Cook for 15 minutes, or until eggs are set. To check, insert a toothpick in the centre of the frittata. The eggs are set if it comes out clean.

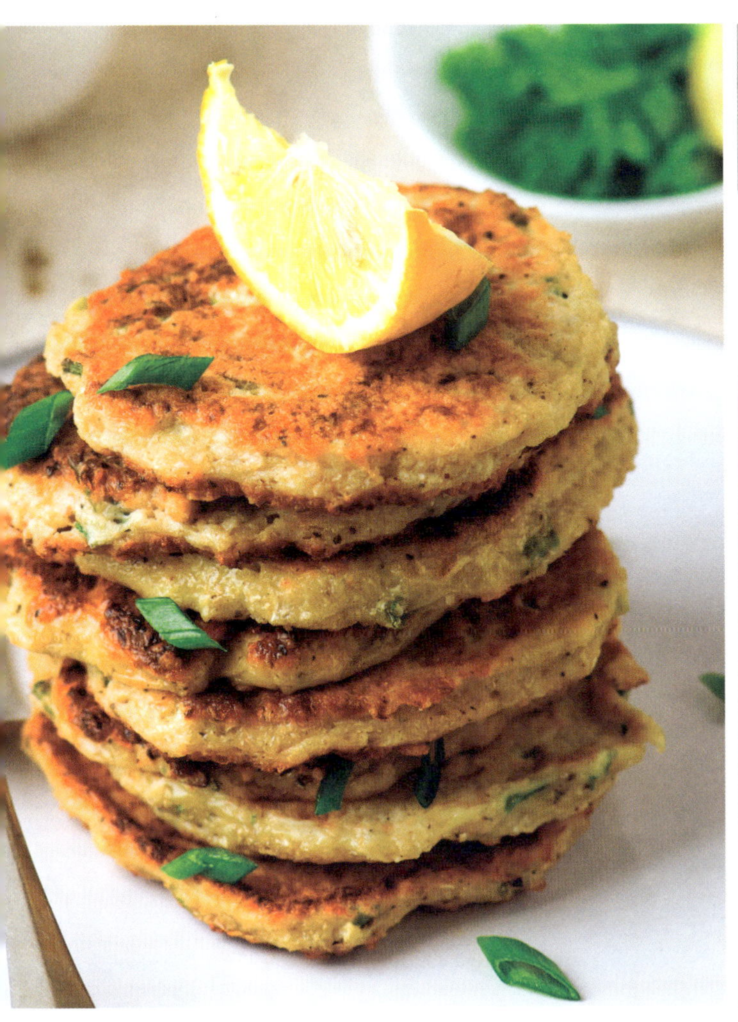

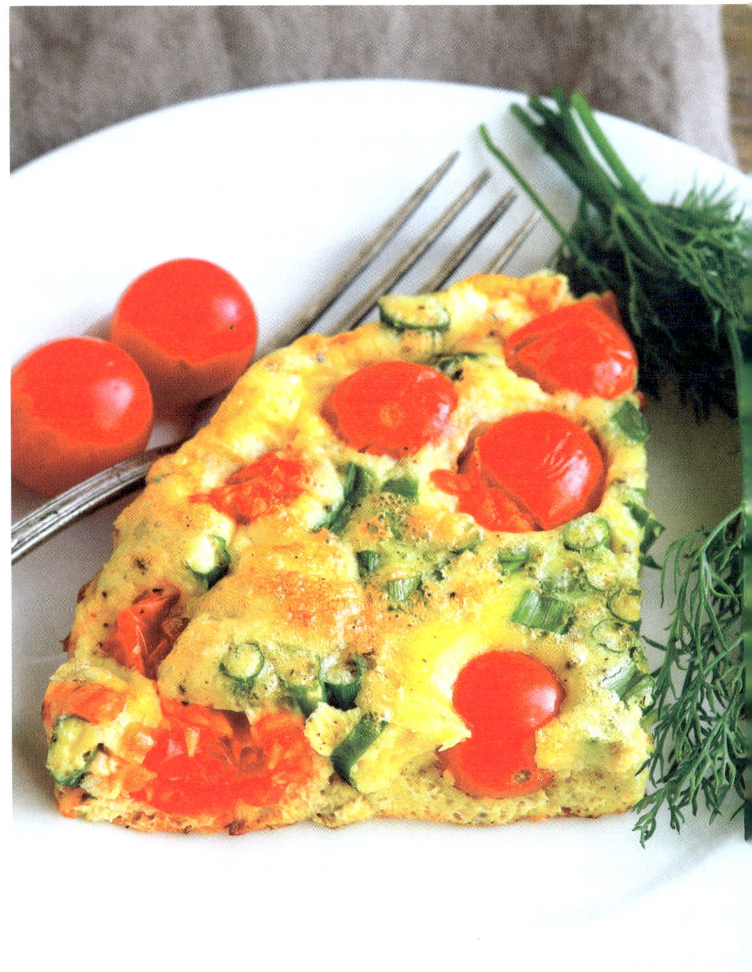

Cauliflower Hash Browns

SERVES 4

PREP + COOK TIME: 20 MINS + FREEZING

VEG • GLUTEN FREE

Breakfast Frittata

SERVES 2

PREP + COOK TIME: 20 MINS

VEG • GLUTEN FREE

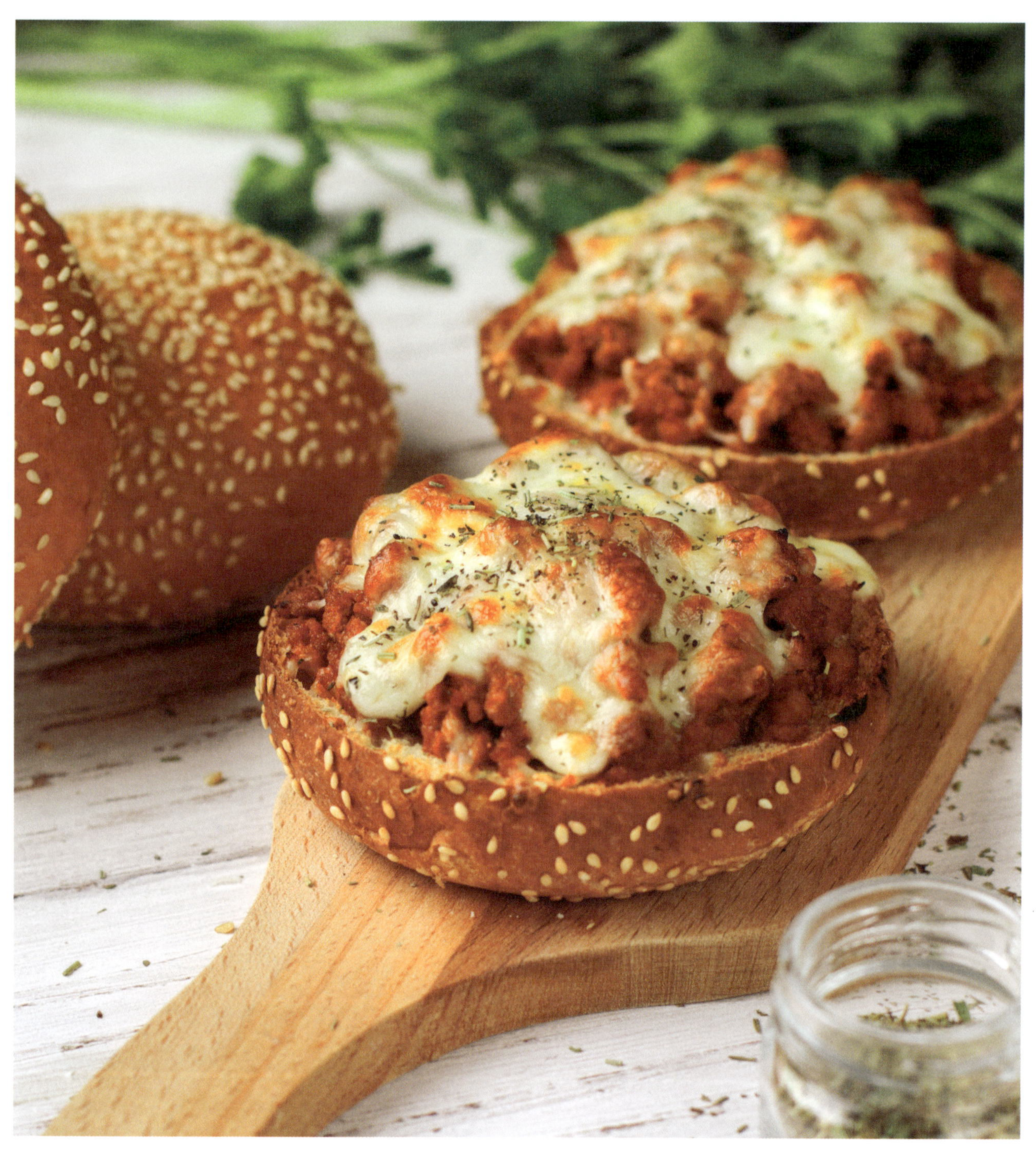

Cheesy Sloppy Joes

SERVES 4

PREP + COOK TIME: 45 MINS

CHEESY SLOPPY JOES

1 tbsp olive oil
1 onion, finely chopped
1 red capsicum, finely chopped
3 cloves garlic, minced
500g beef mince
150g tomato paste
1 tsp brown sugar
1 tbsp English mustard
1 tsp chilli powder
1 tbsp apple cider vinegar
¼ cup (60ml) Worcestershire sauce
Salt and pepper to taste
4 sesame seed burger buns
1 cup (125g) shredded mozzarella
1 tsp Italian seasoning

Heat olive oil in a large frying pan over medium heat. Add the onions and cook for 5-7 minutes until soft and translucent. Stir in the capsicum and cook for 3-4 minutes more until starting to soften. Add the garlic and cook for 1 minute until fragrant. Add the beef mince and cook, breaking up with a spoon, for 3-5 minutes until browned. Stir in the tomato paste, sugar, mustard, chilli powder, vinegar and Worcestershire sauce. Season with salt and pepper and simmer for 10-15 minutes.

Preheat the air fryer to 180°C.

Spoon the meat sauce onto four burger bun bottoms and top each one with shredded cheese and Italian seasoning. Air fry for 3 minutes until the cheese is melted. Remove from the air fryer and set aside.

Place the burger bun tops in the air fryer and cook for 3 minutes.

Place the burger bun tops on the sloppy joes to serve.

Mini Ham, Pea & Corn Frittatas

MAKES 6
PREP + COOK TIME: 20 MINS
GLUTEN FREE

6 large eggs
2 tbsps milk or cream
Salt and pepper to taste
100g thick-cut ham, chopped
½ cup (80g) peas
½ cup (85g) corn kernels
½ cup (60g) grated Cheddar cheese
¼ cup (30g) grated mozzarella cheese
Muffin tray or silicone moulds

Place eggs in a large bowl with milk or cream. Season with salt and pepper and whisk to combine. Add remaining ingredients into the bowl and stir well.

Place 6 silicone muffin moulds or an air fryer muffin tray filled with paper liners into air fryer basket. Pour egg mixture into each of the moulds.

Cook for 12-15 minutes at 175°C until egg is set.

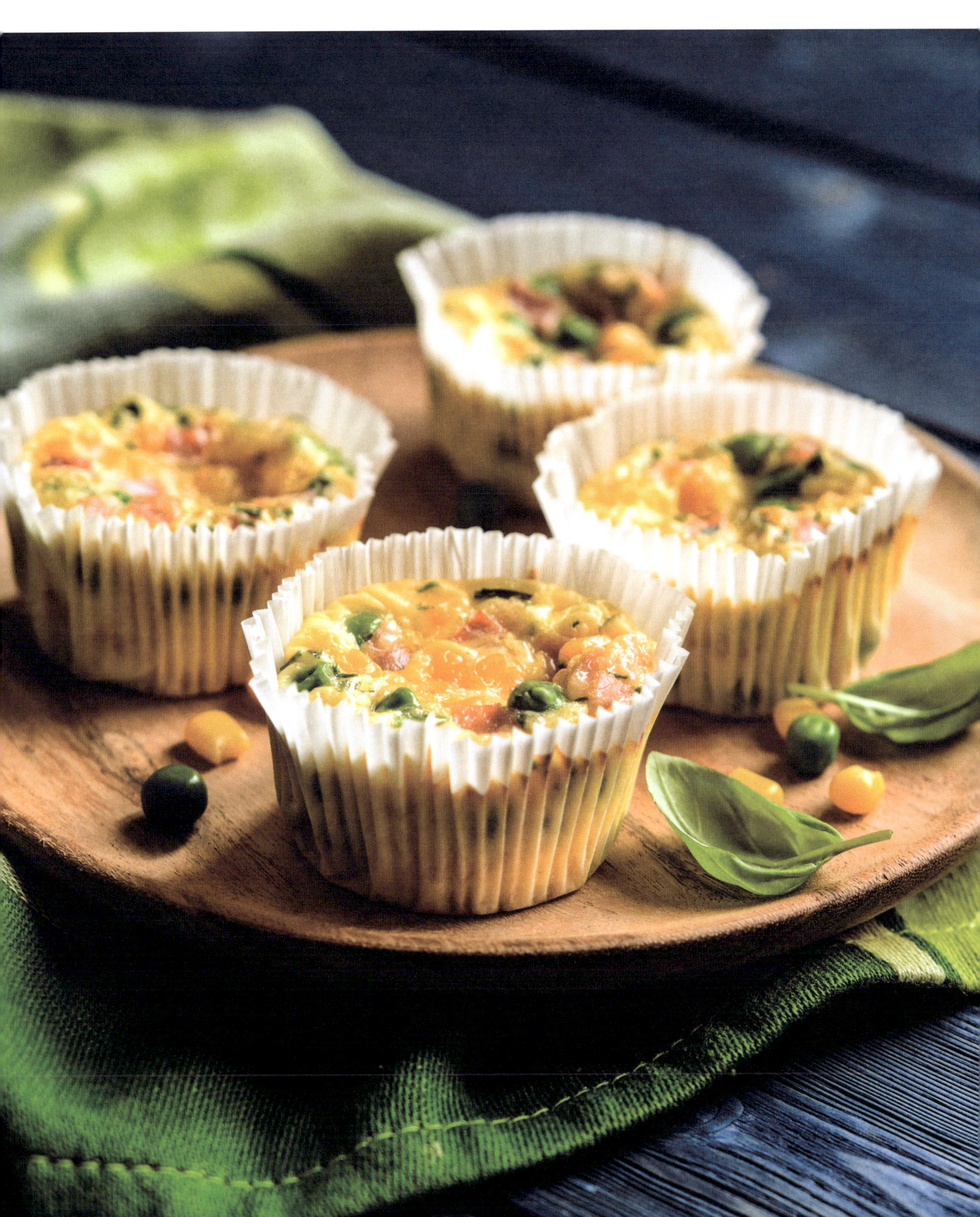

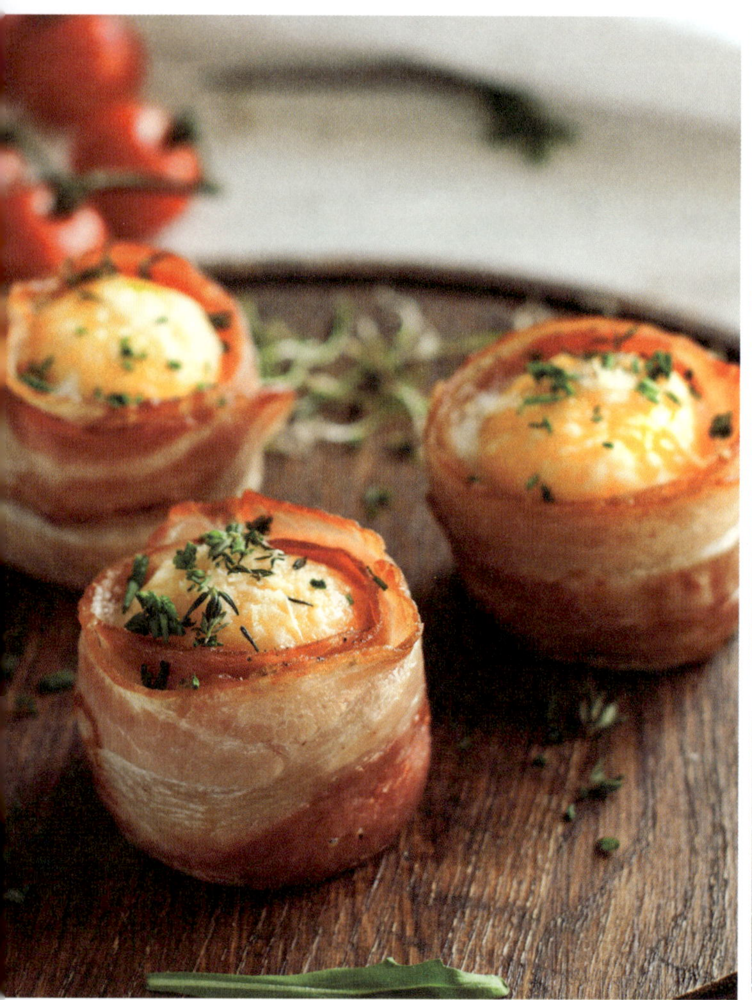

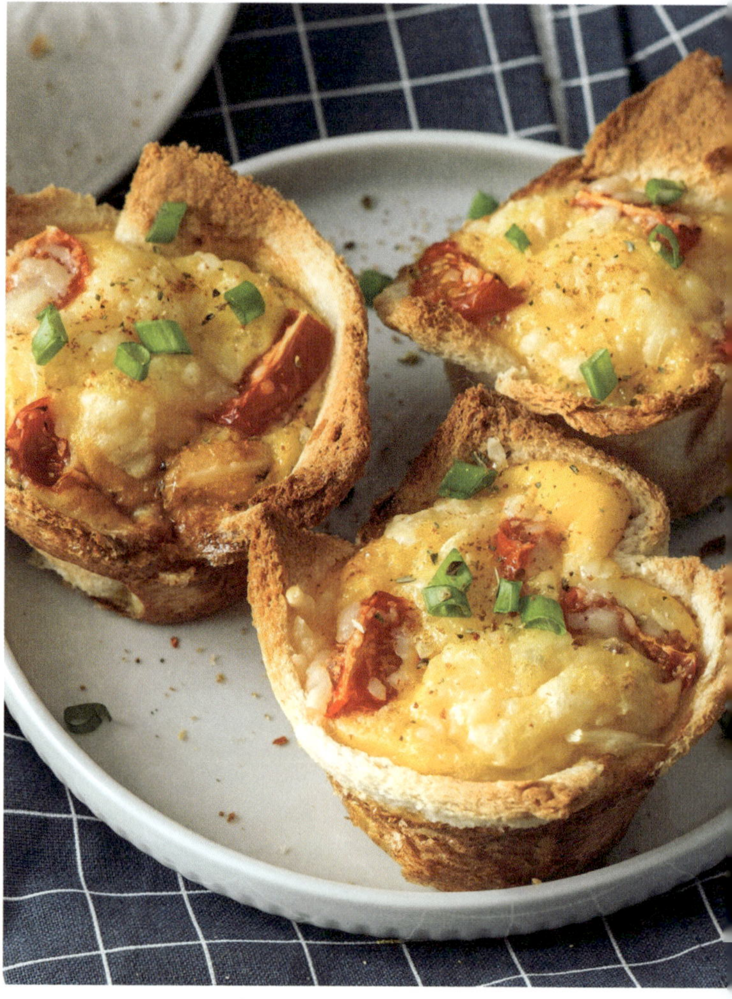

Bacon & Egg Roll-Ups

MAKES 4

PREP + COOK TIME: 20 MINS

GLUTEN FREE

Toast & Egg Cups

SERVES 4

PREP + COOK TIME: 20 MINS

BACON & EGG ROLL-UPS

4 eggs

¼ tsp salt

1 tsp thyme leaves + more to serve

1 tsp chopped chives + more to serve

½ tsp paprika

1 tbsp butter

150g rashers streaky bacon

4 ramekins or muffin moulds

Preheat air fryer to 180°C.

In a mixing bowl beat the eggs. Add salt, thyme, chives and paprika. Mix well.

Spread the ramekins or muffin moulds with butter.

Use the bacon to line the ramekins or muffin moulds in a cup shape.

Pour the egg mix into the bacon cups.

Place into air fryer and cook for 15 minutes.

Sprinkle with fresh herbs to serve.

TOAST & EGG CUPS

3 tbsps butter

4 slices bread

4 eggs

60g ham, chopped

¼ cup (50g) cherry tomatoes, quartered

½ cup (60g) grated cheese

Salt and pepper to taste

Chopped spring onion, to serve

4 small ramekins

Grease the ramekins with some of the butter.

Cut the crusts off the bread and discard or save for another use. Butter one side of each slice of bread. Press bread, buttered-side down, into ramekins.

In a mixing bowl beat eggs. Add ham and tomatoes and mix well. Pour egg mixture into bread cups. Top with grated cheese.

Cook at 190°C for 12-14 minutes.

Run a knife around the sides to transfer to a plate. Season with salt and pepper and scatter with spring onion to serve.

SPINACH & BLUE CHEESE ROLL

150g baby spinach

4 cloves garlic, minced

2 tbsps melted butter

50g feta, crumbled

100g blue cheese, crumbled

Salt and pepper to taste

1 sheet frozen puff pastry, thawed

Bring a large pan of salted water to a boil. Add spinach and blanch for 1 minute then drain and soak in ice water. Drain and then finely chop.

Place spinach in a large bowl and mix with garlic, butter and crumbled cheeses. Season with salt and pepper. Stir to combine.

Spread pastry sheet thinly with spinach and cheese mixture. Roll pastry into a sausage as tightly as possible.

Place rolled pastry, seam-side down, into your air fryer basket.

Cook at 180°C for 25 minutes.

HAM & CHEESE PUFFS

2 sheets frozen puff pastry, thawed

1 ham steak, diced

1⅔ cups (200g) grated Cheddar cheese

Milk, to glaze

Preheat the air fryer to 200°C.

Mix the ham and cheese together in a mixing bowl.

Roll and cut the pastry into squares of 5 x 5cm and scoop a heaped teaspoon of filling onto each square.

Fold over the corners of squares so that they almost meet in the centre.

Place the parcels in the air fryer basket and brush the pastry with milk. Be careful not to overcrowd the basket. Cook in batches or use a double layer accessory if needed.

Slide the basket into the air fryer and cook for 10 minutes until crispy and golden.

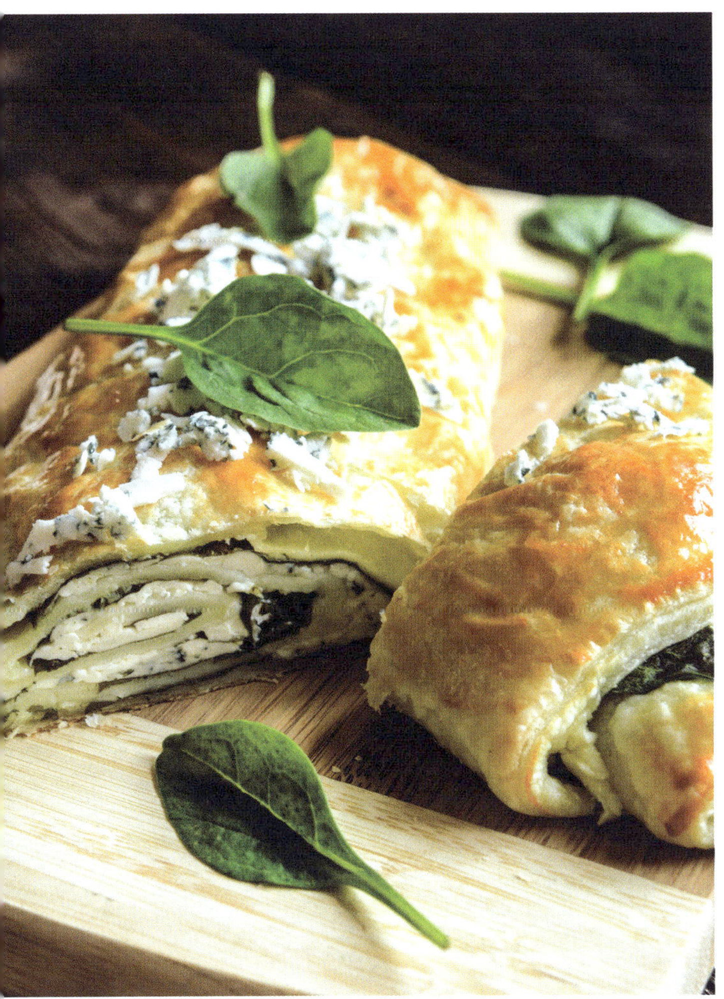

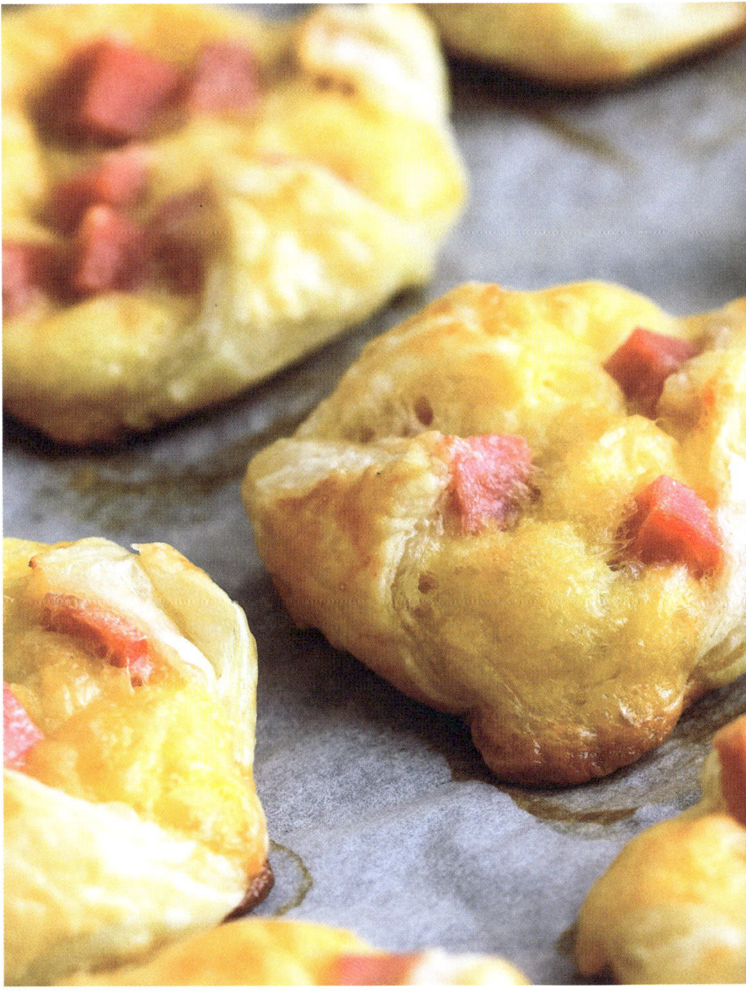

Spinach & Blue Cheese Roll

SERVES 2

PREP + COOK TIME: 35 MINS

VEG

Ham & Cheese Puffs

SERVES 2

PREP + COOK TIME: 20 MINS

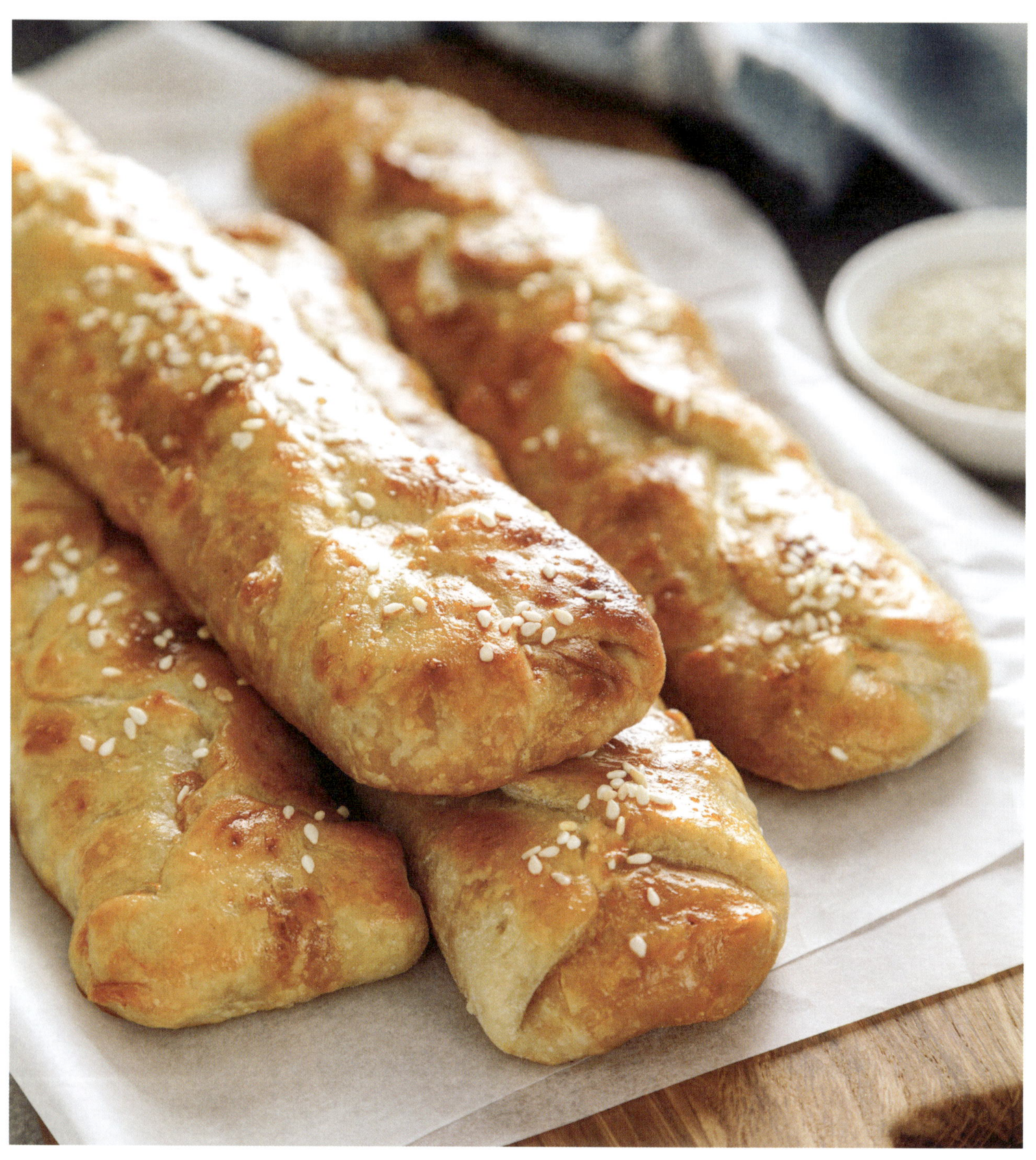

Ricotta & Spinach Rolls

MAKES 8

PREP + COOK TIME: 30 MINS

VEG

RICOTTA & SPINACH ROLLS

1 tbsp olive oil

1 shallot, finely chopped

2 cloves garlic, minced

½ tsp dried chilli flakes

150g baby spinach

½ tsp salt + more to taste

½ tsp pepper + more to taste

½ cup (125g) ricotta cheese

2 sheets frozen puff pastry, thawed

1 egg, beaten

1 tbsp sesame seeds

Heat olive oil in a pan over medium heat. Add shallot and cook for 3-5 minutes until soft and translucent. Add garlic and chilli flakes. Cook for 1 minute until fragrant. Add the spinach leaves and salt and pepper. Stir for 2 minutes until the leaves wilt. Remove from heat and set aside for 5 minutes to allow to cool. Squeeze out any excess liquid from the spinach. Transfer to large bowl and mix in ricotta. Season with salt and pepper to taste.

Cut each sheet of pastry into four equal squares.

Scoop about 1½ tablespoons of the spinach ricotta filling onto the centre-left of a pastry square and roughly shape the filling into a log. Fold the upper and lower sides in.

Brush the folded edges with a little bit of water then roll the pastry into a sausage. Repeat with the remaining filling and pastry squares. Brush the pastries with beaten egg and sprinkle with sesame seeds.

Preheat the air fryer to 180°C. Spray the air fryer basket with cooking spray.

Place pastries into the air fryer basket in one single layer, working in batches if needed, and cook for 10-12 minutes, flipping over halfway through cooking, until golden brown and crisp.

Scotch Eggs

SERVES 3
PREP + COOK TIME: 20 MINS
GLUTEN FREE

500g sausage meat
¼ cup (25g) grated Parmesan cheese
1 tsp onion powder
¼ tsp dried chilli flakes
Salt and pepper to taste
6 eggs, hard-boiled and peeled

Place meat in a bowl. Add the Parmesan, onion powder, dried chilli flakes, salt and pepper and mix with your hands to combine.

Preheat the air fryer to 200°C.

Divide the meat into six even portions. Flatten each portion into a thin patty. Place a hard-boiled egg in the middle of each patty and wrap the meat around the egg, sealing all sides. Repeat with all six eggs and patties and set aside.

Spray the basket of the air fryer with cooking spray and place egg patties into the basket. Spritz with oil spray. Be careful not to overcrowd the basket. Cook in batches or use a double-layer accessory if needed.

Cook for 12 minutes, removing the basket and turning eggs over halfway through. Repeat with remaining eggs, if necessary.

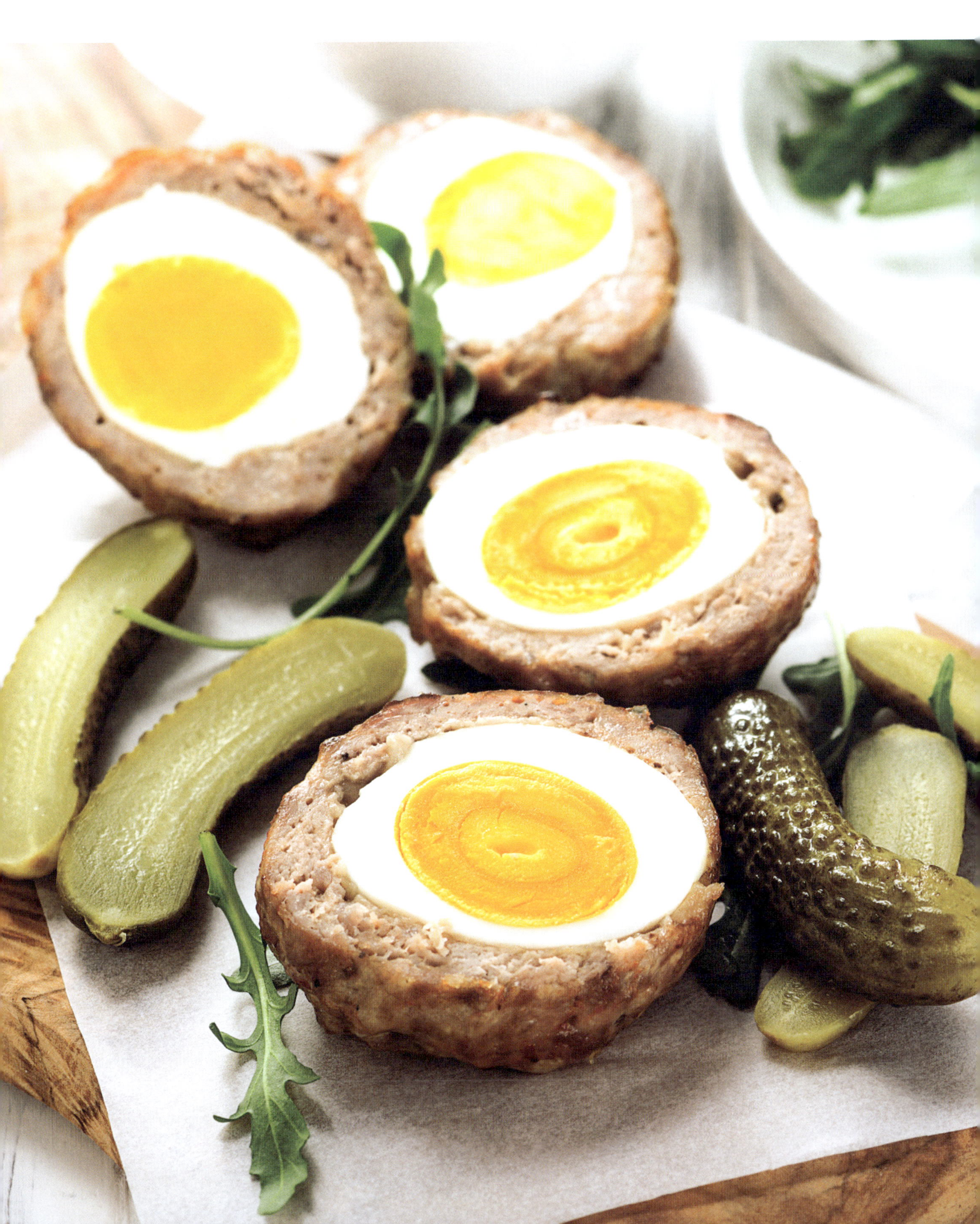

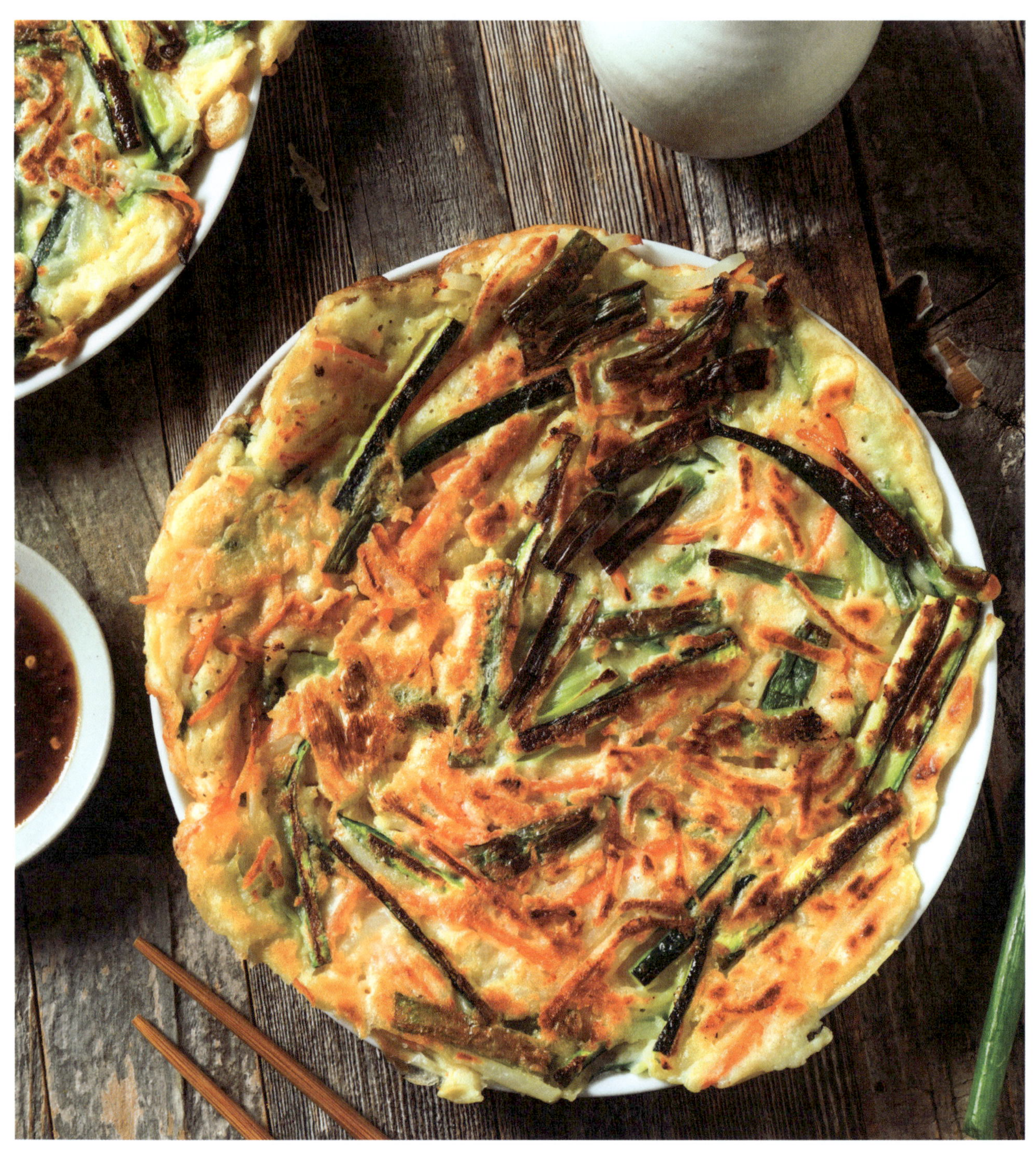

Korean Pajeon (Spring Onion) Pancakes

SERVES 2

PREP + COOK TIME: 30 MINS

VEG • DAIRY FREE

KOREAN PAJEON (SPRING ONION) PANCAKES

DIPPING SAUCE

⅓ cup (80ml) soy sauce

2 tbsps honey

2 tbsps rice wine vinegar

2 tbsps water

1 tbsp toasted sesame oil

2 cloves garlic, minced

½ tsp chilli flakes

PANCAKES

1 cup (125g) plain flour

2 tbsps cornflour

¼ tsp sugar

½ tsp salt

1 cup (250ml) cold sparkling water

1 egg, beaten

2 cloves garlic, minced

8 spring onions, halved lengthways and cut into 5cm pieces

1 carrot, julienned

Combine sauce ingredients in a small pan over medium heat. Bring to a boil, then stir and reduce heat to medium-low. Simmer for 5-7 minutes, until slightly thickened.

In a large mixing bowl, whisk together flour, cornflour, sugar and salt. Make a well in the centre and pour in water, egg and garlic. Stir gently until just combined. Gently fold in spring onions and carrot.

Line base and sides of air fryer basket with greaseproof paper. Spray with cooking spray. Spoon a ladleful of batter onto the paper.

Cook for 6-8 minutes without flipping, at 160°C, until brown. Repeat with remaining batter, spraying each batch.

Spiced Toast Sticks

SERVES 2
PREP + COOK TIME: 20 MINS
VEG

4 slices bread
2 tbsps butter, softened
2 eggs
Pinch of salt
2 tsps ground cinnamon
1 tsp ground nutmeg
½ tsp ground cloves
Icing sugar, to serve
Maple syrup, to serve
Baking pan

Preheat air fryer to 180°C and spray the baking pan with cooking spray.

Butter both sides of the bread slices and cut into thick strips.

In a large mixing bowl, beat together the eggs, salt, cinnamon, nutmeg and cloves.

Dredge each strip in the egg mixture and arrange in a single layer in the pan. Cook in batches or use a double layer accessory with a second pan.

Cook for 2 minutes and then remove. Liberally spray the bread with cooking spray on both sides.

Return pan to the air fryer and cook for a further 4 minutes, checking a few times. Remove when nicely browned.

Sprinkle with icing sugar and serve with a small bowl of syrup for dipping.

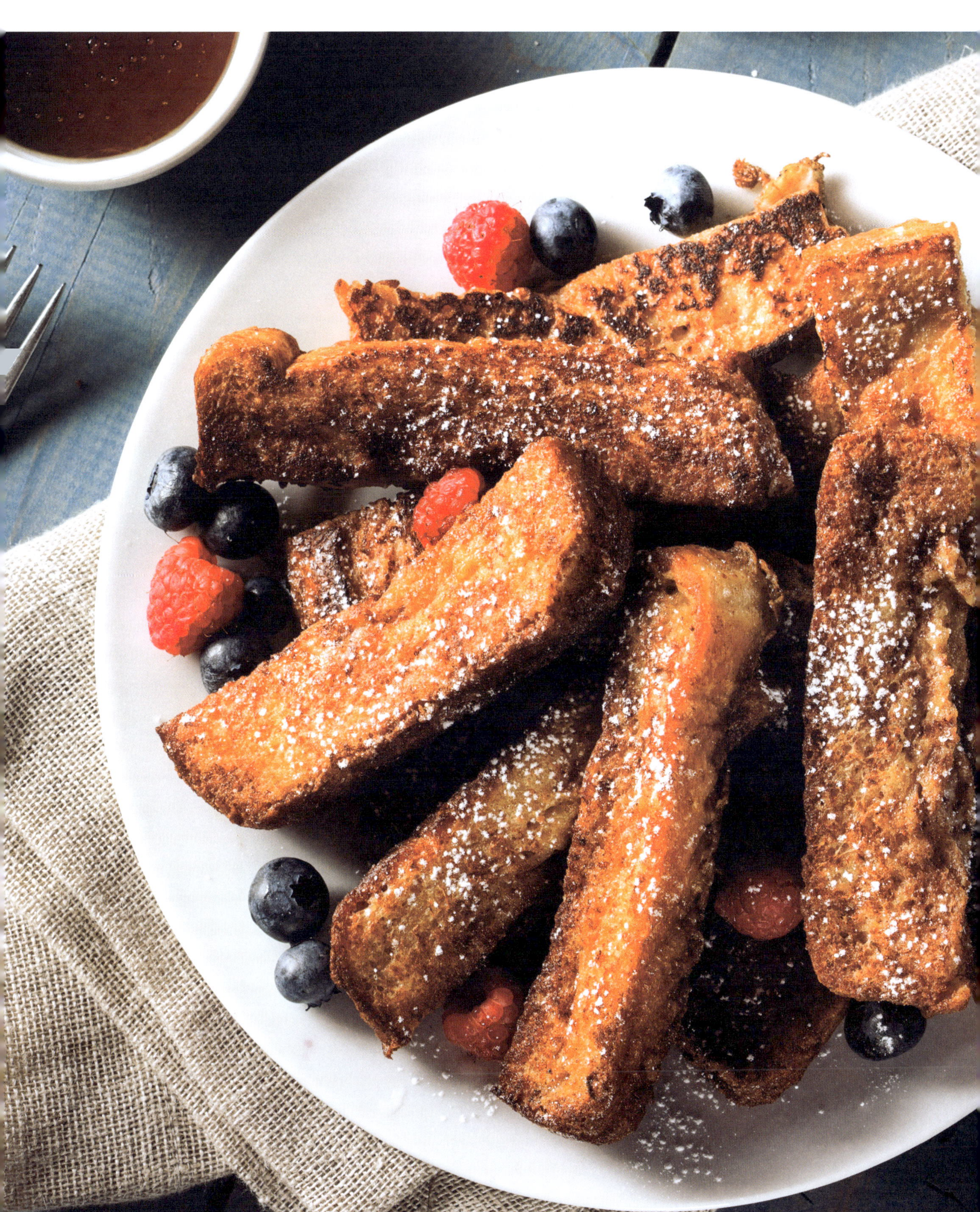

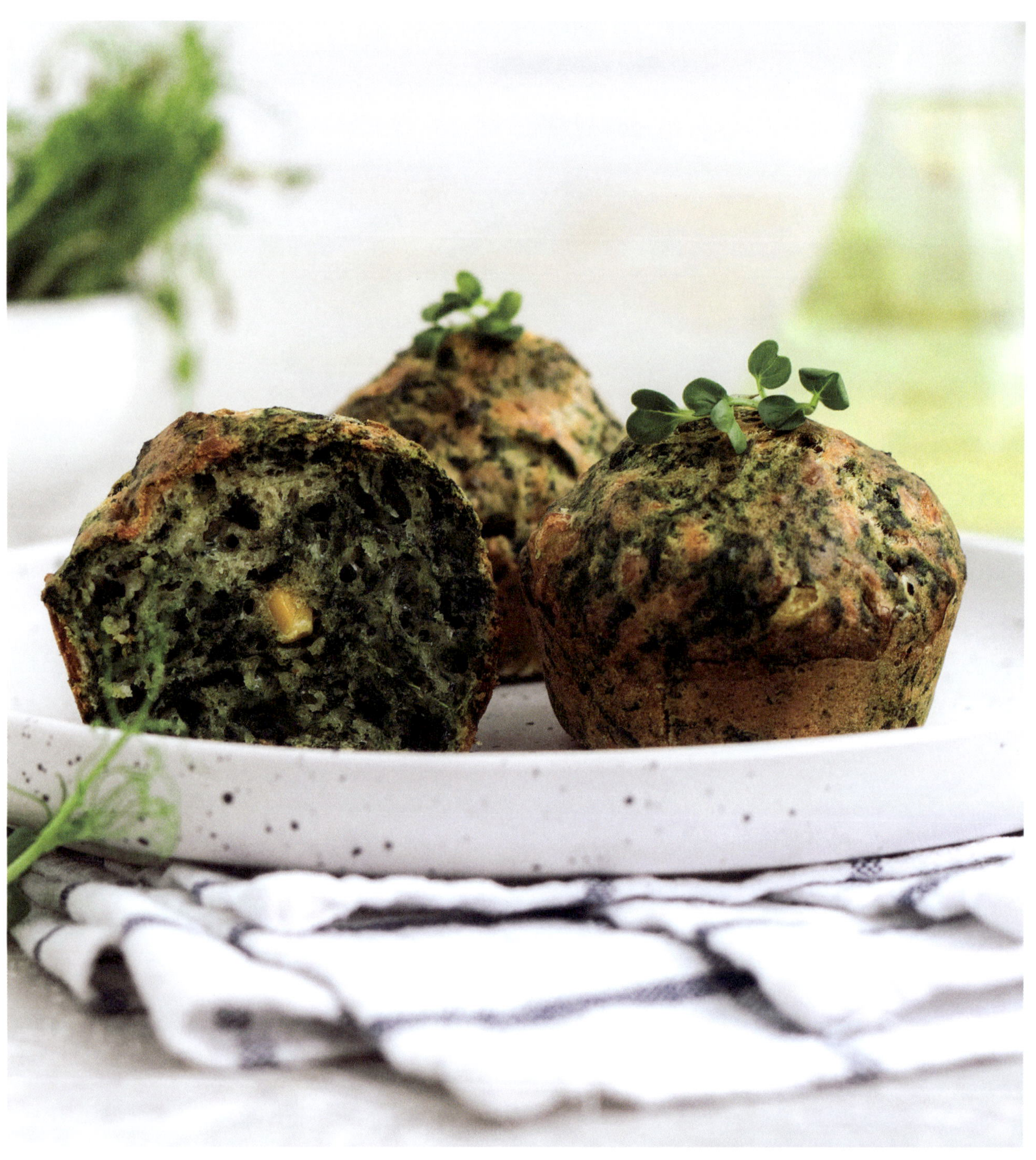

Spinach Muffins

MAKES 12

PREP + COOK TIME: 30 MINS

VEG

SPINACH MUFFINS

350g frozen chopped spinach, thawed and squeezed to remove moisture

2 large eggs

¼ cup (60ml) olive oil

1 cup (250ml) milk

¼ cup (60ml) Greek yoghurt

2 cups (250g) plain flour

2 tsps baking powder

80g feta cheese, crumbled

½ cup (85g) corn kernels

Place spinach, eggs, olive oil, milk and yoghurt in a large bowl. Mix well. Add flour, baking powder, feta and corn. Stir to combine.

Preheat air fryer to 175°C.

Spoon mixture into silicone moulds or an air fryer muffin tray filled with paper liners.

Cook in batches or use a double-layer accessory for 15-20 minutes, until an inserted skewer comes out clean.

Chapter Two

Snacks and Lunchbox

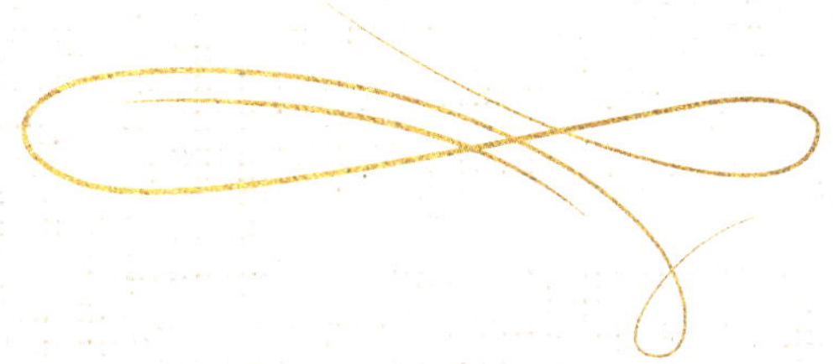

CHINESE CHICKEN WINGS

6 chicken wings

1 tbsp soy sauce

1 tsp mixed spice

1 tbsp Chinese five-spice powder

Pinch of salt and pepper

Combine all the ingredients except for the chicken wings in a small bowl and whisk to combine.

Add the chicken wings and rub the seasoning over the chicken. Massage into the chicken until thoroughly coated.

Place a piece of foil into the bottom of the air fryer. Place the chicken on it and pour over any remaining marinade.

Cook for 15 minutes at 180°C. Remove the chicken and flip it over using tongs then return to the air fryer. Increase the temperature to 200°C and cook for a further 15 minutes.

ASIAN-STYLE CHICKEN MEATBALLS

500g chicken mince

1 cup (125g) breadcrumbs

¼ cup (60ml) chicken stock

1 egg

2 spring onions, finely chopped

2 tsps sesame oil

2 tsps soy sauce

Small piece fresh ginger, minced

1 clove garlic, minced

¼ tsp salt

¼ tsp pepper

¼ tsp brown sugar

Lime wedges, to serve

¼ cup (70g) sweet chilli sauce, to serve

Mix together chicken mince, breadcrumbs, chicken stock, egg, spring onions, sesame oil, soy sauce, ginger, garlic, salt, pepper and brown sugar. Divide into 16 portions. Roll into meatballs.

Preheat air fryer to 175°C.

Place meatballs in single layer in air fryer, working in batches if needed. Cook for 10-12 minutes, turning halfway through cooking, until golden brown and cooked through. Repeat with remaining meatballs.

Serve with lime wedges and sweet chilli sauce.

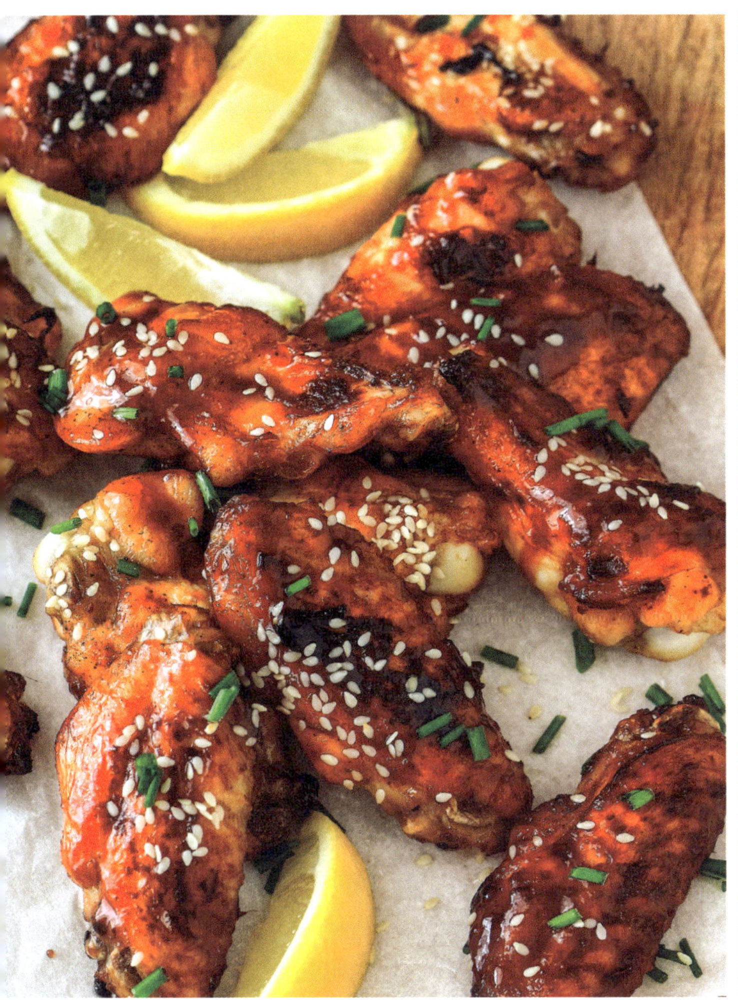

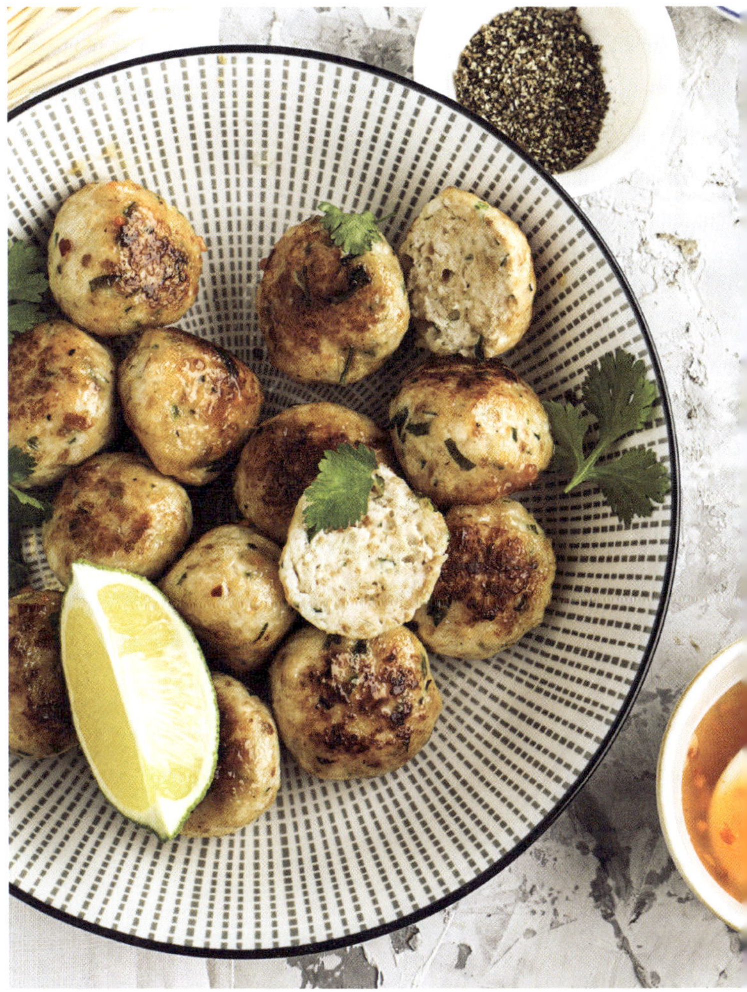

Chinese Chicken Wings

SERVES 2

PREP + COOK TIME: 40 MINS

DAIRY FREE

Asian-Style Chicken Meatballs

SERVES 4

PREP + COOK TIME: 30 MINS

DAIRY FREE

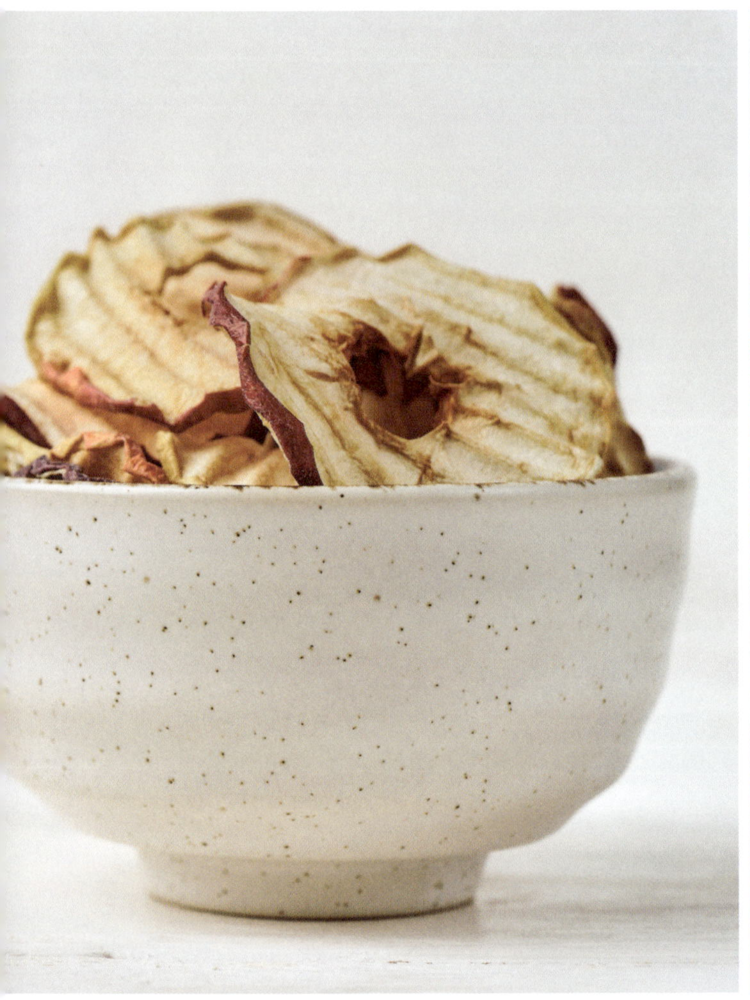

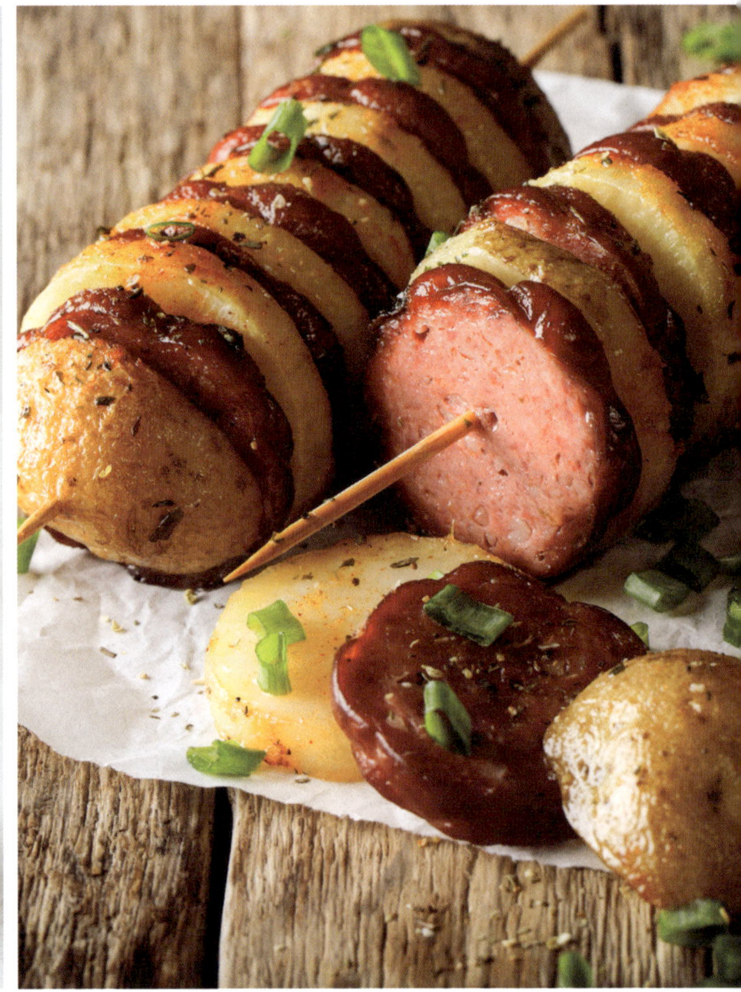

Apple Chips

SERVES 1

PREP + COOK TIME: 30 MINS

VEG • GLUTEN FREE

Potato & Sausage Skewer

SERVES 4

PREP + COOK TIME: 35 MINS

GLUTEN FREE

APPLE CHIPS

1 large apple

Preheat air fryer to 150°C.

Thinly slice apple with a mandoline or sharp knife.

Place apple slices in air fryer and spray with cooking spray.

Cook for 20-25 minutes, shaking every 5 minutes, until the apples are completely dried out.

For crispy apple chips increase the temperature to 160°C and cook for a further 5 minutes, shaking every 90 seconds.

POTATO & SAUSAGE SKEWERS

2 tbsps melted butter

2 tbsps olive oil

½ tsp garlic powder

1 tsp mixed herbs

4 medium potatoes

150g smoked sausage

Salt to taste

Chopped spring onions to serve

Skewer rack

In a small bowl, mix the melted butter, olive oil, garlic powder and mixed herbs. Set aside.

Using a sharp knife cut the potatoes and sausages into 5mm-thick slices.

Alternating between sausage and potato, carefully push the slices onto skewers.

Brush the melted butter over the potato and sausage skewers paying attention to getting it in between the potato slices.

Place the skewers in the air fryer basket, set the temperature to 200°C and cook for 20-22 minutes until the potatoes are crispy and golden.

Sprinkle with salt and spring onions to serve.

Crab Bites

MAKES 36

PREP + COOK TIME: 30 MINS

½ cup (120g) mayonnaise

1 egg

2 tbsps chopped fresh chives

1 tsp Worcestershire sauce

1 tsp Dijon mustard

1 tsp paprika

1 tsp fresh lemon juice

450g refrigerated crabmeat

⅔ cup (80g) panko breadcrumbs

SAUCE

1 cup (245g) mayonnaise

2 tsps Dijon mustard

1 clove garlic, finely chopped

2 tsps fresh lemon juice

¼ tsp salt

1 tbsp chopped dill

Lemon wedges, to serve

Preheat air fryer to 180°C.

To make the crab bites stir together mayonnaise, egg, chives, Worcestershire sauce, Dijon mustard, paprika and lemon juice. Fold in crabmeat and breadcrumbs. Using a tablespoon, shape mixture into 36 balls.

Working in batches place in one layer in the air fryer. Cook for 12-16 minutes or until lightly browned and hot in the centre. Cool for 5 minutes.

Meanwhile, in small bowl, combine sauce ingredients and stir well. Serve bites with sauce and lemon wedges.

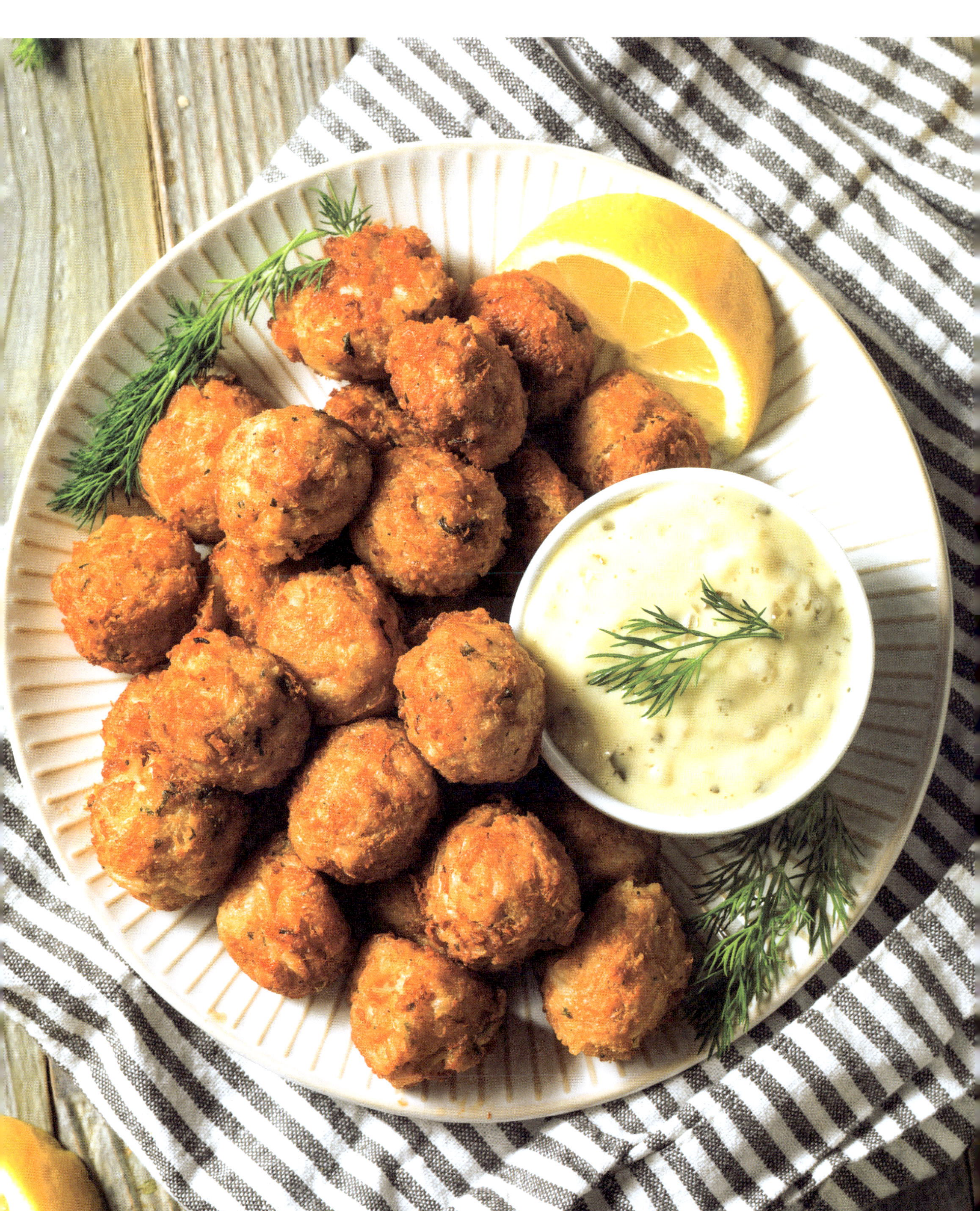

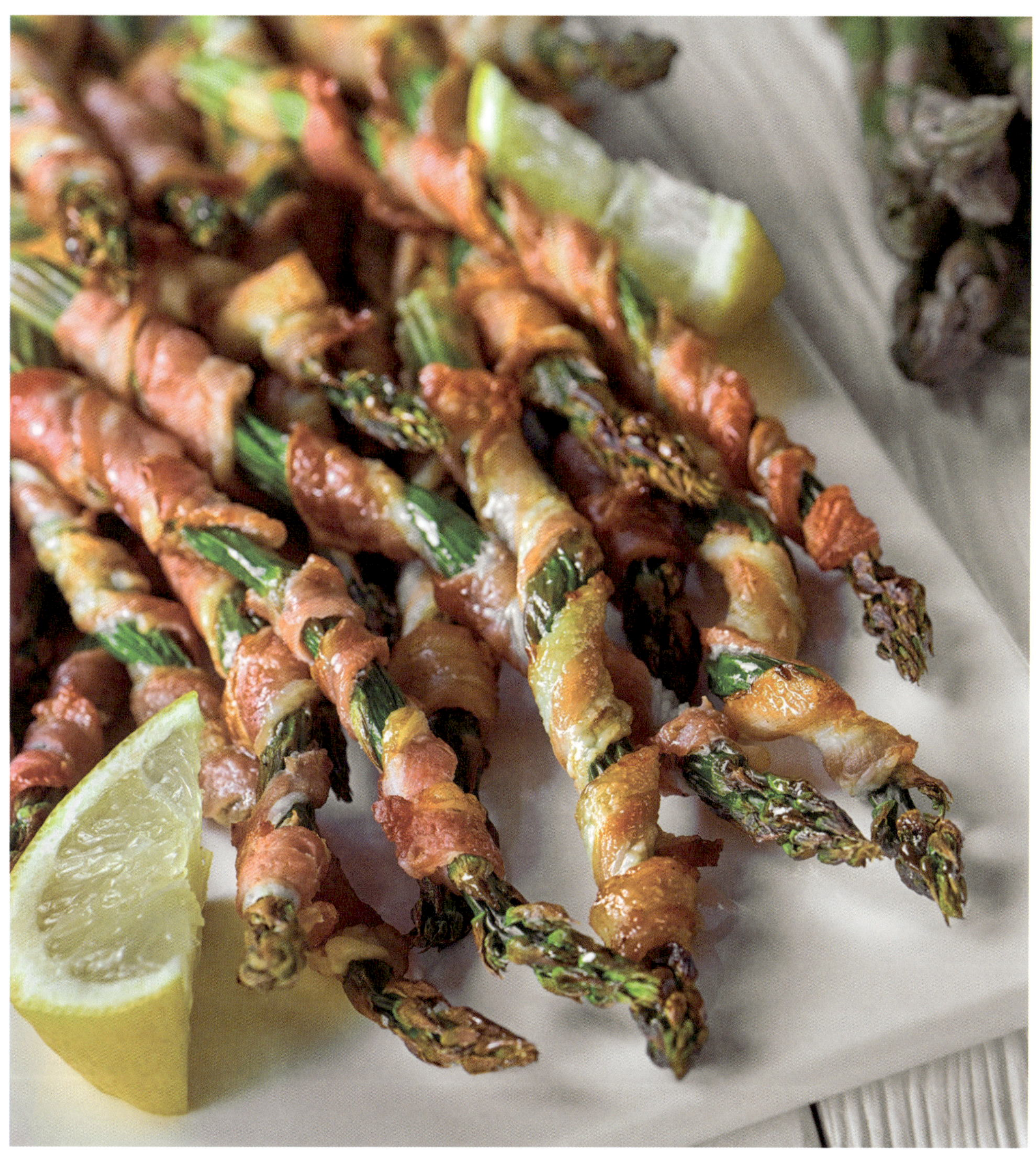

Asparagus in Bacon

SERVES 4

PREP + COOK TIME: 20 MINS

GLUTEN FREE

ASPARAGUS IN BACON

500g asparagus
12 rashers streaky bacon
2 tbsps butter, melted
1 tbsp brown sugar
⅛ tsp salt
⅛ tsp pepper
Lemon wedges, to serve

Wrap asparagus stalks with pieces of bacon. If using thin asparagus spears, cut bacon rashers in half lengthwise before wrapping the asparagus.

In a small bowl, mix butter, brown sugar, salt and pepper.

Spray air fryer basket with cooking spray. Brush brown sugar mixture on each asparagus bacon bundle.

Place 5-6 asparagus spears in air fryer basket at a time and cook at 200°C for 10 minutes.

Serve with lemon wedges.

RADISH CHIPS

6 radishes

1 tbsp balsamic vinegar

½ tsp salt

Wash and pat dry radishes. Using a sharp knife or mandolin, finely slice.

Place the radishes in the air fryer basket and spread out in an even layer. (Be careful not to overcrowd the basket. Cook in batches or use a double layer accessory if needed.)

Lightly spritz with olive oil, drizzle over the balsamic vinegar and sprinkle with salt.

Cook in the air fryer for 10 minutes at 190°C, shaking the basket halfway through.

Spritz with a little more oil and cook for a further 6 minutes, again shaking the basket halfway through.

SWEET POTATOES WITH SPICED CHICKPEAS

2 sweet potatoes

1 tbsp lime juice

1 clove garlic, minced

1 cup (250ml) plain yoghurt

2 tbsps fresh coriander, chopped

½ tsp salt

1 cup (160g) spiced chickpeas (see recipe page 77)

Preheat the air fryer to 200°C.

Scrub clean and pat dry the sweet potatoes. Spritz lightly with cooking spray. Pierce sweet potato skin with a fork and transfer to the air fryer.

Cook 40 minutes until tender.

To make the dressing combine lime juice, garlic, yoghurt, coriander and salt in a sealable jar. Close the lid tightly and shake to combine.

To serve, cut open the potatoes and top with spiced chickpeas and yoghurt dressing.

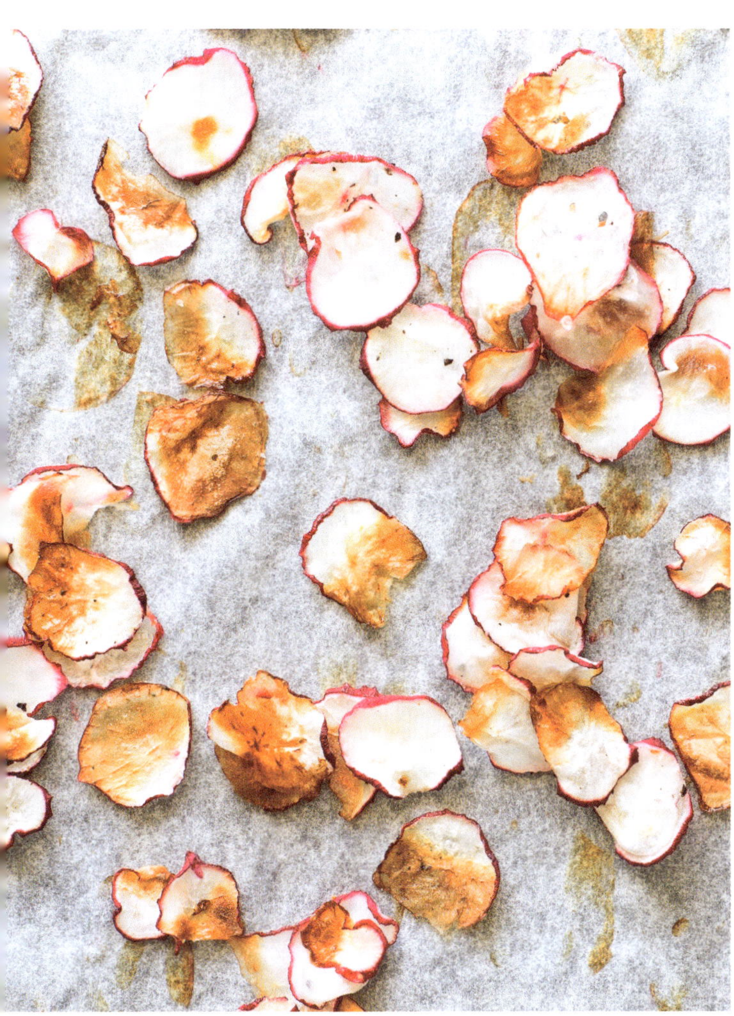

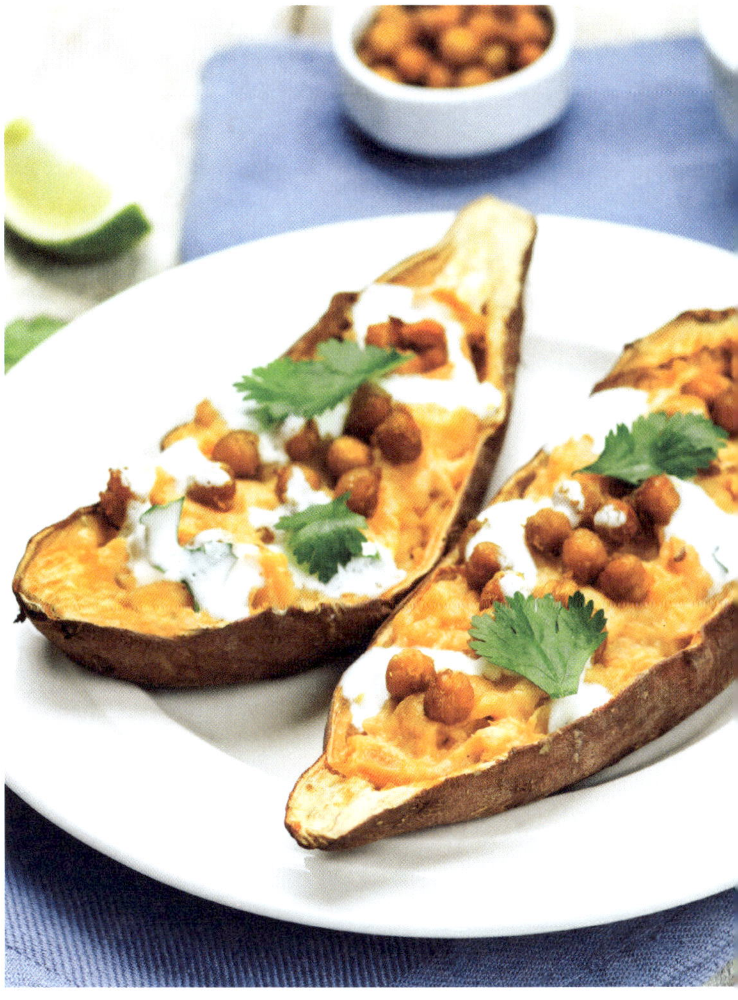

Radish Chips

SERVES 2

PREP + COOK TIME: 20 MINS

VEG • GLUTEN FREE • DAIRY FREE

Sweet Potatoes with Spiced Chickpeas

SERVES 2

PREP + COOK TIME: 50 MINS

VEG • GLUTEN FREE

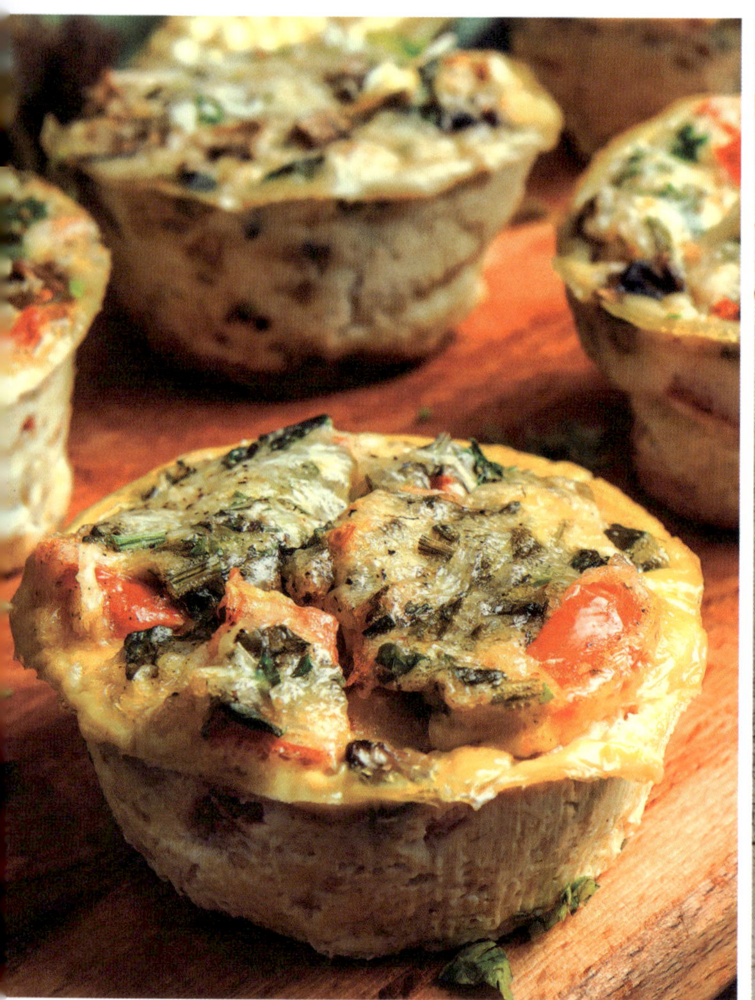

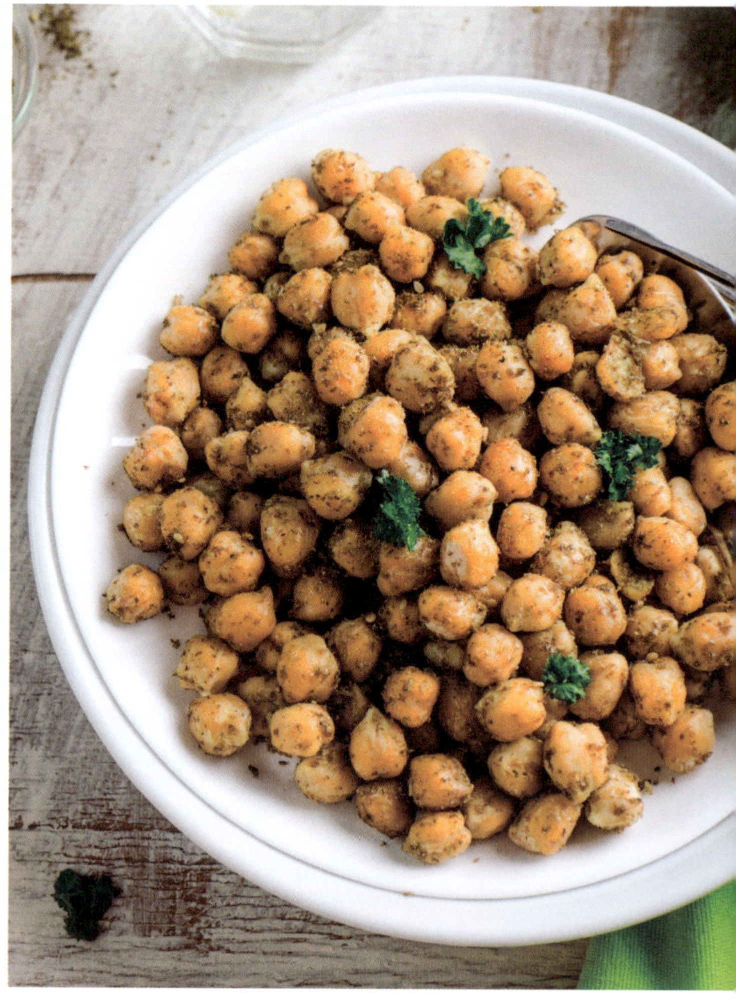

Egg & Veggie Cups

MAKES 6

PREP + COOK TIME: 20 MINS

VEG • GLUTEN FREE

Spiced Chickpeas

SERVES 2

PREP + COOK TIME: 25 MINS

VEG • GLUTEN FREE • DAIRY FREE

EGG & VEGGIE CUPS

6 eggs
2 tbsps milk
Pinch of salt and pepper
½ cup (15g) fresh spinach, finely chopped
¼ cup (45g) red capsicum, finely diced
¼ cup (35g) onion, finely diced
½ cup (60g) grated Cheddar cheese
¼ cup (30g) grated mozzarella cheese
6 silicone moulds

Lightly spray the moulds with oil and transfer to the air fryer.

Place the eggs, milk, salt and pepper in a large mixing bowl and whisk to combine. Sprinkle in spinach, capsicum, onion and Cheddar cheese and stir to combine.

Pour the egg mixture into the silicone moulds.

Sprinkle the mozzarella cheese over the top. Cook for 15 minutes at 160°C.

SPICED CHICKPEAS

1 x 400g can chickpeas
2 tsps olive oil
1 tsp ground coriander
1 tsp garlic powder
1 tsp ground cumin
Pinch of ground ginger
½ tsp salt

Drain and rinse the chickpeas. Place into a large bowl and add all the remaining ingredients. Toss to coat.

Preheat the air fryer to 190°C.

Transfer the mixture into the air fryer basket and cook for 20 minutes, removing the basket and stirring three times at regular intervals during cooking. Continue to cook at 1 minute intervals until the chickpeas are golden and crunchy.

Red Onion Tartlets

MAKES 9

PREP + COOK TIME: 30 MINS

VEG

2 tbsps olive oil

2 large red onions, thinly sliced

1 tbsp caster sugar

1 cup (50g) sun-dried tomatoes, finely chopped

1 sheet frozen puff pastry, thawed

50g goat's cheese, sliced

Muffin tray or silicone moulds

Heat oil in a large frying pan over high heat. Add onions and sugar and cook, stirring, for 3 minutes or until soft. Reduce heat to medium-high and cook, stirring, for 3-4 minutes or until caramelised. Transfer to a large bowl.

Add chopped sun-dried tomatoes and mix to combine.

Cut pastry sheet into 9 even squares.

Press pastry squares into the holes of the muffin tray. Work in batches if necessary.

Place a slice of goat's cheese in the bottom of each pastry case.

Spoon equal amounts of red onion mixture on top of the goat's cheese.

Transfer to the air fryer and cook for 10 minutes at 180°C until golden brown and crisp.

Repeat with remaining tartlets.

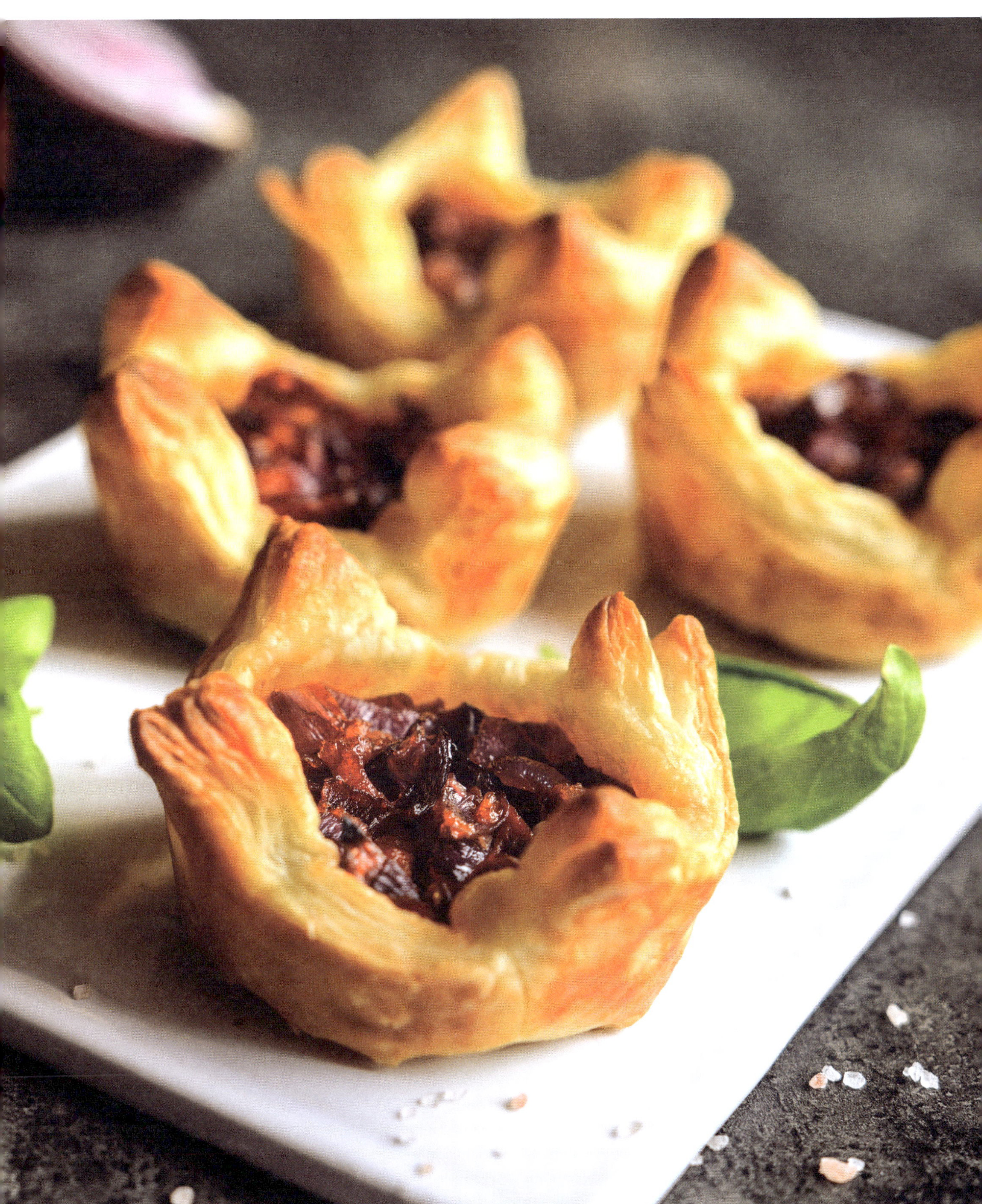

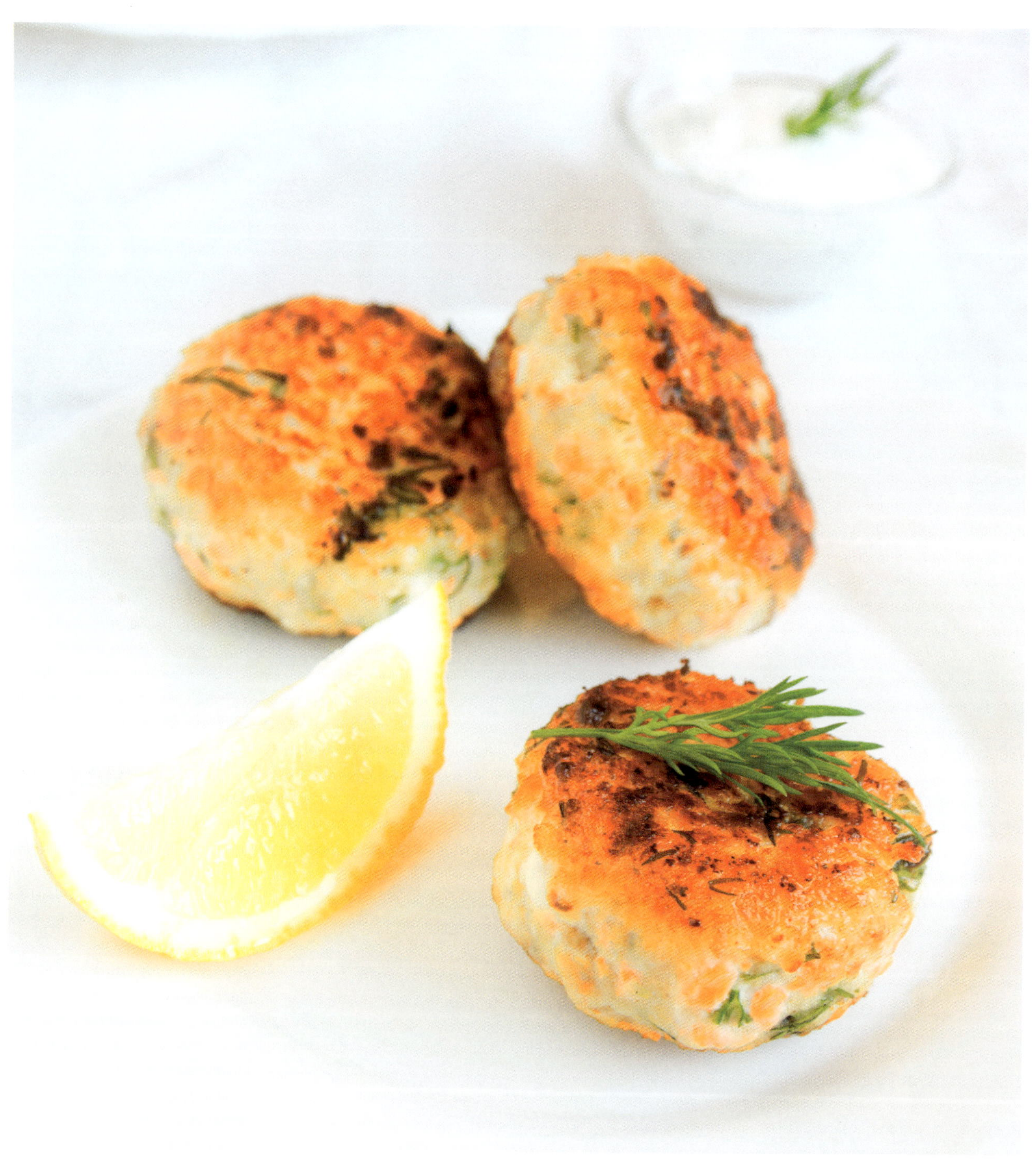

Crab Cakes

SERVES 4

PREP + COOK TIME: 20 MINS

DAIRY FREE

CRAB CAKES

250g crab meat

½ cup (60g) breadcrumbs

2 spring onions, chopped

1 tbsp fresh dill, chopped

1 egg

3 tbsps mayonnaise

2 tsps Dijon mustard

Juice of 1 lemon

Salt and pepper to taste

In a large bowl break up the crab meat with a fork. Add breadcrumbs, spring onions, dill, egg, mayonnaise, mustard, lemon juice, salt and pepper. Stir well then use hands to form mixture into eight small or four large patties.

Spray air fryer baskets and crab cakes with cooking spray.

Cook crab cakes in air fryer for 10 minutes at 180°C until golden brown, turning halfway through.

Salmon & Ricotta Puff Pastry Bites

MAKES 16

PREP + COOK TIME: 25 MINS

¾ cup (200g) ricotta

100g smoked salmon

1 tbsp chives, finely chopped

4 sheets frozen puff pastry, just thawed

3 tbsps milk

2 tbsps sesame seeds

Preheat the air fryer to 200°C.

Combine the ricotta, smoked salmon and chives in a mixing bowl.

Cut each pastry sheet into four squares.

Place a heaped teaspoon of filling onto each square.

Fold the squares into triangles and moisten the edges with water. Press the edges firmly together using a fork.

Place four parcels in the basket and brush with half the milk. Sprinkle with half the sesame seeds.

Slide the basket into the air fryer and cook for 10 minutes, or until golden brown.

Repeat the process for the remaining parcels.

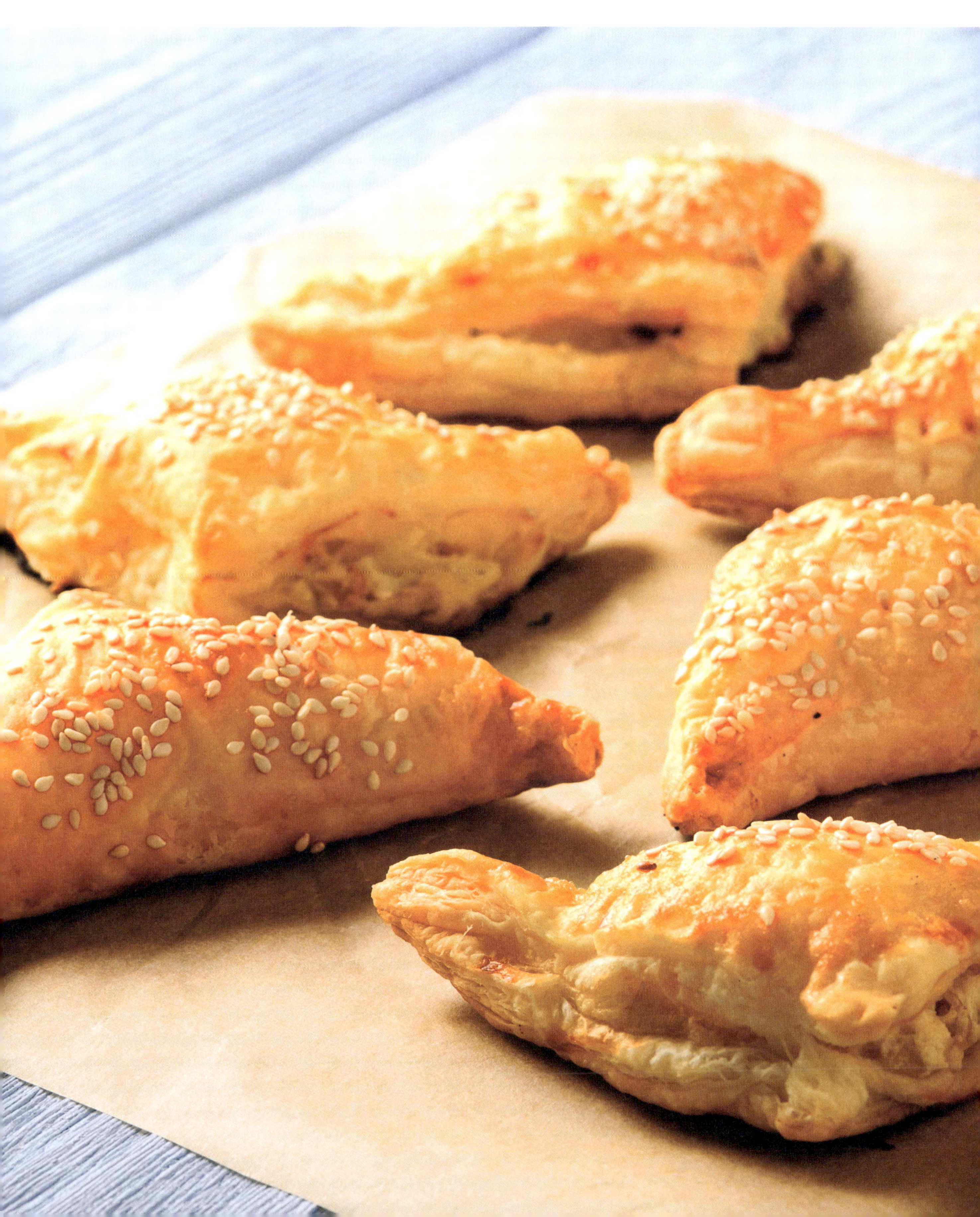

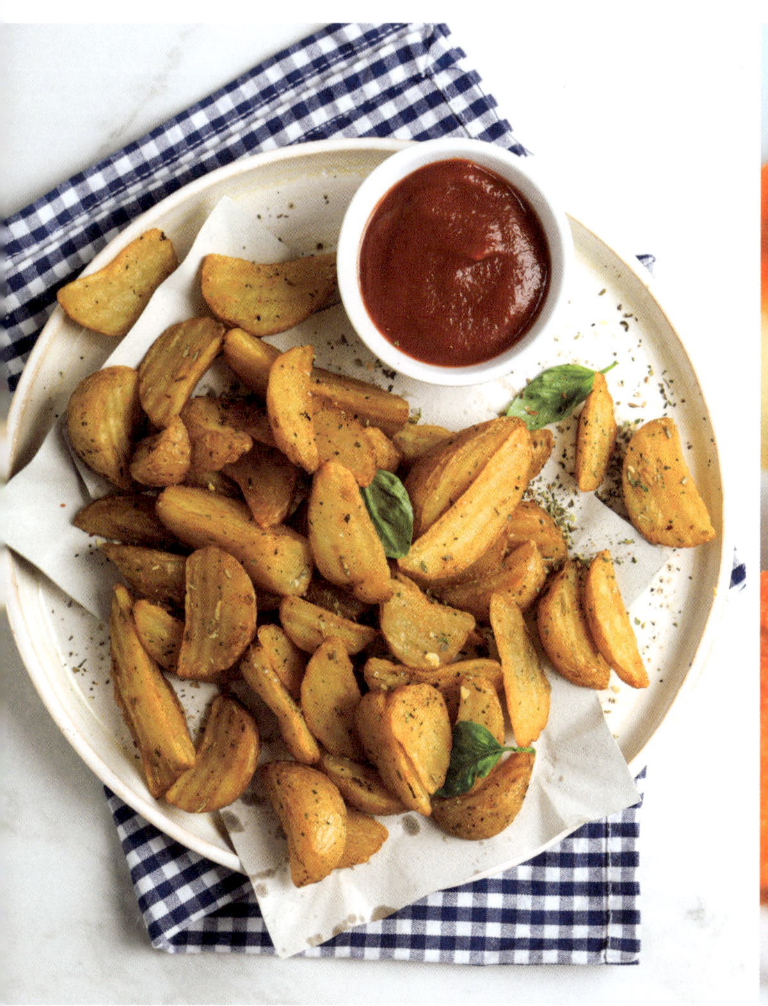

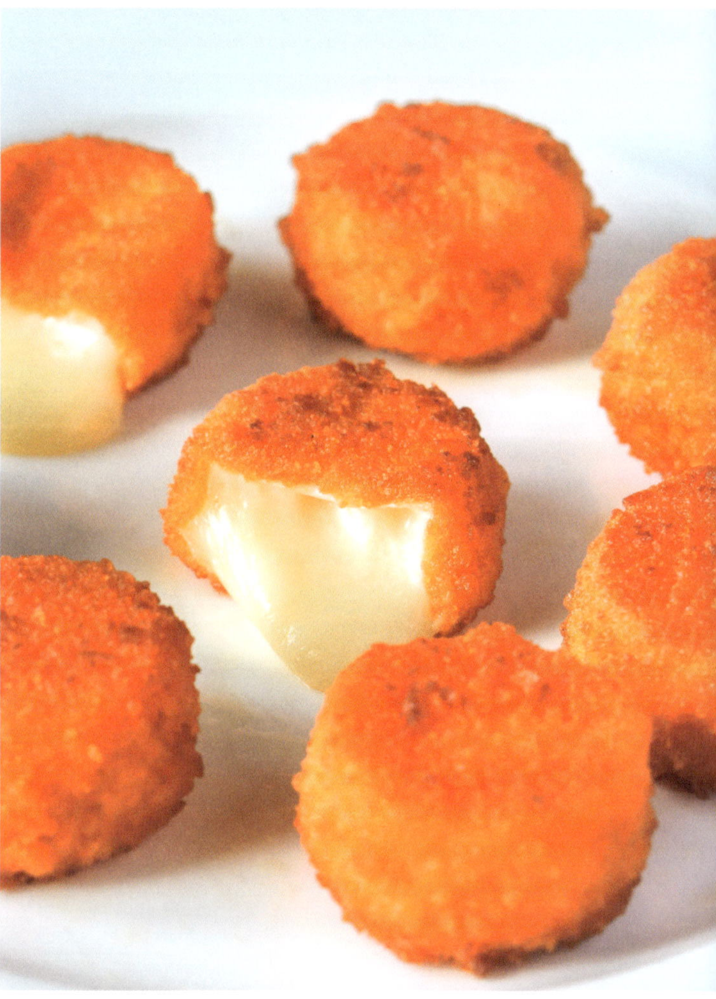

Herbed Potato Wedges

SERVES 4

PREP + COOK TIME: 25 MINS

VEG • GLUTEN FREE

Cheese Balls

SERVES 4

PREP + COOK TIME: 15 MINS

VEG

HERBED POTATO WEDGES

1 tbsp olive oil

1 tbsp lemon juice

½ tsp lemon zest

500g baby potatoes, quartered

½ tsp dried oregano

½ tsp salt

¼ tsp pepper

Mix the olive oil, lemon juice and zest in a large bowl.

Add the potatoes, season with oregano, salt and pepper and stir to coat.

Place potatoes in a single layer in the air fryer basket, working in batches if needed.

Air fry potatoes for 10 minutes at 200°C. Shake the basket and cook for a further 8-10 minutes at 200°C, until crispy.

Eat on their own or with your favourite dipping sauce.

CHEESE BALLS

300g packet frozen cheese (or macaroni cheese) balls

Preheat the air fryer to 200°C.

Place the balls in the air fryer basket and spread evenly over the base.

Cook for 12 minutes, removing and shaking the basket halfway.

Continue to cook for a few extra minutes if needed to crisp up.

TUNA MELT PASTRIES

1 medium potato

1 tbsp olive oil

Salt and pepper to taste

2 sheets frozen puff pastry, thawed

1 x 185g can tuna, drained

1 cup (30g) baby spinach

150g mozzarella cheese, sliced

1 egg, beaten

2 tbsps pepitas

Cut the potato into very thin slices using a mandoline or very sharp knife. Toss potatoes with olive oil and season with salt and pepper.

Transfer to air fryer basket and cook for 10-12 minutes at 200°C, shaking the basket halfway through cooking.

Set aside to cool slightly.

Reduce the air fryer temperature to 160°C.

Cut each pastry sheet into four even squares.

Arrange equal amounts of potato, tuna, spinach and mozzarella in a diagonal lines across the centre of each pastry square.

Bring two opposite corners of pastry over filling, sealing with beaten egg. Brush tops with remaining egg, scatter with pepitas and season with salt and pepper.

In batches, place in a single layer on a greased tray in the air fryer basket. Cook for 8-10 minutes until golden brown.

ZUCCHINI CHIPS

1 cup (125g) breadcrumbs

¾ cup (75g) grated Parmesan cheese

Pinch of salt and pepper

1 large egg

1 medium zucchini, thinly sliced

Preheat air fryer to 175°C.

Combine breadcrumbs, cheese, salt and pepper on a plate.

Lightly whisk egg in a small bowl.

Dip each zucchini slice firstly into the beaten egg and then into breadcrumb mixture, pressing to coat.

Place in a single layer in the air fryer and spray with cooking spray.

Cook for 10 minutes.

Use tongs to flip, then cook for a further 2 minutes. Remove chips with tongs.

Repeat with remaining zucchini slices.

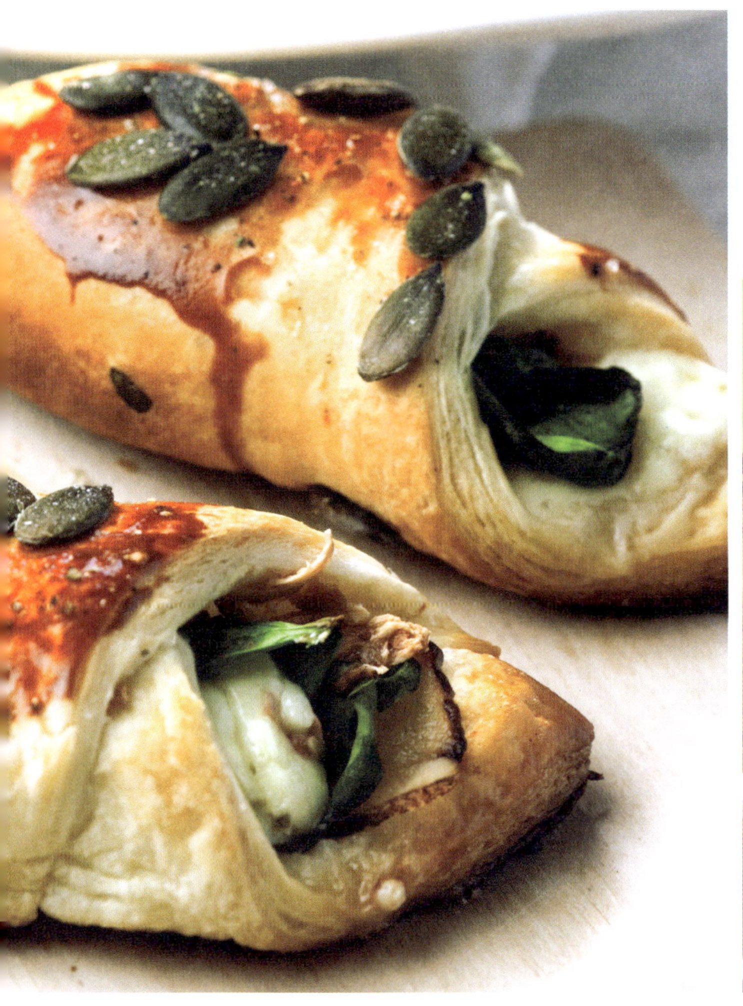

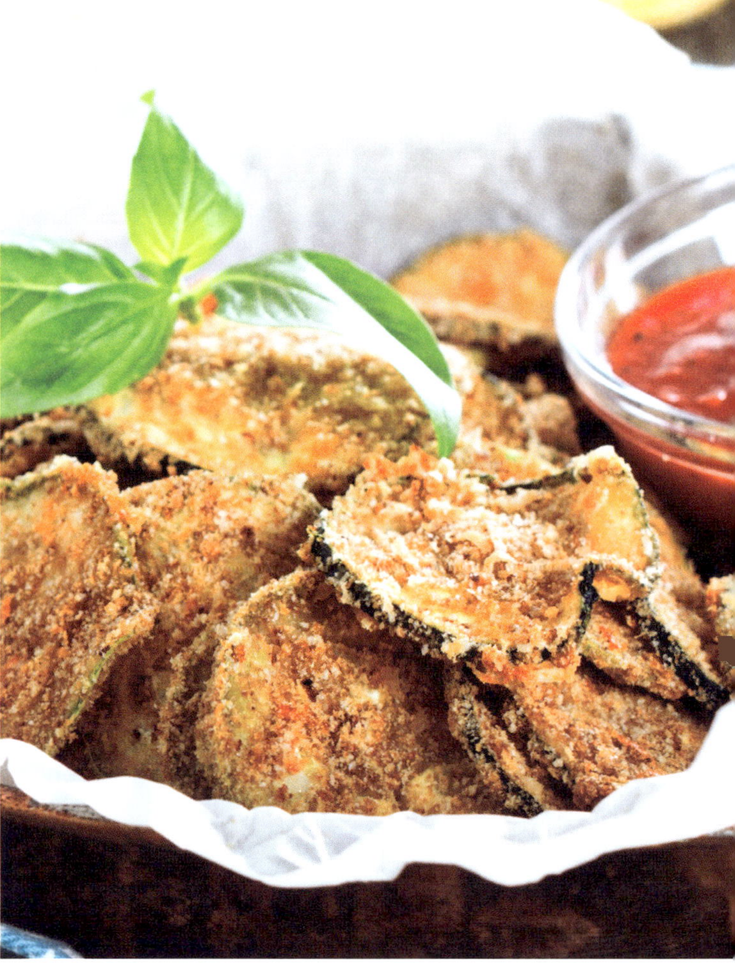

Tuna Melt Pastries

MAKES 8

PREP + COOK TIME: 25 MINS

Zucchini Chips

SERVES 2

PREP + COOK TIME: 20 MINS

VEG

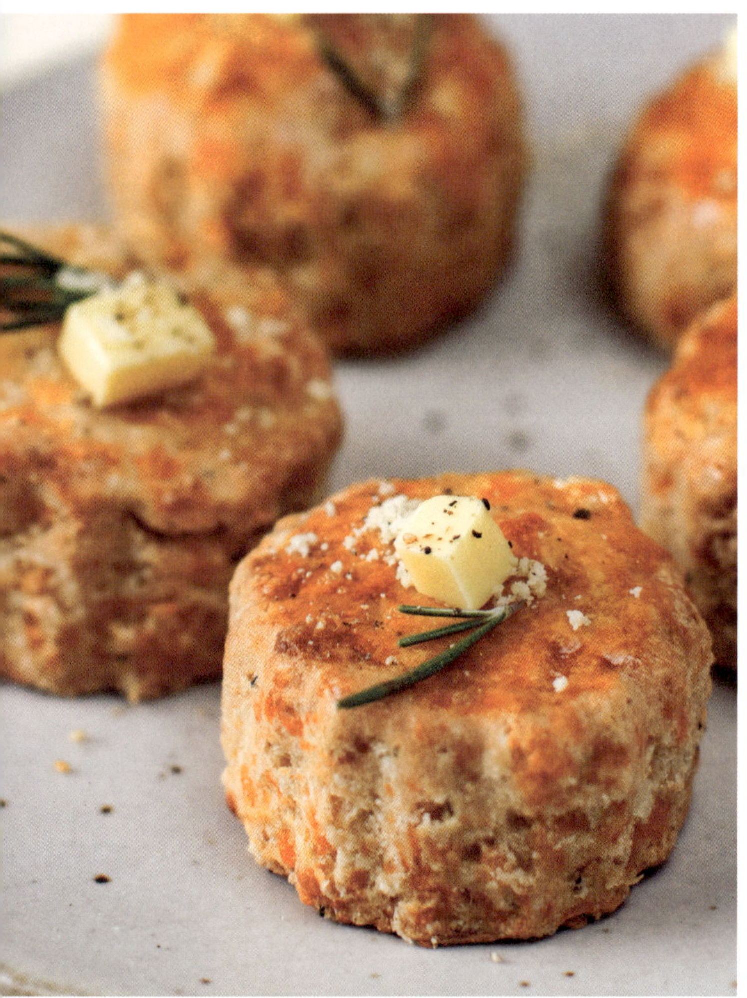

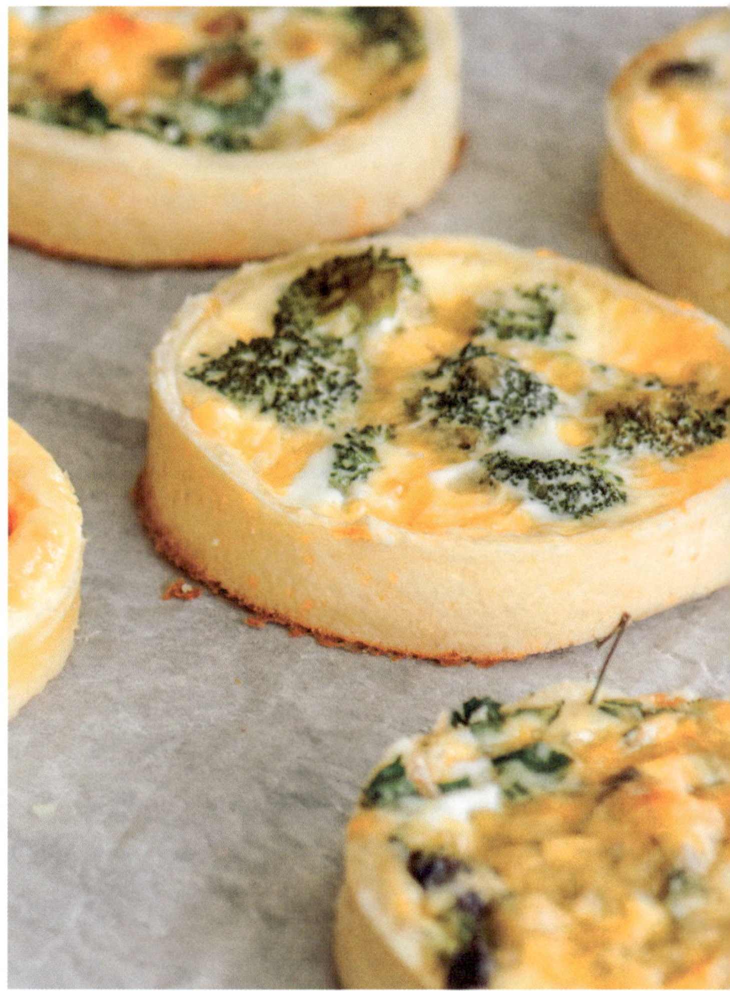

Mini Cheese Scones

MAKES 10

PREP + COOK TIME: 40 MINS

VEG

Mini Quiches

SERVES 2

PREP + COOK TIME: 25 MINS

VEG

MINI CHEESE SCONES

1½ cups (175g) self-raising flour

25g butter

⅔ cup (75g) grated Cheddar cheese

Pinch of salt and pepper

1 tbsp milk (more as needed)

1 egg

Baking pan

Preheat the air fryer to 180°C. Lightly spray and line a baking pan with greaseproof paper and set aside.

Place flour in a large mixing bowl. Add butter and rub into the flour using fingertips until it reaches a breadcrumb consistency. Add two-thirds of the cheese, salt and pepper and mix well. Add the milk and egg and stir until the mixture forms a soft dough (add more milk if needed).

Roll out the dough to a thickness of around 1½ cm and then cut out 10 rounds using a cookie cutter. Place remaining cheese into the middle and then roll into balls.

Place scones into the pan and cook for 20 minutes.

MINI QUICHES

1 shortcrust pastry sheet

1 egg

3 tbsps thickened cream

⅓ cup (40g) grated tasty cheese

Pinch of salt and pepper

1 cup (165g) broccoli, cooked and chopped

2 pie moulds (or use ramekins)

Preheat the air fryer to 200°C and lightly spray the moulds with oil.

Cut two rounds of approximately 7cm from the pastry sheet. Press down into the moulds. Transfer to the air fryer.

Beat the egg, cream, cheese, salt and pepper together until combined. Pour the mixture into the pastry moulds and add the broccoli.

Cook for 12 minutes until firm and golden.

Remove the quiches from the moulds before serving.

VEGETABLE CHIPS

1 parsnip, peeled
1 large carrot, peeled
1 medium beetroot, peeled
1 small sweet potato
2 tbsps olive oil
¼ tsp salt
¼ tsp pepper

Use a mandoline or sharp knife to thinly slice the vegetables, slicing the parsnips and carrots lengthways. Place in a large bowl and drizzle with oil. Sprinkle with salt and pepper and toss to coat.

Arrange in a single layer in the air fryer. Cook in batches or use a double layer accessory if necessary.

Air fry at 180°C for 12-15 minutes. Shake the basket halfway through cooking and check after 12 minutes to ensure the chips are not burning.

Remove the chips with tongs and place on a cooling rack to cool slightly before serving.

POPCORN

¼ cup (50g) popcorn kernels
1 tbsp oil
½ tsp salt

Line the air fryer with foil or create a foil pouch.

Place the corn kernels in a bowl and toss with the oil. Place on the foil or in the pouch inside the air fryer.

Cook at 200°C for 8-10 minutes or until the popcorn stops popping. Remove from the air fryer and season with salt.

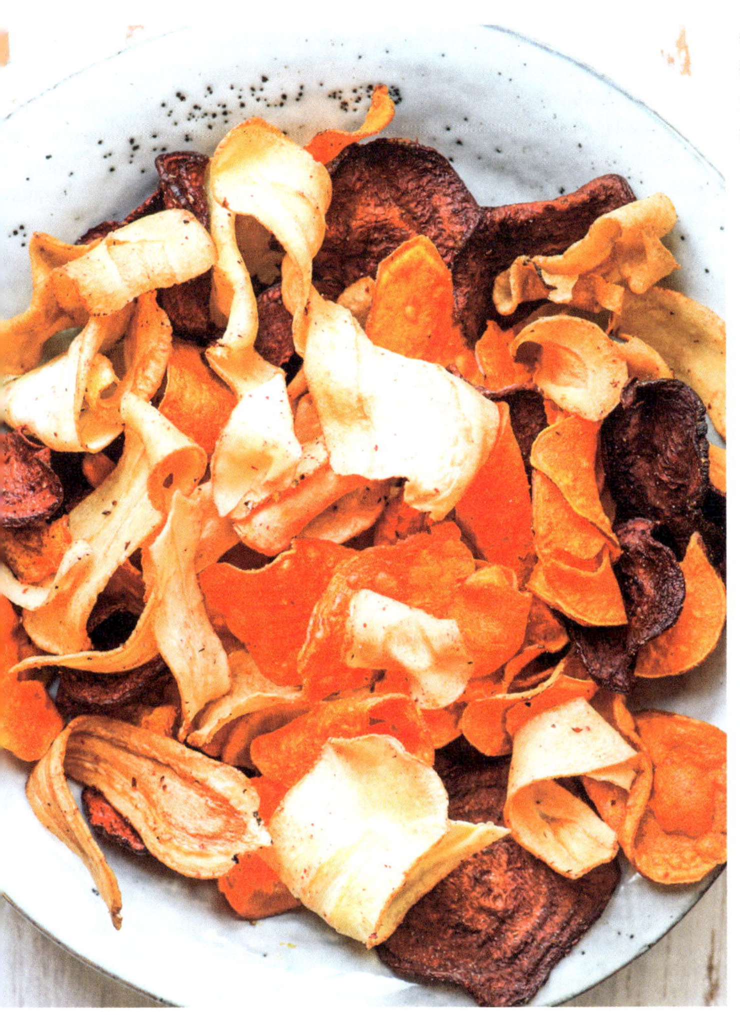

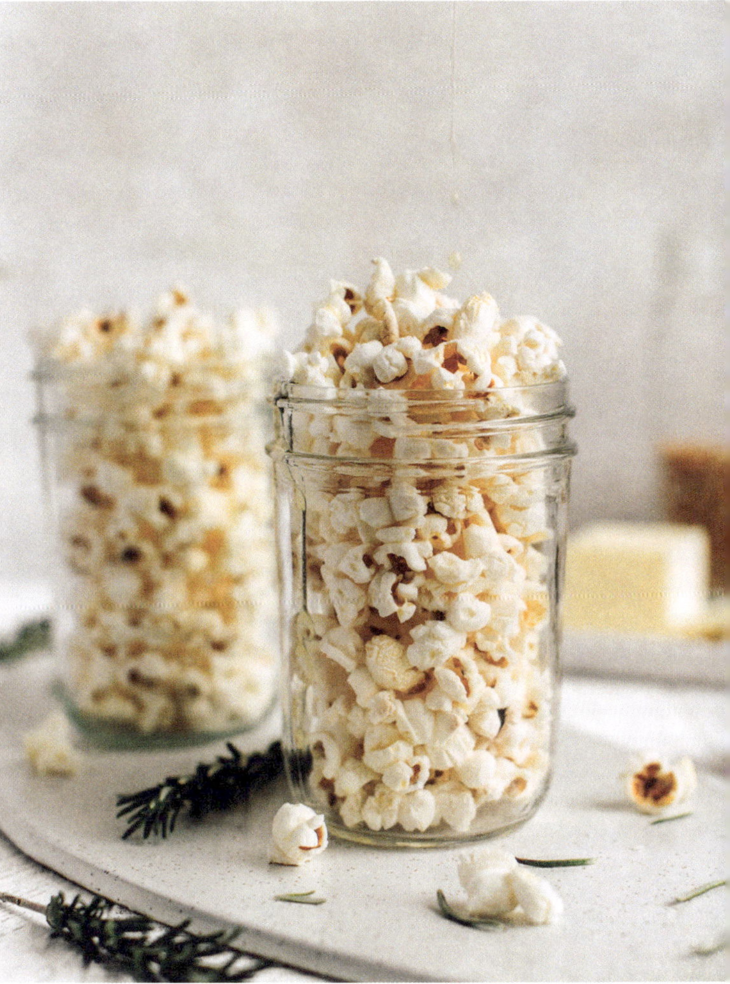

Vegetable Chips

SERVES 4

PREP + COOK TIME: 40 MINS

VEG • GLUTEN FREE • DAIRY FREE

Popcorn

SERVES 2

PREP + COOK TIME: 25 MINS

VEG • GLUTEN FREE

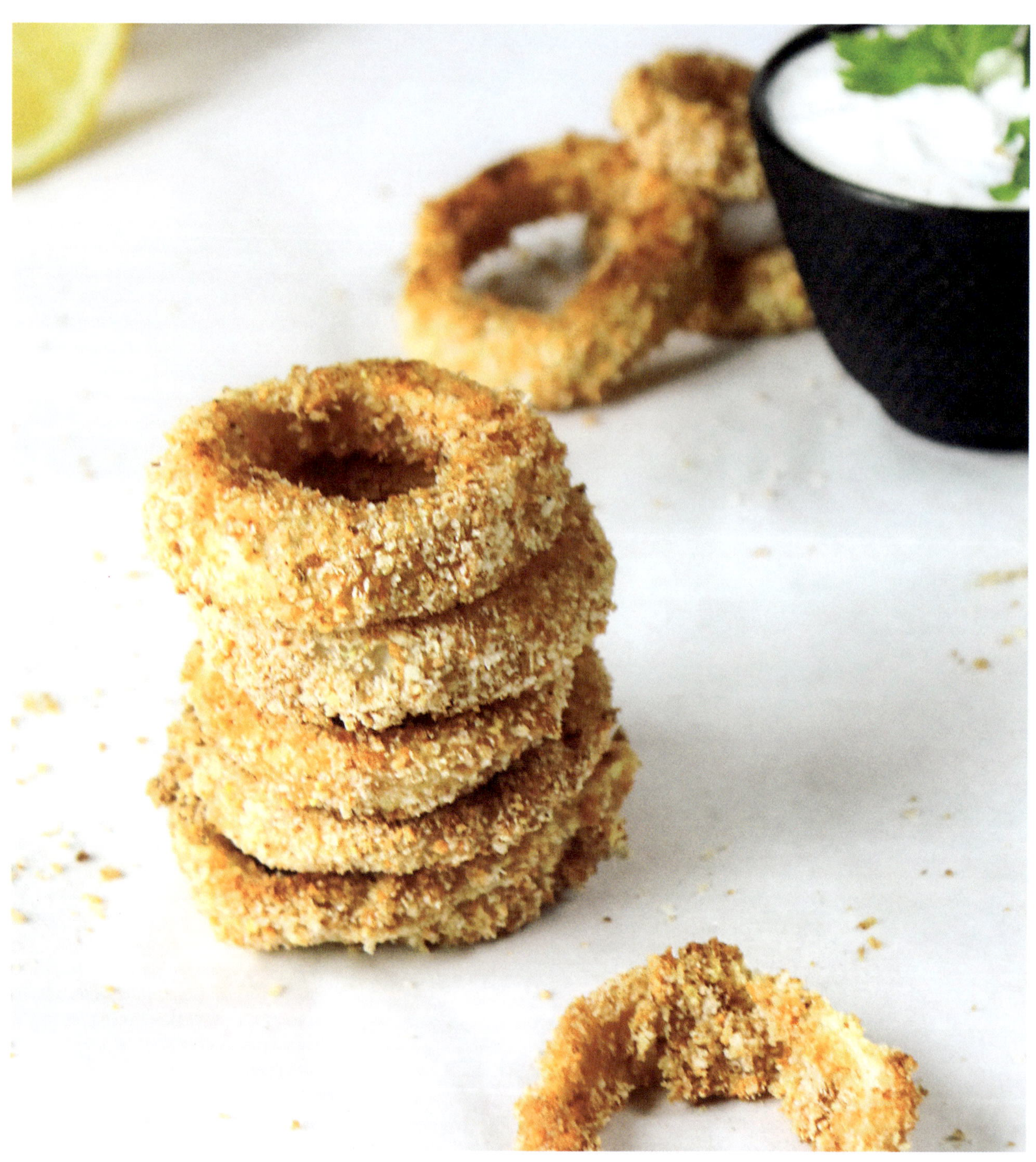

Onion Rings

SERVES 2

PREP + COOK TIME: 20 MINS

VEG

ONION RINGS

1 large onion
½ cup (60g) plain flour
1 tbsp baking powder
1 tsp salt
1 egg
1 tsp pepper
1 cup (125g) breadcrumbs

Preheat the air fryer to 190°C.

Cut the onion into thick slices. Separate each slice into multiple rings.

Combine the flour, baking powder and salt together in a shallow bowl. Beat the egg and pepper together in another shallow bowl. Place the breadcrumbs in a third shallow bowl.

Take an onion ring and dredge it in the flour mixture, then dip in the egg, shaking off any excess. Press into the breadcrumbs and turn to coat fully.

Spritz the air fryer basket with cooking spray. Lay the rings in the basket in an even layer (cook in batches if needed) and spray the tops with oil. Cook for 7 minutes until golden and crispy.

Zucchini & Feta Slice

SERVES 4

PREP + COOK TIME: 35 MINS

VEG

5 eggs

1 cup (125g) self-raising flour

3 large zucchinis, grated

3 spring onions, chopped

80g soft feta, cut into small pieces

½ cup (125ml) oil

Pinch of salt and pepper

½ cup (60g) grated tasty cheese

Cake tin

Preheat the air fryer to 180°C.

Whisk the eggs in large bowl. Add the flour and beat until smooth, then add the zucchini, spring onion, feta, oil, salt and pepper and stir to combine.

Pour the mixture into the cake tin and sprinkle with the tasty cheese. Transfer to the air fryer.

Cook for 30 minutes.

Note:

When cooked, a skewer inserted in the centre should come out clean.

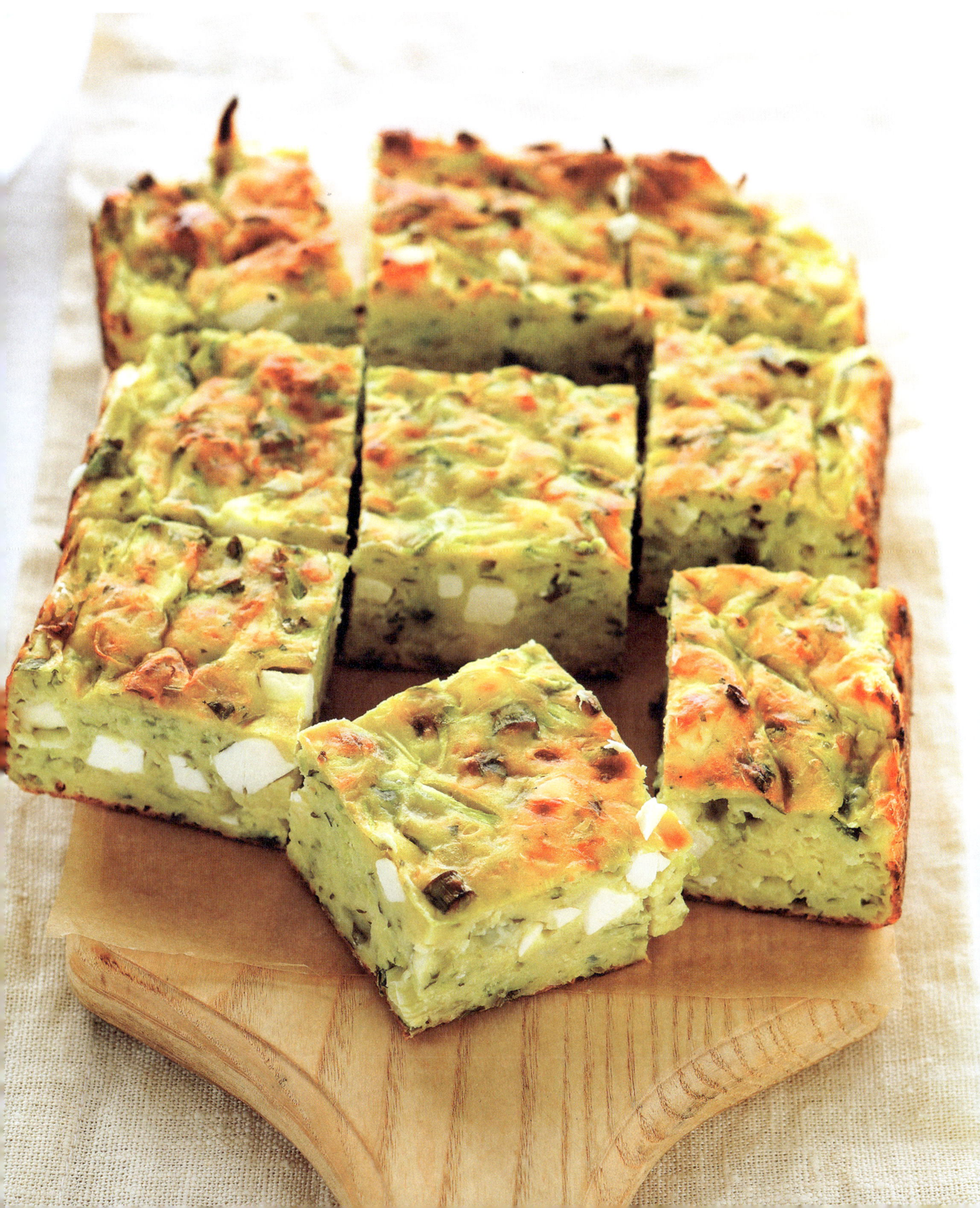

CHEESE CRACKERS

1 cup (150g) plain flour
2 tbsps self-raising flour
⅛ tsp cayenne pepper
125g butter, chopped
2 tbsps grated Parmesan cheese
1 cup (120g) grated Cheddar cheese
1 tbsp water
1 tbsp sesame seeds

Places the two types of flour and cayenne pepper into a bowl. Rub in the butter to form a crumbly mixture. Stir in the cheeses. Add the water and bring the mixture together into a dough.

Knead the dough on a floured surface until smooth. Cover and refrigerate for 30 minutes.

Roll the dough into a ½ cm-thick disc. Scatter with sesame seeds.

Cut dough into wedges, then cut out small circles, if desired, using the large end of a piping nozzle (to resemble slices of Swiss cheese).

Cook in batches in a single layer in the air fryer for 14-16 minutes at 170°C, until golden brown.

PARMESAN CHICKEN NUGGETS

1 chicken breast
½ tsp salt
Pinch of pepper
115g butter
½ cup (60g) breadcrumbs
2 tbsps grated Parmesan cheese
1 tbsp chicken seasoning

Preheat the air fryer to 200°C.

Trim any excess fat from the chicken breast, then cut into thick slices. Cut each slice into three or four nuggets. Season with salt and pepper.

Melt the butter in a small saucepan over medium heat (or in the microwave). Place melted butter in a small, shallow bowl. Combine the breadcrumbs, Parmesan and chicken seasoning and place in a second shallow bowl.

Dredge each piece of chicken in butter, then breadcrumbs.

Place in a single layer in the air fryer basket. (You may need to do multiple batches.)

Cook for 12 minutes, removing and shaking the basket halfway through.

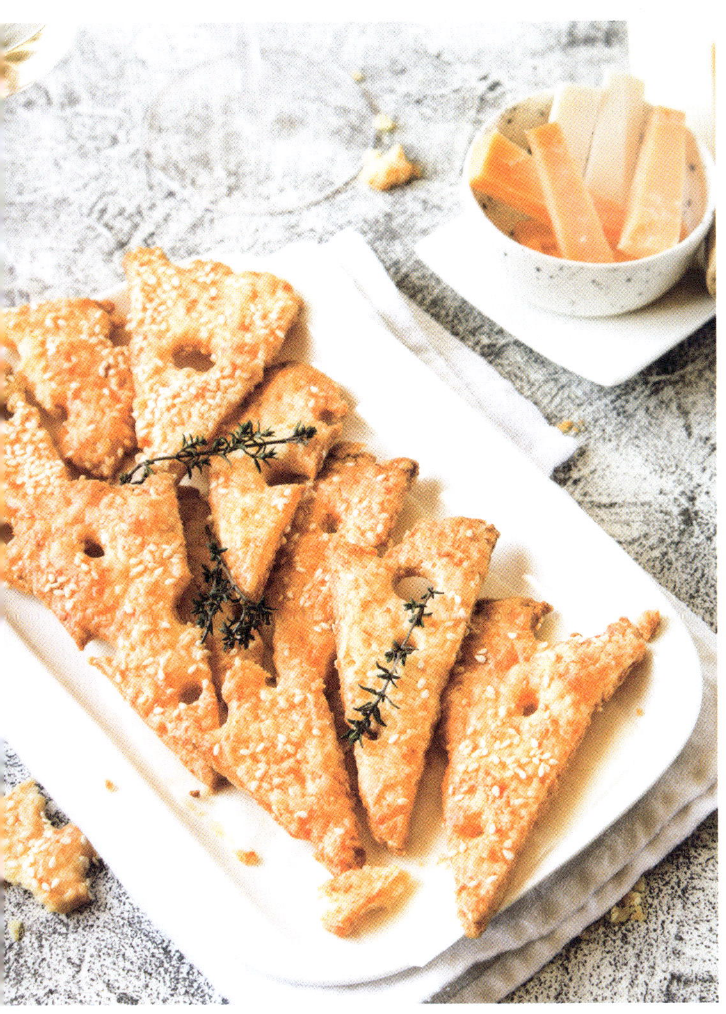

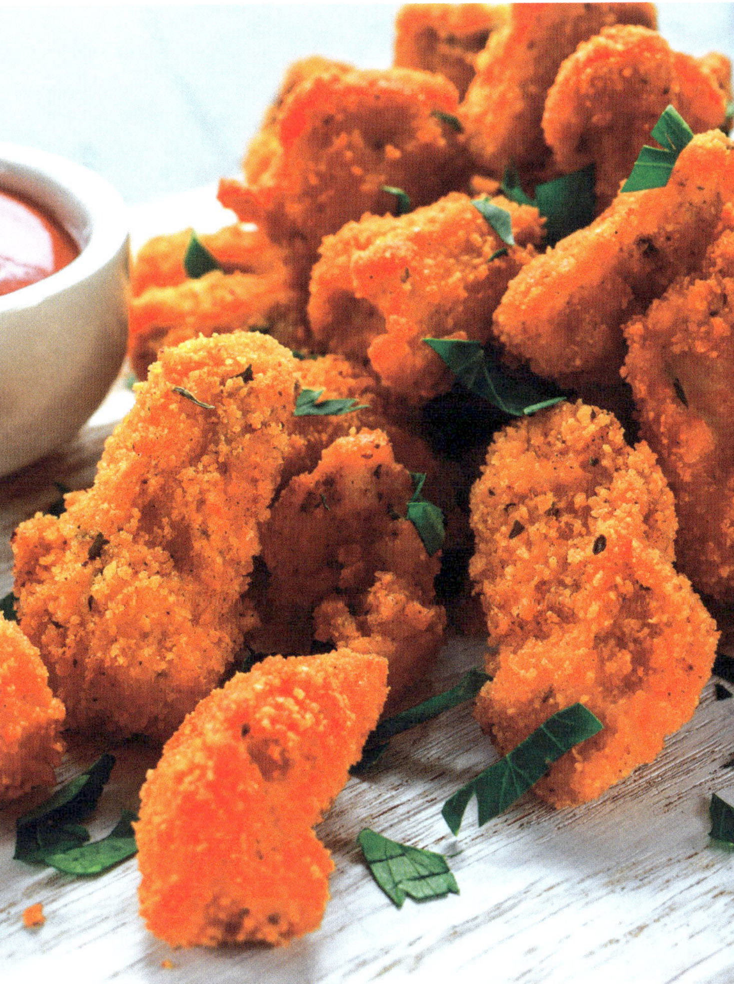

Cheese Crackers

SERVES 4

PREP + COOK TIME: 25 MINS + 30 MINS CHILLING

VEG

Parmesan Chicken Nuggets

SERVES 2

PREP + COOK TIME: 30 MINS

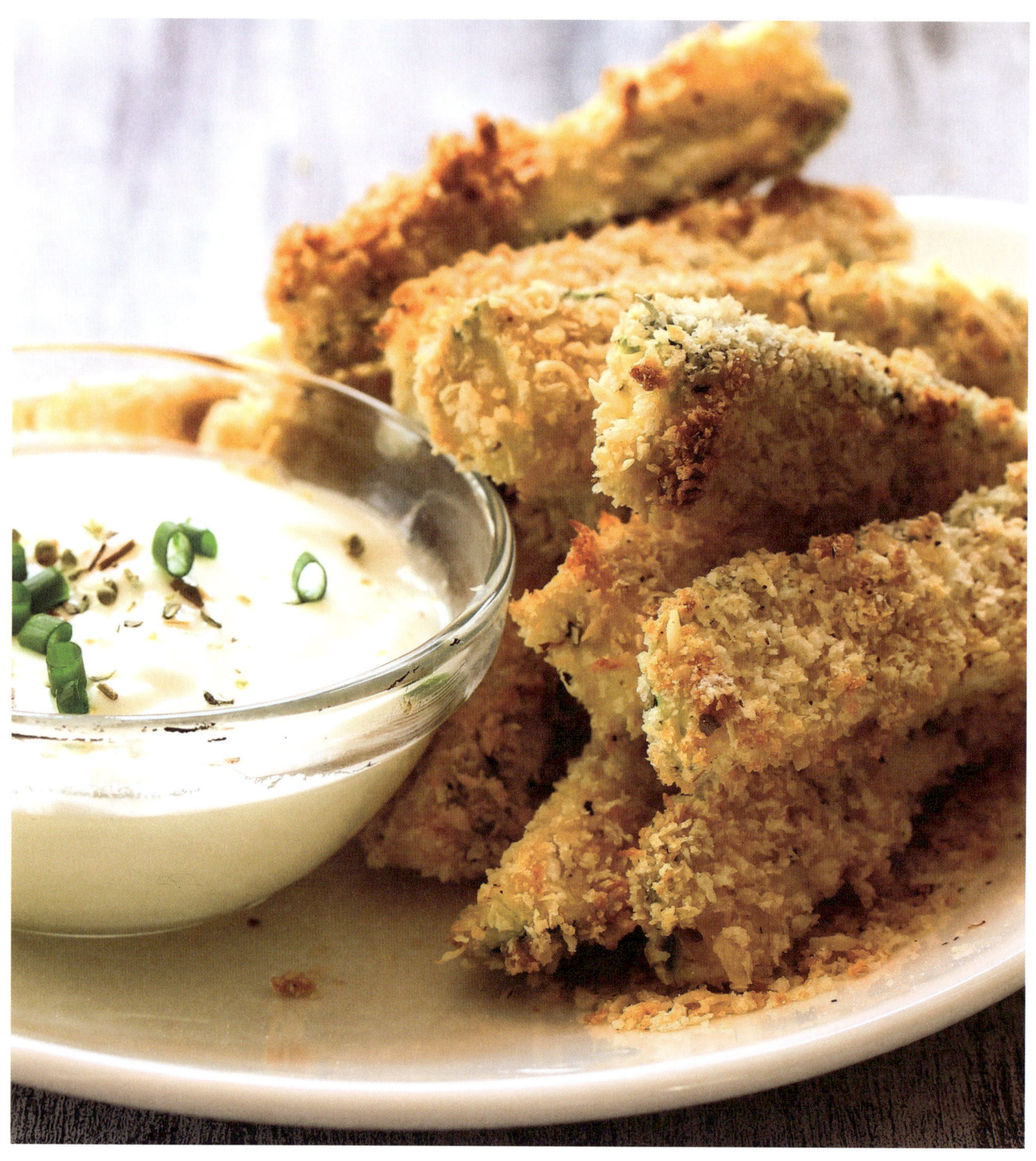

Baked Zucchini Fries

SERVES 2

PREP + COOK TIME: 30 MINS

VEG

BAKED ZUCCHINI FRIES

3 medium zucchinis

2 egg whites

Pinch of salt and pepper

½ cup (60g) panko breadcrumbs

¼ tsp garlic powder

¼ cup (25g) grated Parmesan cheese

Cut the zucchinis into sticks.

Preheat the air fryer to 200°C. Spritz the air fryer basket with cooking spray.

Beat the egg whites in a small bowl and season with salt and pepper.

Place the panko, garlic powder and cheese into a second bowl and mix well.

Dip the zucchini sticks into the egg whites then into the panko and cheese mixture, a few at a time, ensuring that each is well coated.

Spray all sides of the zucchini sticks with oil.

Place the zucchini sticks in a single layer in the basket. (Be careful not to overcrowd the basket. Cook in batches or use a double layer accessory if needed.)

Bake for 20 minutes, or until crisp and golden.

VEGETABLE SAMOSAS

10 frozen vegetable samosas

Preheat the air fryer to 190°C.

Lightly spray each frozen samosa with oil and place in the air fryer basket.

Cook for 20 minutes, removing the basket and shaking halfway. Cook a few minutes longer, if needed, until browned to your liking.

Using a double layer accessory, you should be able to cook in one batch. Otherwise, repeat the process.

KALE CHIPS WITH VEGAN CHEESE

2 tbsps olive oil

1 small bunch kale, leaves picked

1 tbsp nutritional yeast flakes

¼ tsp salt

Place all the ingredients in a mixing bowl and toss to fully coat. Transfer to the air fryer basket and slide into the air fryer. Cook for 5 minutes on 190°C.

Check regularly after 2 minutes cooking as they can burn quickly.

Notes:

Use the leaves of the kale only and discard the stems, as the stems will not cook without the leaves burning.

Use grated Parmesan instead of yeast flakes if you prefer (and are not vegan).

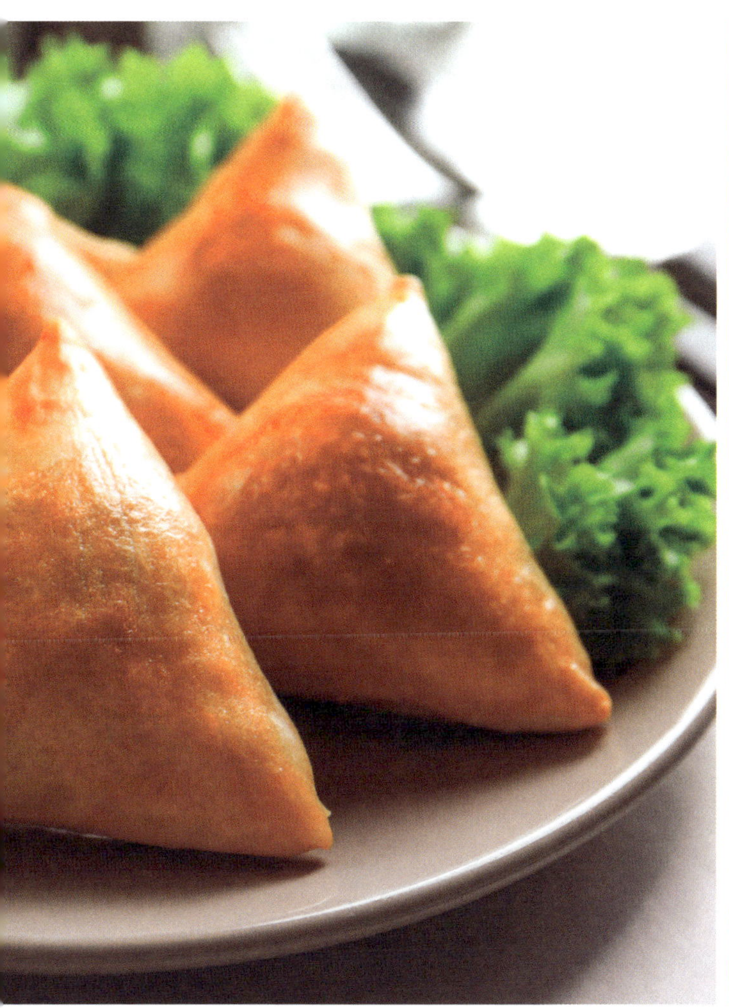

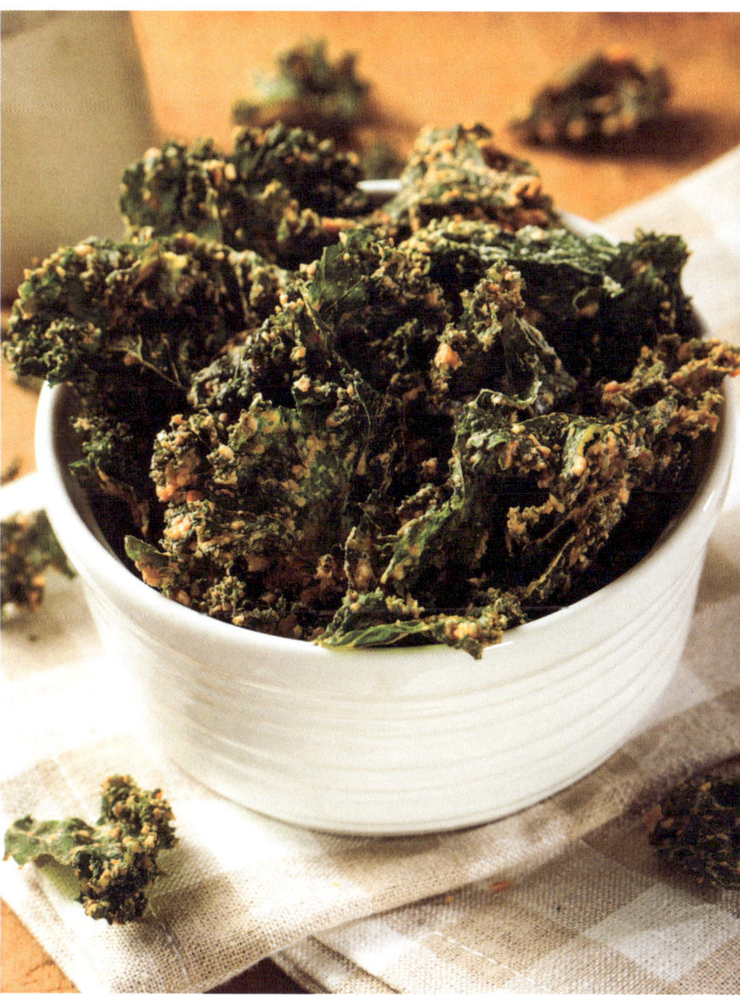

Vegetable Samosas

SERVES 4

PREP + COOK TIME: 25 MINS

VEG • DAIRY FREE

Kale Chips with Vegan Cheese

SERVES 3

PREP + COOK TIME: 10 MINS

VEG • GLUTEN FREE • DAIRY FREE

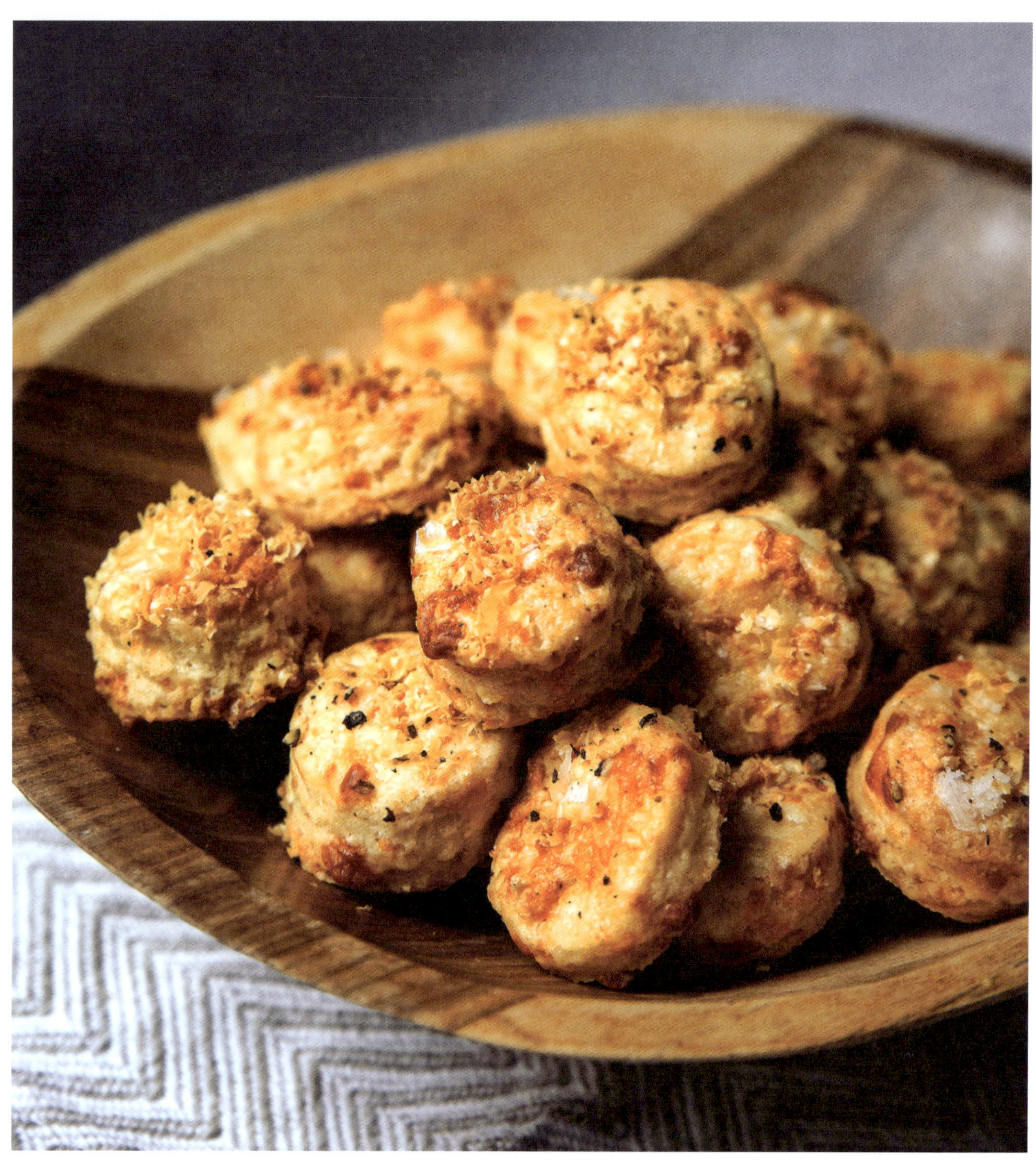

Cheese Puffs

SERVES 10

PREP + COOK TIME: 30 MINS + 1 HOUR CHILLING

VEG

CHEESE PUFFS

2 cups (250g) grated Cheddar cheese
5 tbsps unsalted butter
½ tsp garlic powder
½ tsp onion powder
1 tsp salt
2 cups (250g) plain flour
1-2 tbsps water
½ cup (50g) grated Parmesan cheese
¼ tsp pepper

In a food processor, add the Cheddar cheese, butter, garlic powder, onion power and ½ teaspoon salt. Pulse to combine. Add the flour and pulse a few times. Add water 1 tablespoon at a time and pulse until a dough forms. You may not need the second tablespoon water.

Divide the dough into three. Cover and refrigerate for 1 hour.

Remove one piece of dough from the fridge. Place on a lightly floured work surface and roll out to ½ cm thickness. Use a small round cutter to cut out circles of dough. Sprinkle with Parmesan cheese, salt and pepper.

Put the cheese puffs in the air fryer basket. Bake at 190°C for 6 minutes. Remove cheese puffs. Let them cool and dry on a wire cooling rack.

Repeat this process with the two other balls of dough, rerolling and cutting out the scraps.

JALAPENO CHEESE CRISPS WITH YOGHURT DIP

2 jalapeno chillies, sliced horizontally
1 cup (100g) grated Parmesan cheese
½ cup (60g) grated Cheddar cheese
Salt and pepper to taste

YOGHURT DIPPING SAUCE

⅓ cup (80ml) Greek yoghurt
1 clove garlic, minced
1 tsp lemon juice
1 tsp olive oil
¼ tsp smoked paprika
Pinch of salt
Cake tin or baking pan

Place jalapeno slices into air fryer basket and spray with cooking spray. Cook for 5 minutes at 170°C, turning halfway through cooking. Remove jalapenos from air fryer basket.

Line a cake tin or baking pan that will fit into your air fryer with greaseproof paper.

In a large bowl combine the two cheeses and salt and pepper.

Using 2 tablespoons at a time place small mounds of cheese on the paper about 4cm apart. Cook in batches if necessary. Top each mound with two slices of jalapeno and press down slightly.

Cook for about 10 minutes at 170°C until golden brown.

Allow to cool slightly before peeling off the greaseproof paper. Repeat with remaining cheese and jalapenos.

Combine all the ingredients for the dipping sauce in a medium bowl. Mix well to combine. Serve the cooled crisps with the yoghurt dip on the side.

AVOCADO FRIES

½ cup (60g) flour
½ tsp salt
1 egg
½ cup (125ml) milk
½ cup (60g) almond meal
½ tsp garlic powder
3 large avocados, peeled and cut into 2cm-thick slices

Preheat air fryer to 200°C.

Combine flour and ¼ teaspoon salt in a shallow dish. Beat together egg and milk in a bowl. Combine almond meal, garlic powder and remaining salt in another dish.

Dip each avocado slice first into seasoned flour, then egg mix, and finally almond meal mix, pressing gently to coat.

Spray basket and avocados with cooking spray. Arrange avocados in a single layer. Cook in batches if necessary.

Cook for 8-10 minutes until crispy. Serve with dip of choice.

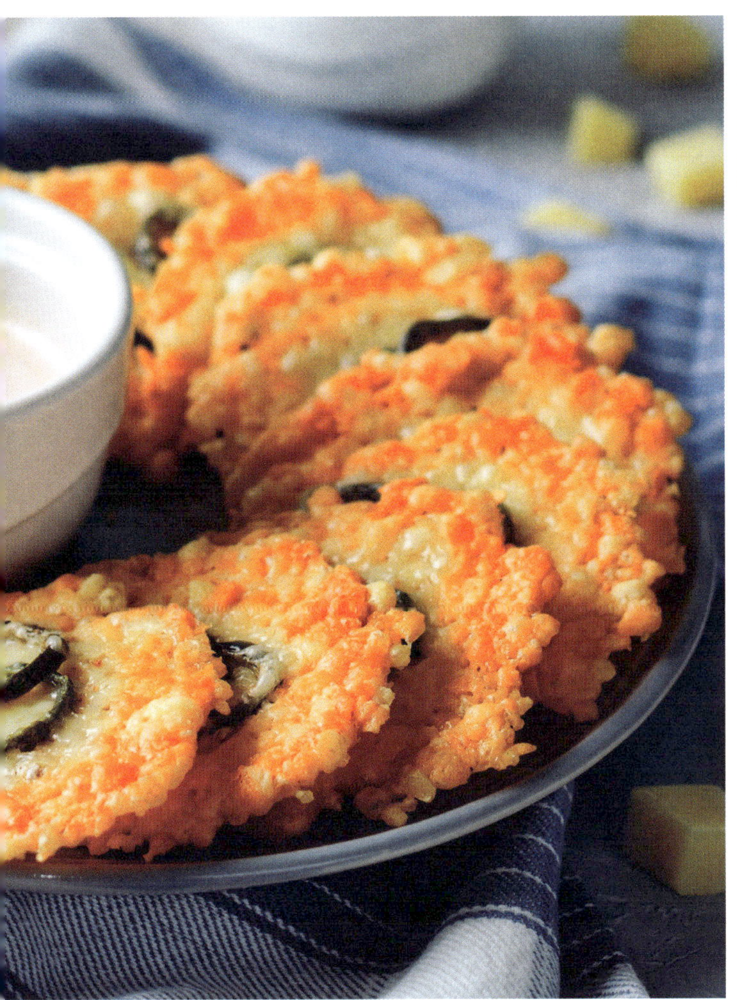

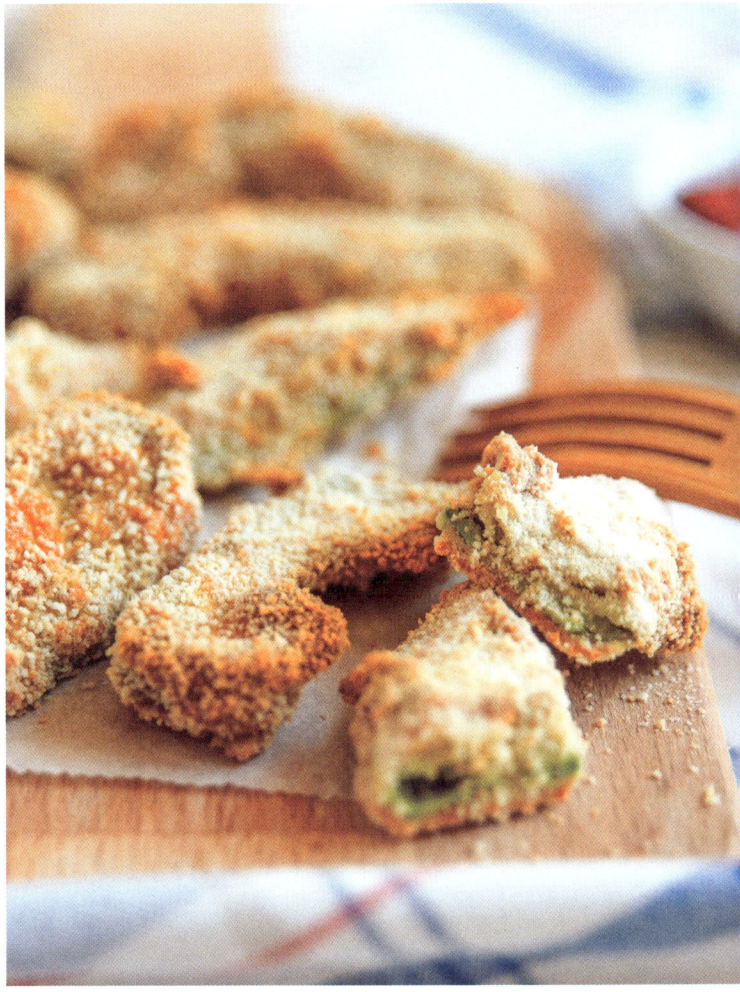

Jalapeno Cheese Crisps with Yoghurt Dip

SERVES 4

PREP + COOK TIME: 25 MINS

GLUTEN FREE

Avocado Fries

SERVES 4

PREP + COOK TIME: 20 MINS

VEG • GLUTEN FREE

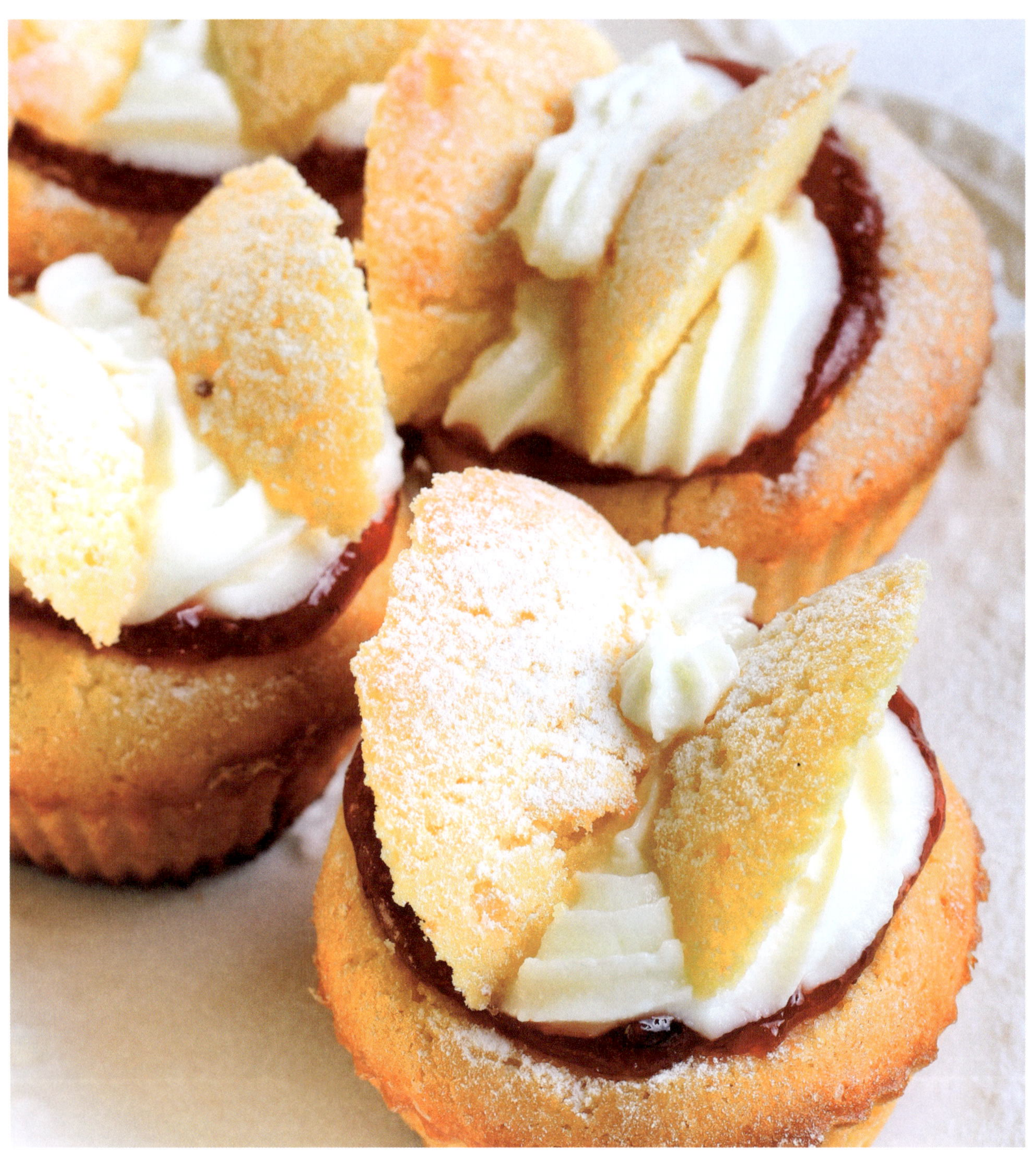

Lemon Butterfly Cakes

MAKES 6

PREP + COOK TIME: 30 MINS + COOLING

VEG

LEMON BUTTERFLY CAKES

150g butter, softened, divided
½ cup (100g) caster sugar
1 tsp vanilla essence
2 eggs
¾ cup (100g) flour
1 tsp baking powder
⅔ cup (100g) icing sugar
½ lemon, juiced and zested
⅔ cup (200g) strawberry jam
Muffin tray or silicone moulds

Place 100g of the butter and the caster sugar in a large bowl and beat with an electric mixer until pale and fluffy. Add the vanilla essence and briefly beat to combine.

Add in the eggs, one at a time, beating well after each addition. Gently fold in the flour and baking powder with a wooden spoon.

Preheat the air fryer to 170°C. Line a muffin tray with patty pans.

Spoon the mixture into the patty pans leaving room for them to rise. Place the muffin tray into the air fryer. Cook for 8 minutes. Remove and set aside to cool.

Meanwhile, make the buttercream icing. Cream the remaining 50g of butter in the mixer, and gradually add in the icing sugar until softly whipped. Add the lemon juice and zest and mix to combine.

Using a sharp knife, cut out a circle from the top of each of the cupcakes. Cut the circles into halves.

Fill the holes with strawberry jam and then spoon over the buttercream. Place the cut out pieces as 'wings' on top of the cupcakes.

Note:

If you have a small air fryer you could put the patty pans directly into the air fryer basket. Fill the basket with as many as you can and cook in batches.

Cranberry Pecan Scones

SERVES 6-8
PREP + COOK TIME: 30 MINS
VEG

¾ cup (185ml) milk

1 tsp white vinegar

1¾ cups (215g) plain flour

½ cup (45g) oats

¼ cup (55g) white sugar

2 tsps baking powder

½ tsp bicarbonate of soda

½ tsp salt

½ tsp grated nutmeg

115g butter, chilled and cut into small pieces

1 cup (160g) dried cranberries

½ cup (75g) chopped pecans

1 egg white, beaten

ICING

1½ cups (235g) icing sugar

2 tbsps milk

Preheat air fryer to 180°C.

Combine milk and vinegar in a bowl. Set aside for 5 minutes until milk is curdled.

Combine flour, oats, sugar, baking powder, bicarb, salt and nutmeg in a large bowl. Cut in butter with a knife. Stir in milk mixture, cranberries and pecans. Knead until dough comes together in a ball.

Place dough onto a floured work surface. Shape into a large round and roll out with a rolling pin to 3cm thickness. Cut round into triangular wedges. Brush tops with egg white.

Transfer to the air fryer.

Bake for 10-12 minutes until tops are golden brown.

Combine icing sugar and 2 tablespoons milk in a small bowl mix well to combine. Drizzle over scones to serve.

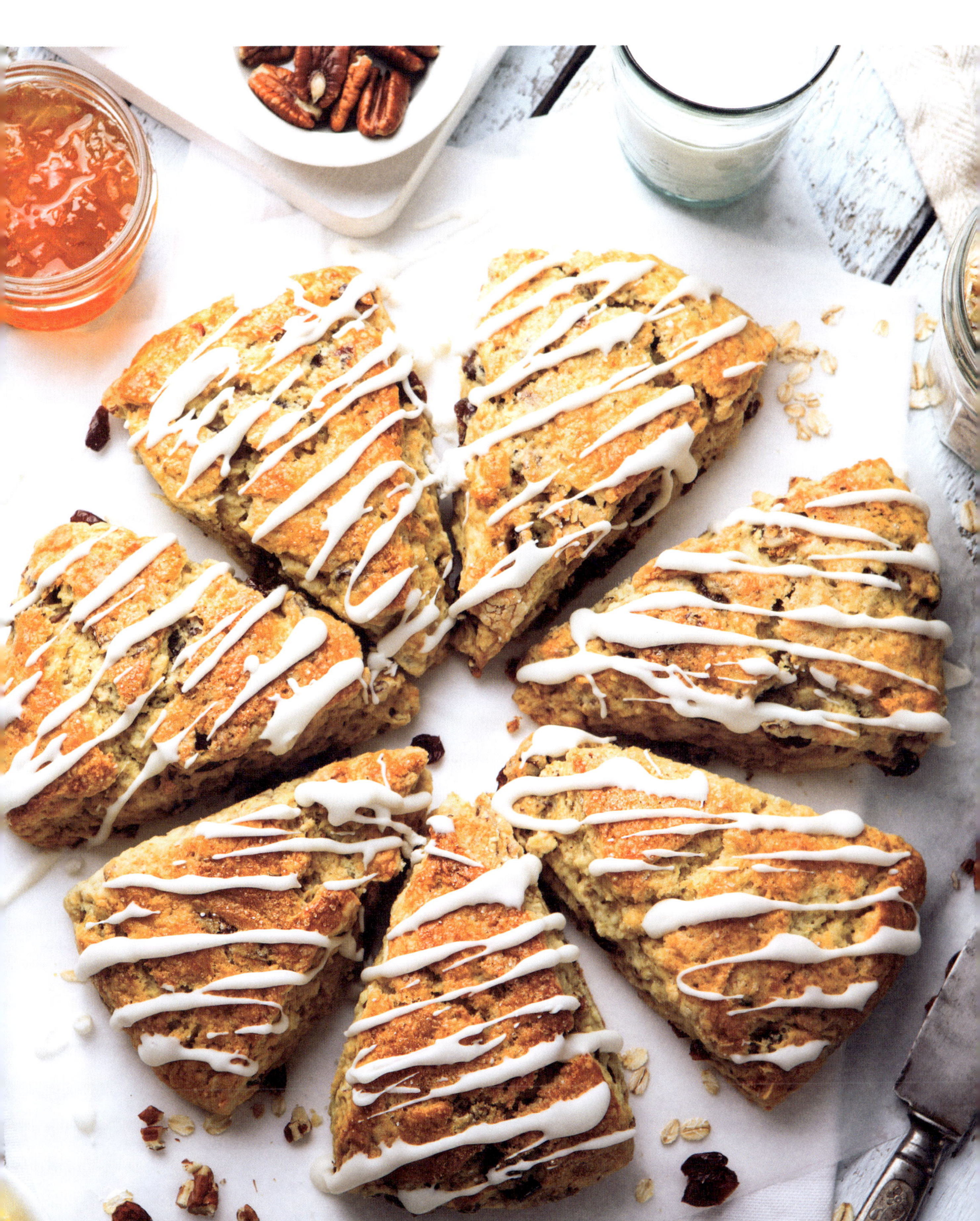

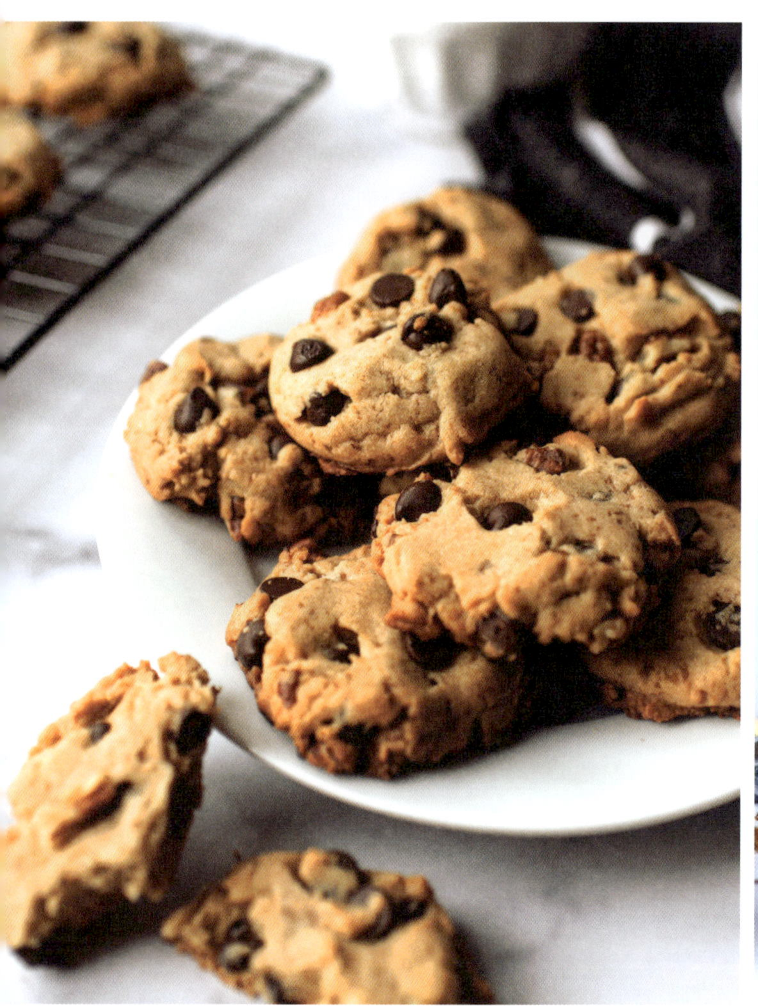

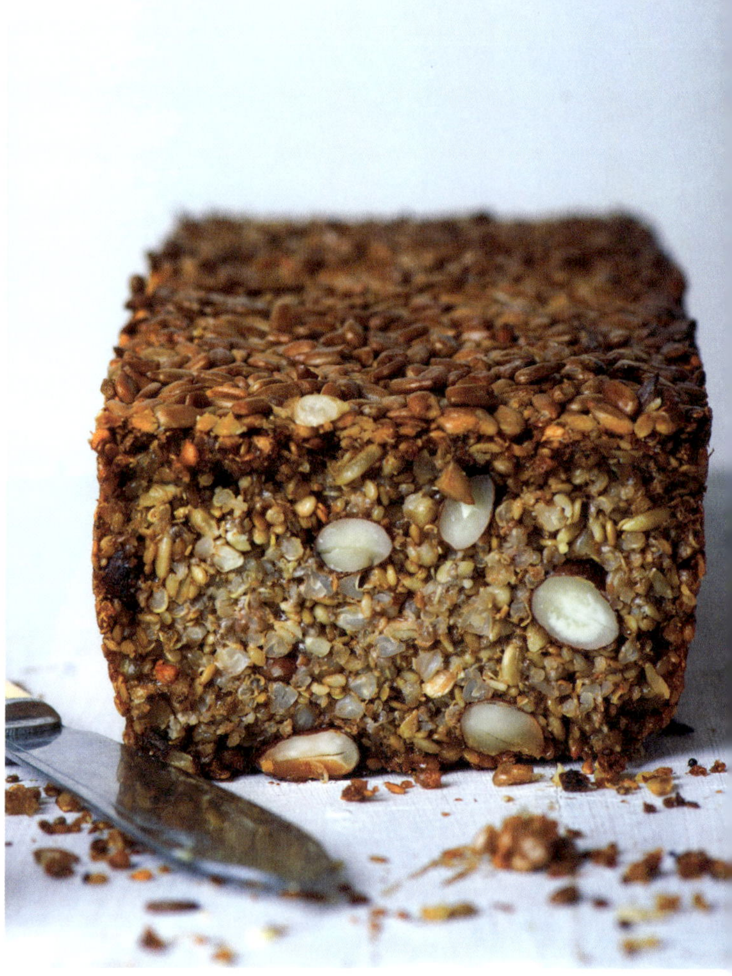

Choc Chip Cookies

MAKES 20

PREP + COOK TIME: 20 MINS

VEG

Seed Bread

SERVES 10

PREP + COOK TIME: 1 HOUR

VEG • GLUTEN FREE

CHOC CHIP COOKIES

115g butter, softened
1 cup (155g) packed brown sugar
2 eggs
1 tsp vanilla extract
1½ cups (210g) flour
½ tsp salt
½ tsp bicarbonate of soda
½ tsp baking powder
1 cup (155g) chocolate chips

Using a mixer, cream together the butter and sugar until light and fluffy.

Stir in the eggs, vanilla, flour, salt, bicarb and baking powder. Fold in the chocolate chips.

Form the mixture into balls and flatten each one gently. Transfer to the air fryer.

Air fry for 8-10 minutes at 150°C.

SEED BREAD

1 cup (125g) almonds
½ cup (75g) flaxseed
½ cup (60g) sunflower seeds
½ cup (80g) sesame seeds
½ cup (80g) hemp seeds
3 eggs
¼ cup (60ml) macadamia or avocado oil
¾ tsp salt
Loaf tin or 2 mini loaf tins

Grease and line a loaf tin (or 2 mini loaf tins).

In a large bowl, combine all the ingredients together, and stir well.

Pour the mixture into greased loaf tin or tins.

Place into the air fryer.

Cook at 160°C for 40 minutes.

Let the bread cool in the tin for 10 minutes, then turn it out onto a wire rack to finish cooling.

Cinnamon Scrolls

MAKES 8
PREP + COOK TIME: 30 MINS
VEG

CINNAMON SCROLLS

1¾ cups (215g) self-raising flour
1 cup (250ml) vanilla yoghurt
2 tbsps butter, melted
¼ cup (40g) brown sugar
2 tsps cinnamon

ICING

60g unsalted butter, softened
4 cups (620g) icing sugar
4 tbsps milk + more if needed
1 tsp vanilla extract

Combine the flour and yoghurt in a large mixing bowl and mix well. Transfer the dough to a lightly floured work surface. Knead the dough several times, then roll out into a large rectangular shape, around 1½ cm thick.

In a small bowl, mix together the melted butter, brown sugar and cinnamon. Use a spatula to spread the cinnamon mixture over the dough, leaving a 1cm border around the sides.

Beginning at the long end, tightly roll up the dough into a log. Use a sharp knife to slice the log into eight portions.

Line air fryer basket with greaseproof paper.

Working in batches place the cinnamon scrolls in one layer in the air fryer basket. Air fry at 180°C for 7-8 minutes, until the edges are golden brown. Repeat with the remaining scrolls. Allow to cool.

In a medium bowl, whisk together butter, sugar, milk and vanilla. Drizzle over the cooled cinnamon scrolls.

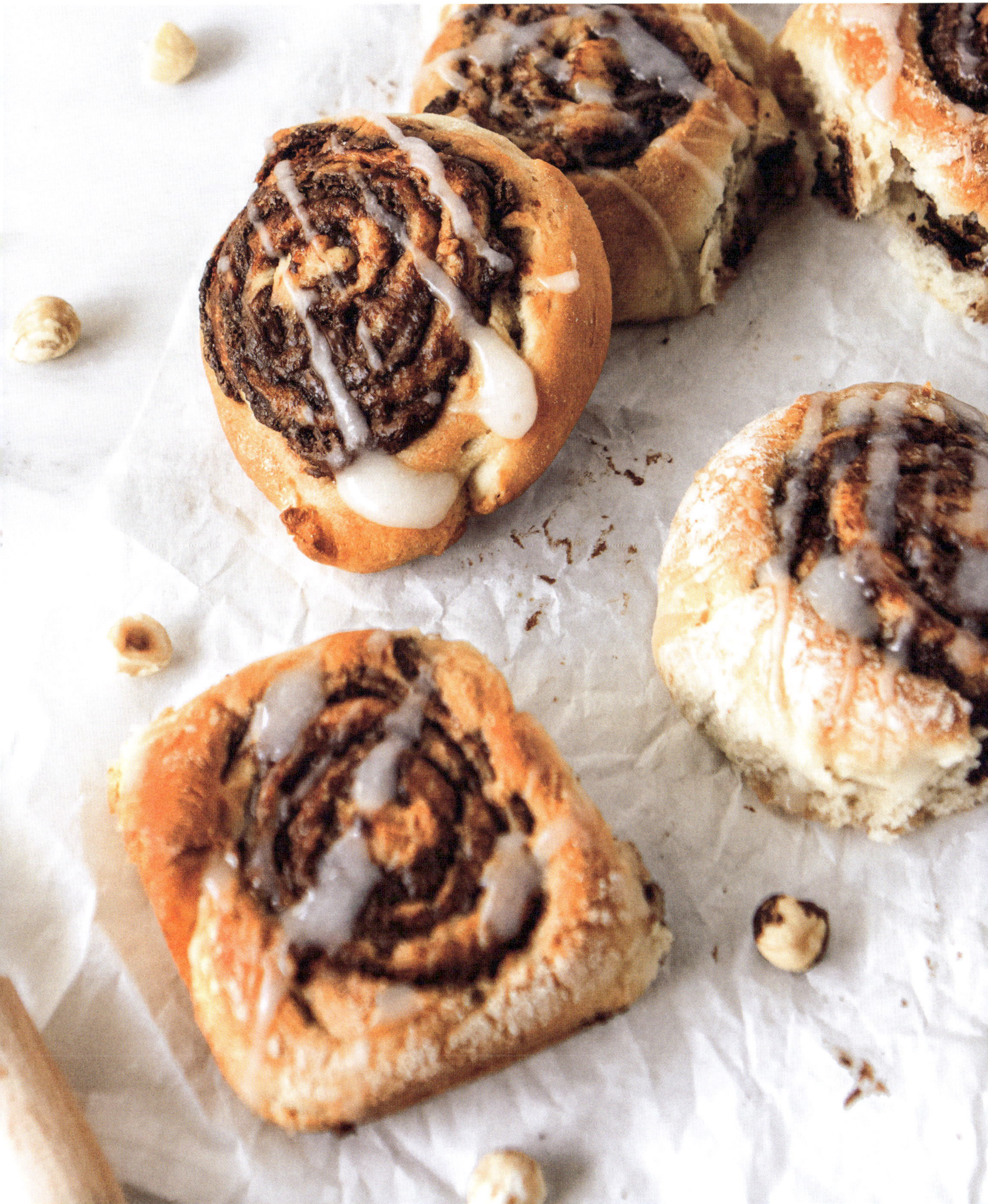

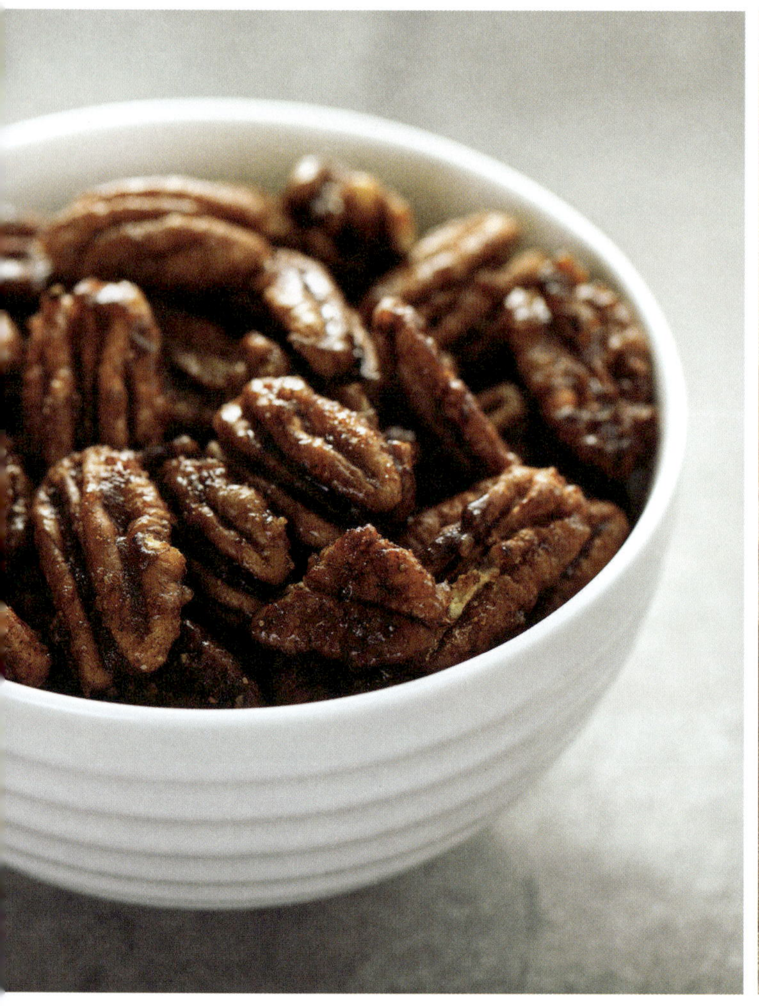

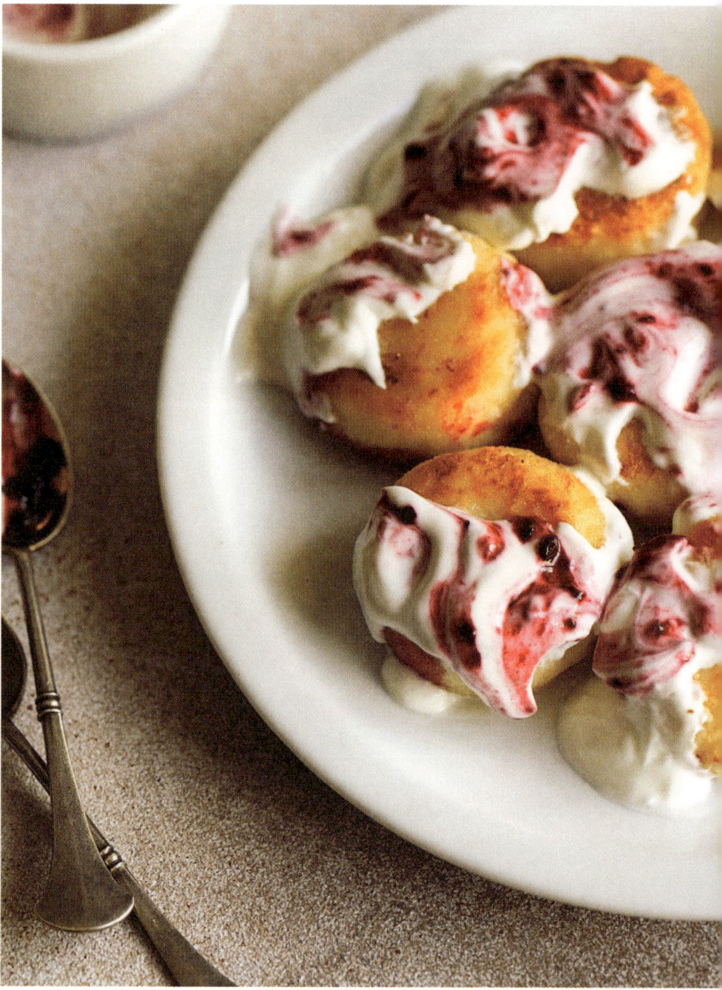

Cinnamon Pecans

MAKES 2 CUPS

PREP + COOK TIME: 25 MINS

VEG • GLUTEN FREE

Ricotta Fritters

MAKES 12

PREP + COOK TIME: 45 MINS

VEG

CINNAMON PECANS

2 cups (250g) pecans

2 tbsps peanut oil or melted ghee

¼ tsp salt

2 tsps cinnamon

2 tbsps maple syrup

Place the pecans in a large bowl. Drizzle with peanut oil or ghee. Sprinkle with salt and cinnamon and toss to combine.

Transfer to the air fryer basket and cook at 160°C for 18-20 minutes, stirring every 5 minutes.

When crispy remove from the air fryer and drizzle with maple syrup. Allow to cool slightly, then serve warm.

RICOTTA FRITTERS

2 cups (250g) ricotta cheese

3 tbsps plain flour

⅓ cup (70g) sugar

1 egg yolk

Zest of 1 lemon

Sour cream and jam to serve

Add the ricotta, flour, sugar, egg yolk and lemon zest into a large bowl and mix well to combine.

With wet hands, divide the ricotta mixture into 12 portions and shape into balls.

Cover and refrigerate for 15 minutes.

Arrange the ricotta balls in the air fryer basket.

Cook for 12 minutes at 180°C, turning halfway through cooking.

Serve with sour cream and jam.

HONEY MUFFINS

2 cups (280g) gluten-free flour

1 tsp xanthan gum (omit if your flour already contains it)

1½ tsps baking powder

¼ tsp bicarbonate of soda

½ tsp salt

¼ tsp ground cinnamon

½ cup (110g) sugar

¾ cup (185ml) milk

6 tbsps butter, melted and cooled

¼ cup (90g) honey

2 eggs, beaten

1 tsp vanilla extract

2 tsps sesame seeds (optional)

Muffin tray or silicone moulds

Preheat your air fryer to 160°C.

In a large bowl, place the flour, xanthan gum, baking powder, bicarb, salt, cinnamon and sugar, and whisk to combine. Create a well in the centre and add the milk, butter, honey, eggs and vanilla, mixing to just combine after each addition.

Pour batter into silicone moulds or paper liners inside an air fryer muffin tray. Sprinkle with sesame seeds, if desired.

Cook for 12-15 minutes until lightly golden brown on top and a toothpick inserted in the centre comes out with no more than a few moist crumbs attached. Allow to cool slightly before serving.

BANANA MUFFINS

3 large bananas

2 large eggs

1 cup (250ml) Greek yoghurt

2 cups (175g) oats

¼ cup (35g) chopped walnuts

1½ tsps baking powder

4 tbsps honey

1 tsp vanilla extract

1 tsp ground cinnamon

¼ cup (30g) flaked almonds

Muffin tray or silicone moulds

Preheat air fryer to 180°C.

Place two of the bananas, the eggs, yoghurt, oats, walnuts, baking powder, honey, vanilla and cinnamon in a food processor and blend until smooth.

Pour into silicone moulds or paper liners inside an air fryer muffin tray. Slice the third banana and top each muffin with a slice.

Working in batches place muffins in the air fryer basket and cook for 13-15 minutes until an inserted skewer comes out clean.

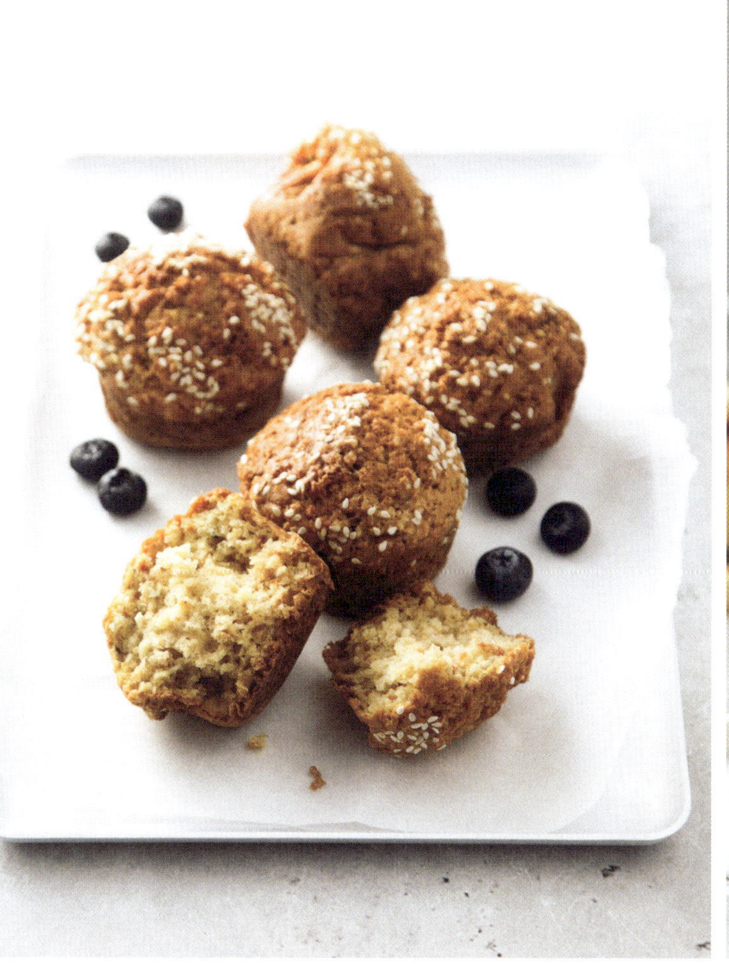

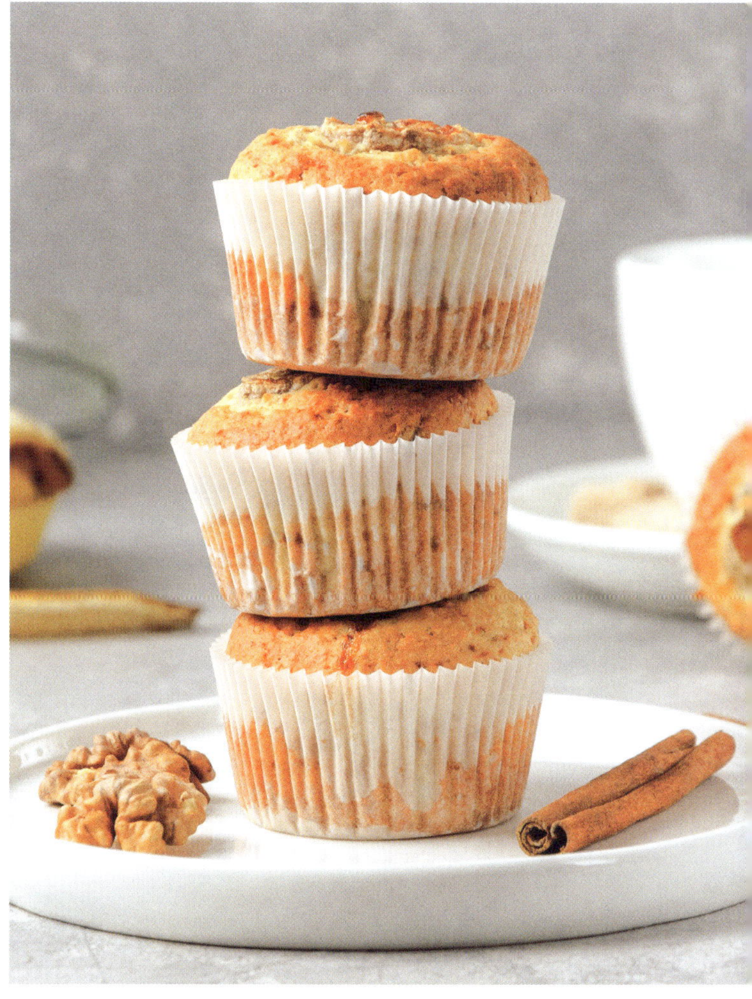

Honey Muffins

MAKES 12

PREP + COOK TIME: 30 MINS

VEG • GLUTEN FREE

Banana Muffins

MAKES 10

PREP + COOK TIME: 20 MINS

VEG

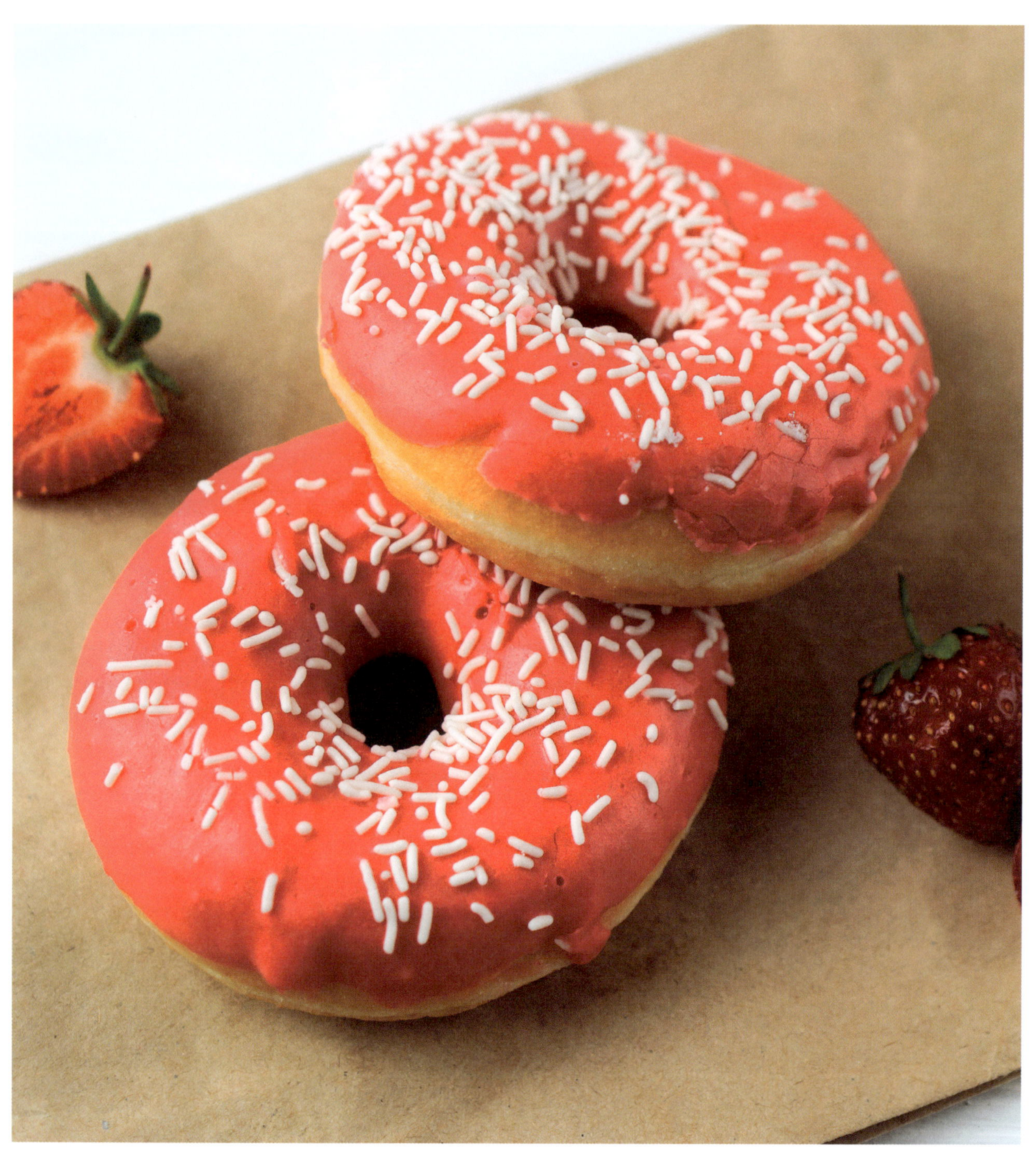

Pink Glazed Doughnuts

MAKES 4

PREP + COOK TIME: 35 MINS + COOLING

VEG

PINK GLAZED DOUGHNUTS

1¾ cups (225g) self-raising flour

1 tsp baking powder

¼ cup (50g) caster sugar

⅓ cup (50g) brown sugar

½ cup (120ml) milk + 3 tbsps milk

70g butter, melted

1 egg

1 cup (155g) icing sugar

½ tsp pink food colouring

Sprinkles, to decorate

Preheat the air fryer to 180°C.

Combine the flour, baking powder, caster sugar and brown sugar in a large mixing bowl.

In a separate bowl whisk together the ½ cup milk, butter and egg.

Pour the wet mixture into the dry ingredients and stir gently until just combined.

Roll dough out onto a floured surface to create a log shape. Slice into disks around 2cm thick. Use a small cookie cutter (or bottle lid) to remove a circle in the centre of the disk. Discard (or see the Doughnut Holes recipe on page 89).

Line the air fryer basket with greaseproof paper. Place the doughnuts inside. (Be careful not to overcrowd the basket. Cook in batches or use a double layer accessory if needed.) Cook for 15 minutes, until they spring back when lightly pressed. Set aside to cool.

Meanwhile, make the icing. Sift the icing sugar over a mixing bowl and whisk in the remaining milk, 1 tablespoon at a time, until the icing reaches a sticky but pourable consistency. Add a couple of drops of pink colouring until the desired colour is achieved.

When the doughnuts have cooled, place the icing over the top, and finish with sprinkles to decorate.

Chocolate Zucchini Bread

SERVES 8
PREP + COOK TIME: 50 MINS
VEG

½ cup (60g) plain flour
¼ cup (30g) cocoa powder
½ tsp bicarbonate of soda
¼ tsp salt
1 egg
¼ cup (80g) maple syrup
4 tbsps butter, melted
½ tsp vanilla extract
¾ cup (170g) packed grated zucchini
½ cup (80g) chocolate chips
70g chocolate, melted, to serve
Flaked almonds, to serve
Mini loaf pan

Preheat air fryer to 150°C. Grease and line the mini loaf pan with greaseproof paper.

In one bowl, whisk together flour, cocoa powder, bicarb and salt. In another bowl, combine egg, maple syrup, melted butter and vanilla. Whisk until smooth. Add dry ingredients to wet mixture and stir to combine. Fold in zucchini and chocolate chips. Transfer to loaf pan.

Cook for 30-35 minutes, or until an inserted skewer comes out clean.

Drizzle with melted chocolate and sprinkle with flaked almonds to serve.

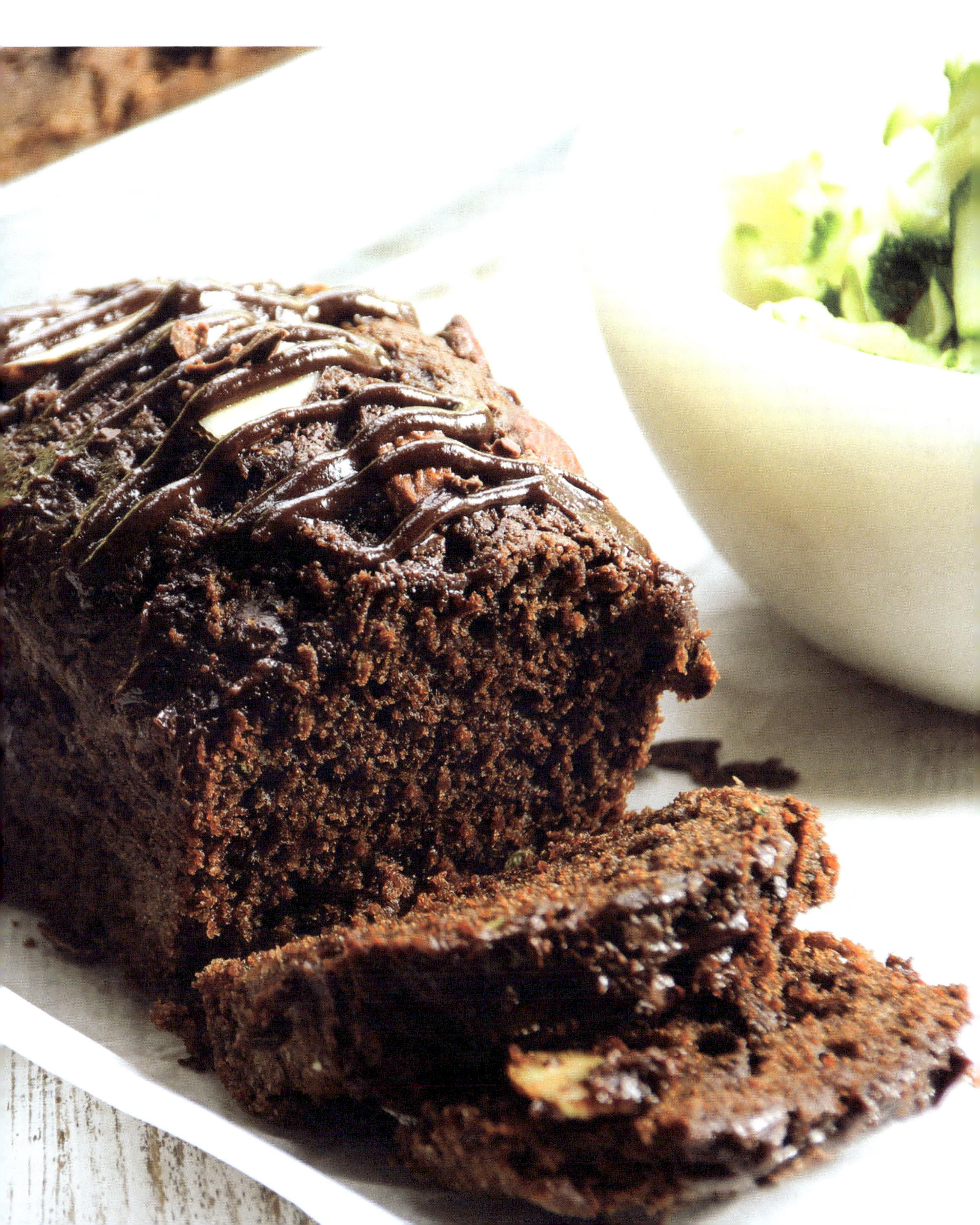

CORNFLAKE COOKIES

100g butter, softened

½ cup (100g) caster sugar

1 egg

1 tsp vanilla extract

1 cup (120g) gluten-free plain flour

1½ tsps baking powder

2½ cups (75g) cornflakes

Preheat air fryer to 160°C.

In a large bowl beat butter and sugar with an electric hand mixer until light and fluffy. Add egg and vanilla and mix to incorporate. Add flour, baking powder and 1 cup of cornflakes. Stir with a wooden spoon to incorporate.

Add remaining 1½ cups of cornflakes to a small bowl and set aside. Spoon heaped tablespoons of dough and roll into balls. Drop the balls one at a time into the bowl of cornflakes and turn to coat.

Place the cookies in the air fryer basket, leaving plenty of room for the cookies to spread. Work in batches, or use a double-layer accessory, if needed. Cook for 8-12 minutes or until golden and set around the edges.

Place onto a wire rack to cool completely.

SCONES WITH STRAWBERRY JAM

1 cup (125g) self-raising flour, sifted

¼ cup (55g) caster sugar

30g chilled butter, cut into pieces

⅓ cup (80ml) milk

Jam and whipped cream to serve

Baking pan

Lightly spray and line the baking pan with greaseproof paper and set aside.

Combine the flour and sugar in a large mixing bowl. Add the butter and rub it into the flour using fingertips until it reaches a breadcrumb consistency.

Make a well in the centre and pour in the milk. Stir until well combined.

Turn the mixture out onto a floured workbench and gently knead the dough until it comes together. Roll out the dough to a thickness of around 1½ cm and then cut out six rounds using a cookie cutter.

Place the rounds into the prepared pan and cook for 12 minutes at 200°C.

Serve with jam and cream.

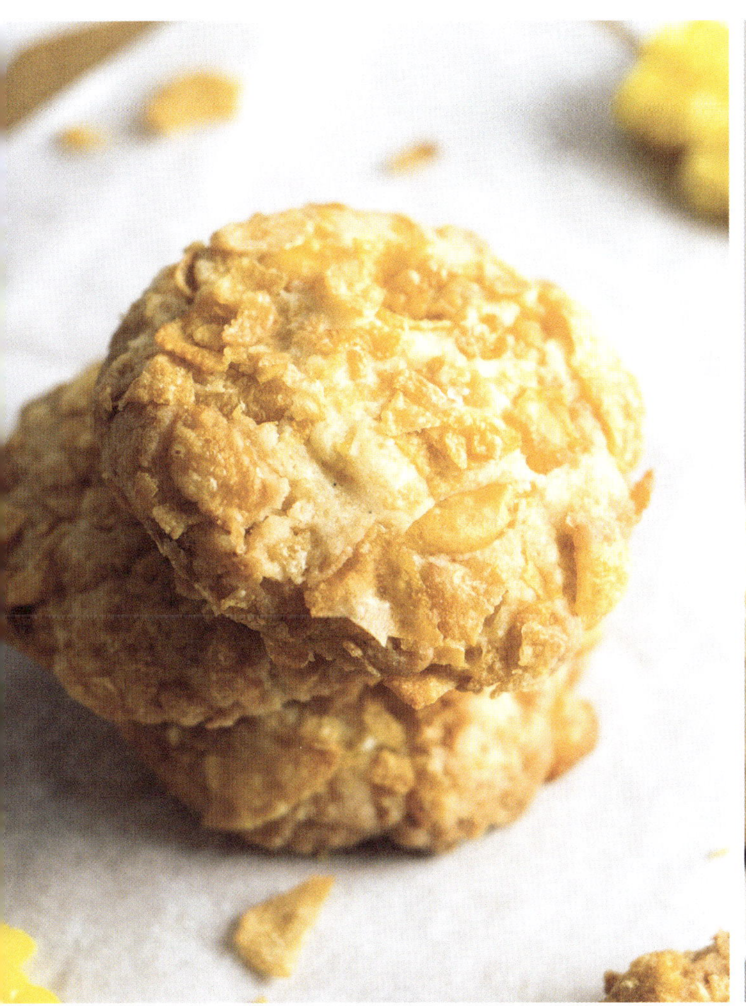

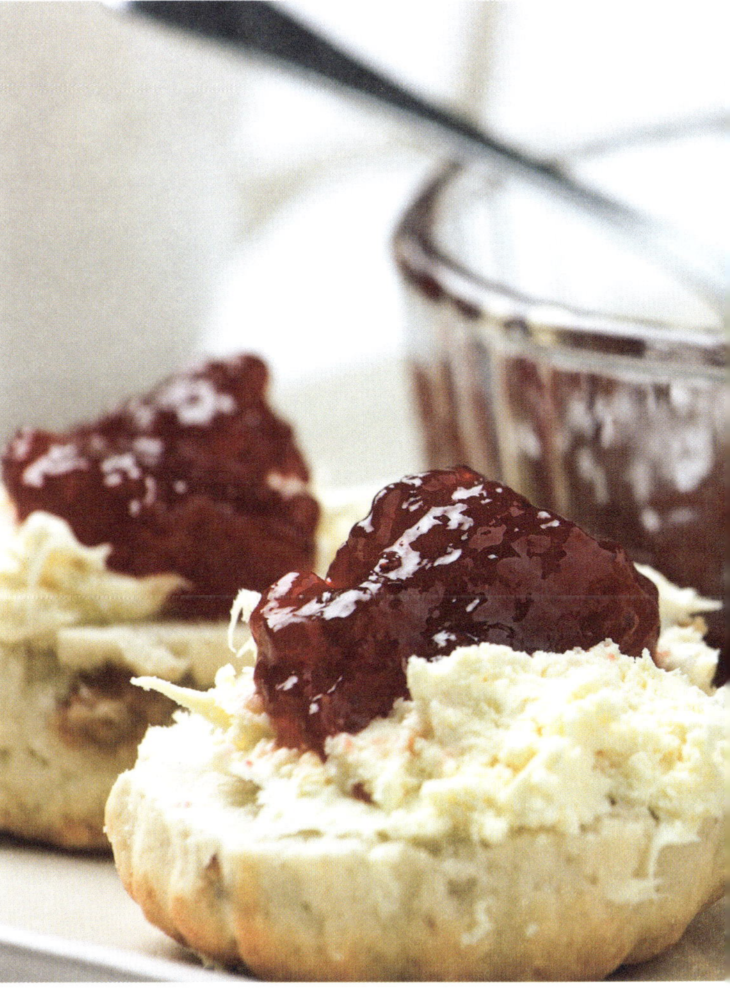

Cornflake Cookies

MAKES 12

PREP + COOK TIME: 30 MINS

VEG • GLUTEN FREE

Scones with Strawberry Jam

MAKES 6

PREP + COOK TIME: 30 MINS

VEG

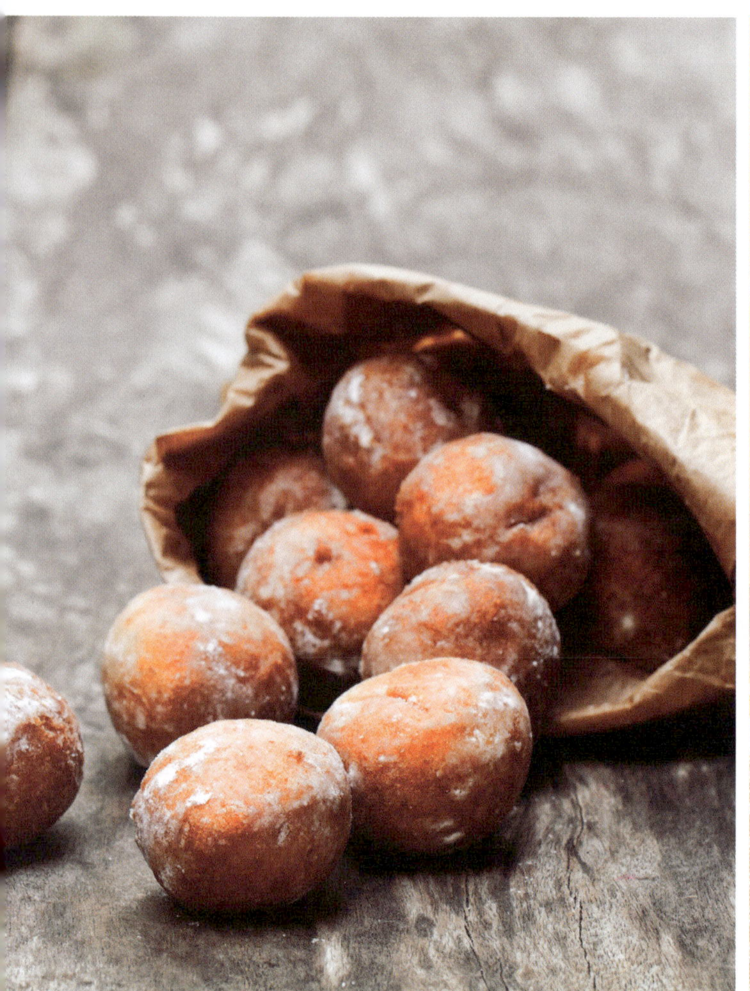

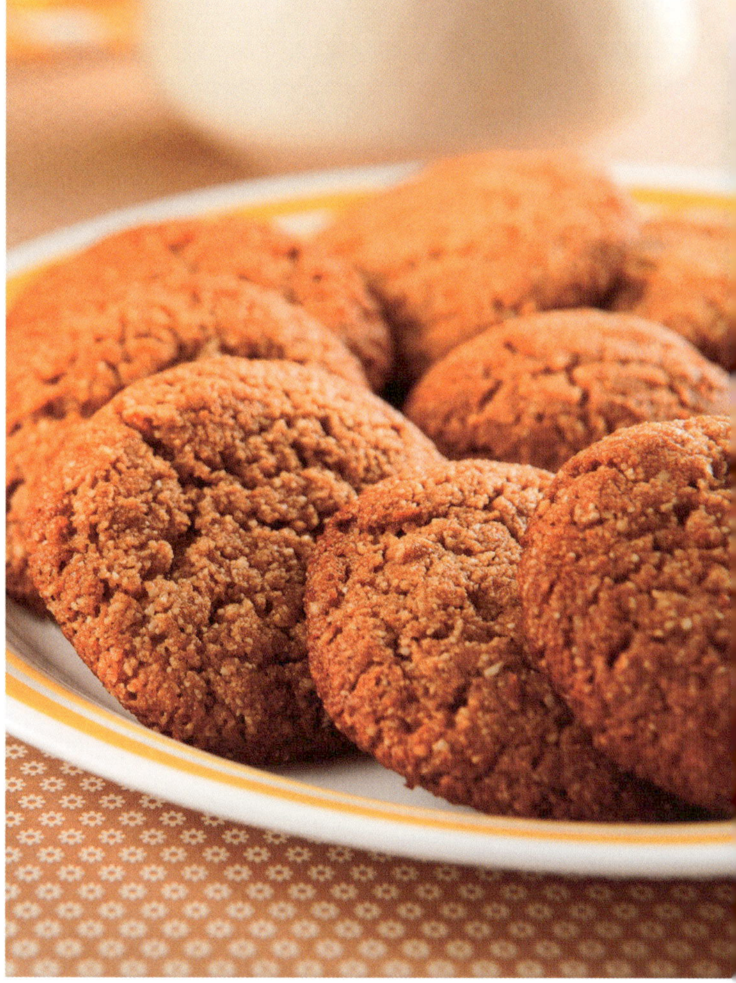

Doughnut Holes

MAKES 12

PREP + COOK TIME: 30 MINS

VEG

Gluten-Free Ginger Biscuits

MAKES 12

PREP + COOK TIME: 20 MINS + CHILLING

VEG • GLUTEN FREE • DAIRY FREE

DOUGHNUT HOLES

1¼ cups (155g) plain flour

2 tbsps caster sugar

¾ tsp baking powder

¼ tsp salt

100g chilled butter, cut into small pieces

¼ cup (60ml) milk

⅓ cup (70g) sugar

1½ tsps cinnamon

Combine the flour, caster sugar, baking powder and salt in a medium bowl and mix together. Cut in the butter and rub using fingertips until a fine crumble forms. Add the milk and stir until coated.

Transfer the mixture to a floured workbench and knead for approximately 1 minute until it forms a smooth dough ball. Cut the dough into equal portions and roll each into a ball.

Line the air fryer basket with greaseproof paper and preheat it to 180°C.

Combine cinnamon and the sugar in a medium bowl. Roll the dough balls in the cinnamon sugar and place in the air fryer basket. (Be careful not to overcrowd the basket. Cook in batches or use a double layer accessory if needed.)

Cook for 8 minutes until puffed and golden.

GLUTEN-FREE GINGER BISCUITS

1 cup (120g) almond meal

¼ cup (30g) tapioca flour

½ cup (80g) coconut sugar

¾ tsp bicarbonate of soda

¼ tsp salt

½ tbsp ground cinnamon

½ tbsp ground ginger

1 egg

2 tbsps molasses

1 tbsp maple syrup

¼ cup (60ml) melted coconut oil

¼ tsp vanilla extract

In a bowl combine almond meal, tapioca flour, coconut sugar, bicarb, salt and spices. Mix well.

In a separate bowl, whisk together egg, molasses, maple syrup, coconut oil and vanilla. Pour wet ingredients into dry ingredients and stir to combine.

Form dough into a ball. Wrap in plastic wrap and refrigerate for 25 minutes.

Roll dough into 12 balls then press gently to flatten.

Cooking in batches if necessary, arrange biscuits in air fryer basket. Cook for 6-8 minutes at 160°C.

Chapter Three

Simple Lunches

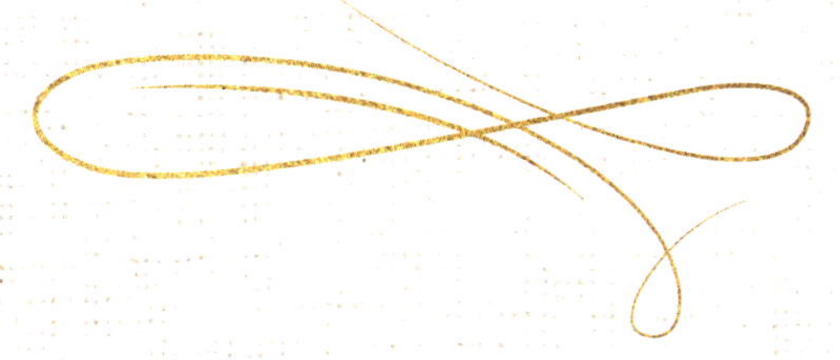

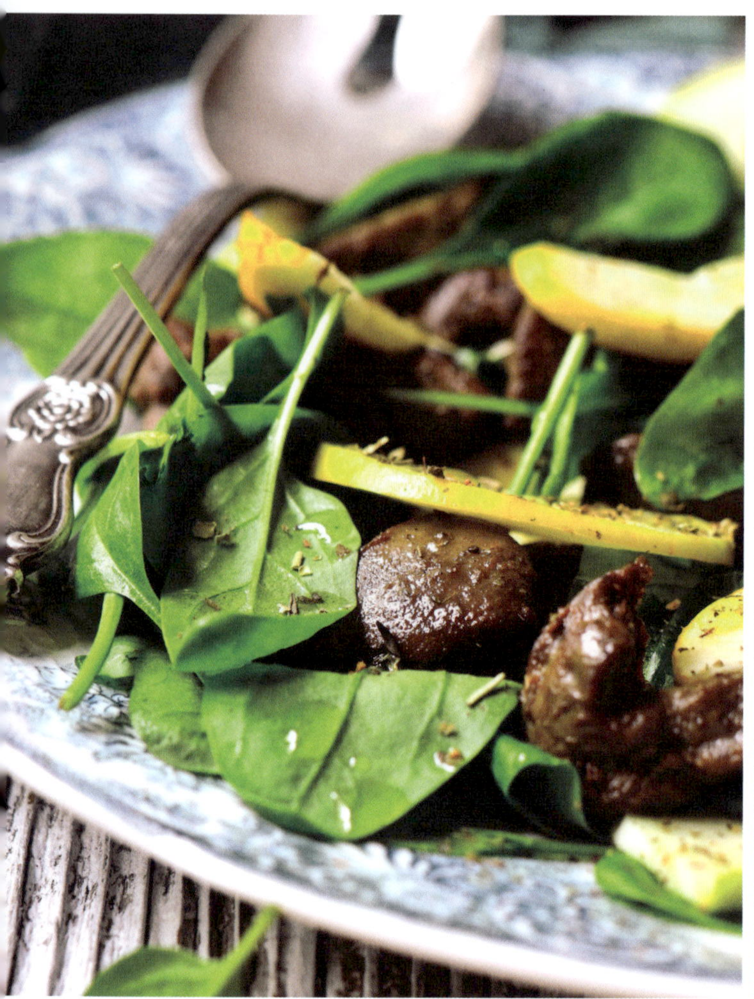

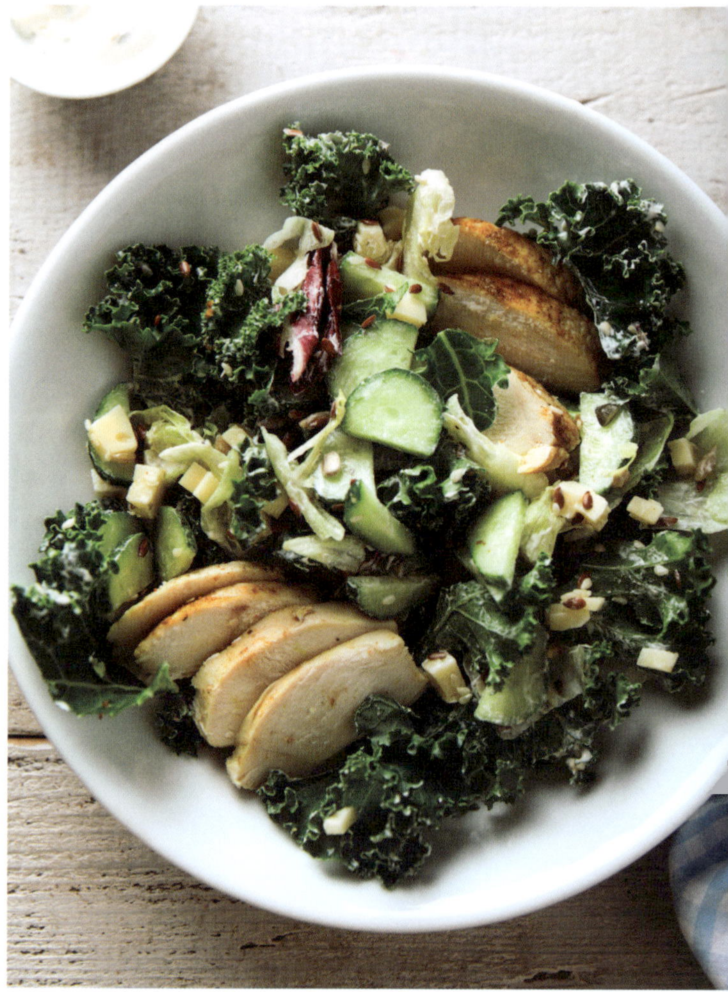

Beef Liver & Apple Salad

SERVES 2

PREP + COOK TIME: 30 MINS

GLUTEN FREE • DAIRY FREE

Kale & Chicken Salad

SERVES 2

PREP + COOK TIME: 25 MINS

GLUTEN FREE • DAIRY FREE

BEEF LIVER & APPLE SALAD

400g beef livers, sliced
Salt and pepper to taste
3 tbsps olive oil
1 tbsp vinegar
¼ tsp mixed herbs
300g baby spinach leaves
1 green apple, sliced
Baking pan

Place livers in a baking pan that will fit into your air fryer. Spray with olive oil cooking spray and toss to coat.

Place in air fryer and cook for 15-20 minutes at 190°C, stirring every few minutes.

Season well with salt and pepper and set aside.

Combine olive oil, vinegar and mixed herbs in a small bowl or sealable jar with a lid. Season with salt and pepper. Stir or shake to combine.

Arrange spinach leaves, apple and cooked liver on two serving plates. Drizzle with dressing and toss to coat.

KALE & CHICKEN SALAD

500g chicken breast
Salt and pepper to taste
¼ cup (60ml) olive oil
1½ tbsps red or white wine vinegar
1 tbsp wholegrain mustard
1 tbsp honey
150g kale, washed and roughly torn
1 cucumber, sliced
1 avocado, diced
¼ cup (25g) red cabbage, chopped
½ bulb fennel, sliced

Place chicken breasts in air fryer. Spray with cooking spray. Season with salt and pepper.

Cook for 14 minutes at 190°C, turning and spraying halfway through. Rest.

Whisk together olive oil, vinegar, mustard and honey.

Slice chicken and arrange with remaining ingredients in serving bowls. Drizzle with dressing and toss to coat.

CHICKEN WALDORF SALAD

500g chicken breast

Salt and pepper to taste

6 tbsps Greek yoghurt

1 tbsp lemon juice

200g mixed salad leaves

¼ cup (30g) walnut pieces

1 apple, julienned

2 stalks celery, chopped

1 spring onion, chopped

Place chicken breasts in air fryer. Spray with cooking spray. Season with salt and pepper.

Cook for 7 minutes at 190°C. Flip over, spray once more and cook for a further 7 minutes until cooked through. Set aside to rest.

Place yoghurt and lemon juice in a bowl. Stir to combine.

Place remaining ingredients in a serving bowl.

Slice chicken and add to bowl along with yoghurt dressing. Toss to combine and serve immediately.

CAULIFLOWER GRATIN

1 head cauliflower, cut into florets

1 tbsp olive oil

Salt and pepper to taste

¾ cup (185ml) thickened cream

½ cup (60g) grated Cheddar cheese

½ cup (60g) grated mozzarella cheese

¼ cup (25g) grated Parmesan cheese

½ tsp garlic powder

Baking pan

Toss the cauliflower florets in olive oil, salt and pepper. Place in air fryer basket and cook for 16-17 minutes at 190°C until just tender.

Meanwhile in a small saucepan over medium-low heat combine cream, cheeses and garlic powder. Cook, stirring until the sauce thickens.

Arrange the cooked cauliflower in baking pan. Pour cheese sauce over cauliflower.

Place pan in air fryer and cook for a 12 minutes at 190°C until sauce is bubbling.

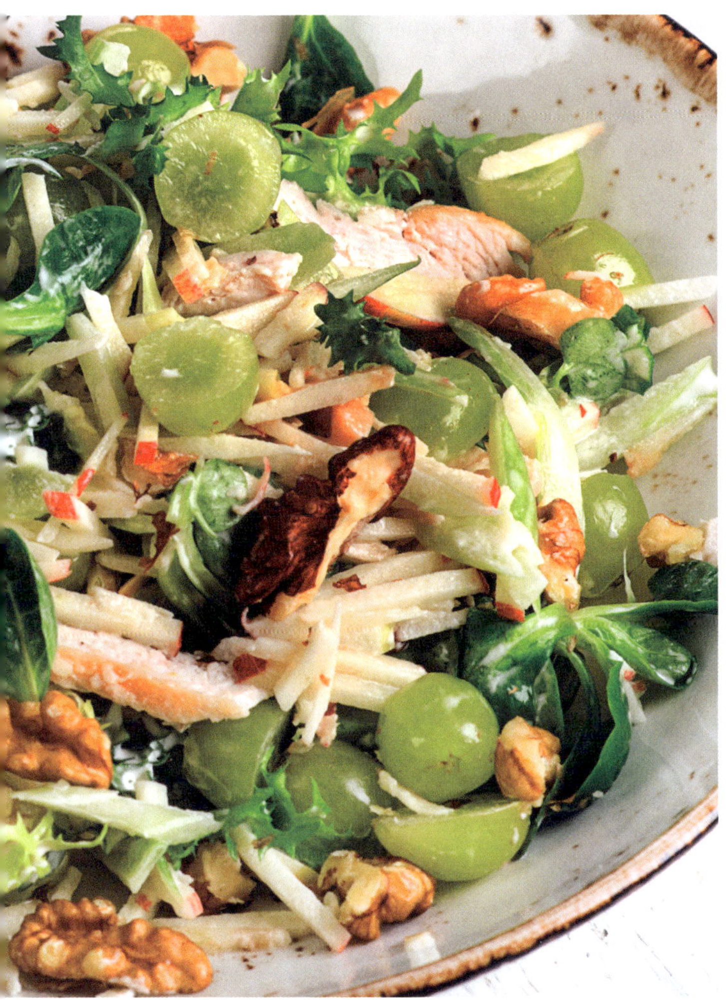

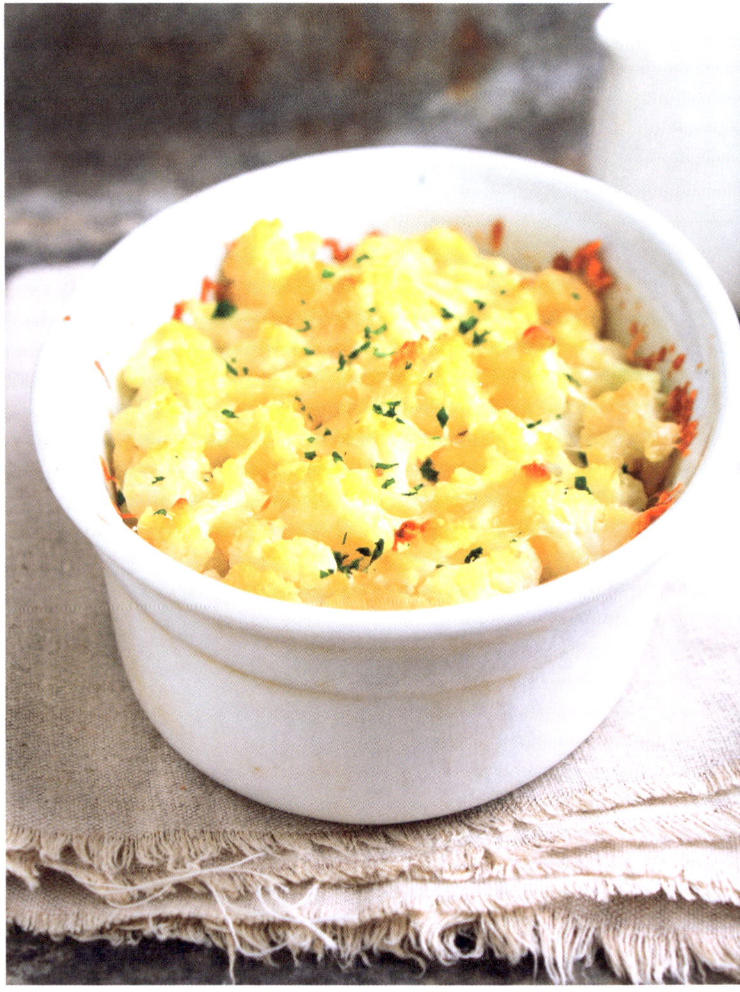

Chicken Waldorf Salad

SERVES 2

PREP + COOK TIME: 25 MINS

GLUTEN FREE

Cauliflower Gratin

SERVES 4

PREP + COOK TIME: 35 MINS

GLUTEN FREE

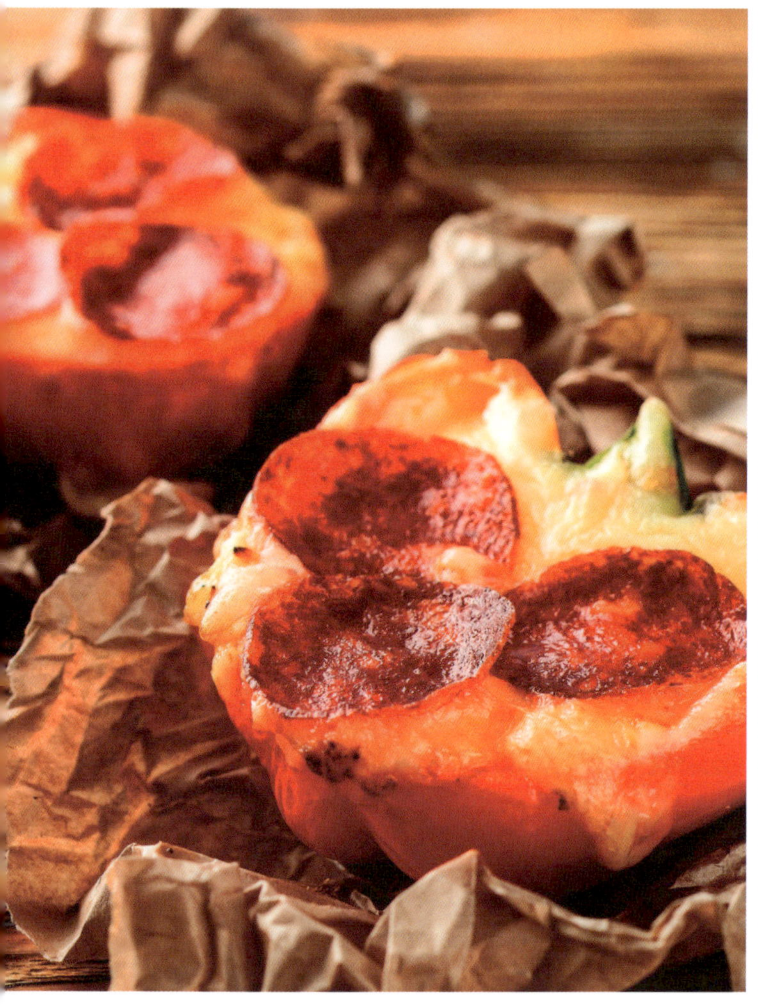

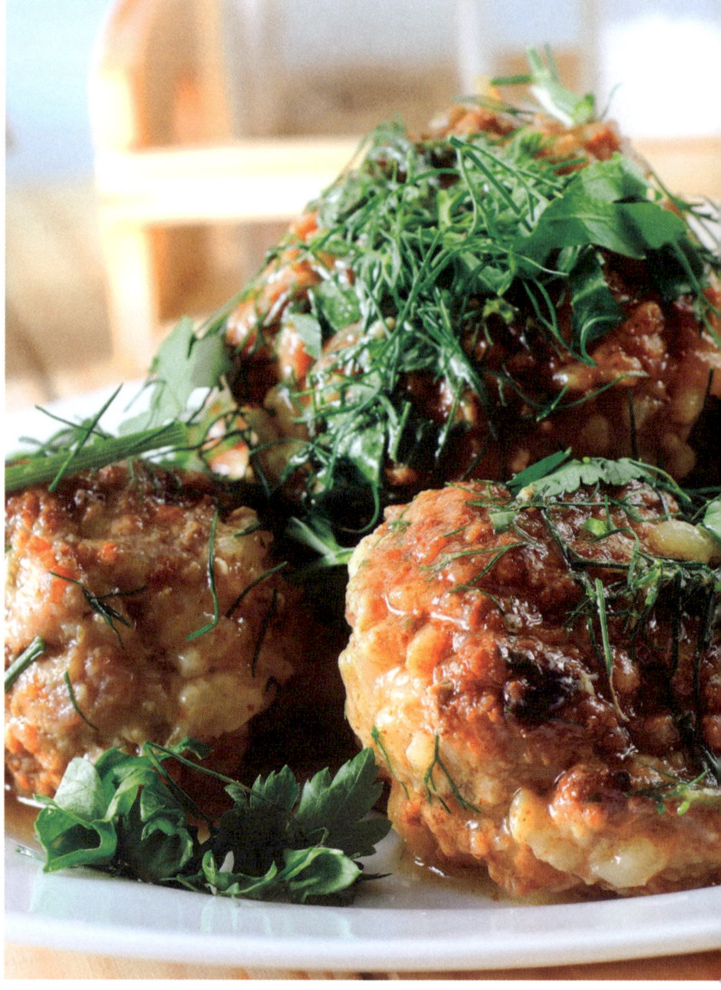

Cheese & Salami Stuffed Capsicums

SERVES 2

PREP + COOK TIME: 20 MINS

GLUTEN FREE

Cheese & Herb Meatballs

SERVES 4

PREP + COOK TIME: 20 MINS

GLUTEN FREE

CHEESE AND SALAMI STUFFED CAPSICUMS

2 red capsicums

Salt and pepper to taste

2 cups (250g) Cheddar cheese, grated

150g salami sausage, thinly sliced

Cut the capsicums in half lengthways and scoop out the seeds and membranes.

Spray inside and out with olive oil cooking spray and season with salt and pepper.

Place capsicums in air fryer basket cut-side up and cook for 6 minutes at 175°C.

Remove from air fryer and when cool enough to handle fill each half with equal amounts of cheese. Top with salami slices.

Return to the air fryer and cook for a further 4-5 minutes at 175°C until the cheese is melted.

CHEESE & HERB MEATBALLS

½ cup (50g) grated Parmesan cheese

½ cup (60g) grated mozzarella cheese

1 large egg, lightly beaten

2 tbsps thickened cream

1 clove garlic, minced

500g beef mince

2 tbsps fresh parsley, chopped + more to serve

2 tbsps fresh dill, chopped + more to serve

Salt and pepper to taste

Cake tin or baking pan

Preheat air fryer to 175°C. Grease cake tin or baking pan.

In a large bowl, combine cheeses, egg, cream and garlic. Add beef and herbs and season with salt and pepper. Use your hands to mix well.

Shape into golf-ball–sized meatballs.

Place in a single layer in the tin and place in air fryer basket. Cook in batches if necessary. Cook for 8-10 minutes until lightly browned and cooked through.

Keep warm while you cook the remaining meatballs.

Sprinkle with fresh herbs to serve.

Prawn Tacos

SERVES 4
PREP + COOK TIME: 15 MINS
GLUTEN FREE • DAIRY FREE

500g peeled, deveined prawns
2 tbsps olive oil
½ tsp garlic powder
¼ tsp ground cumin
¼ tsp onion powder
Salt and pepper to taste
4 flour tortillas, warmed
1 cup (225g) cherry tomatoes, chopped
½ yellow capsicum, diced
1 avocado, sliced
½ red onion, diced
¼ cup (5g) fresh coriander leaves
Juice of 1 lemon
Lemon slices, to serve

Toss prawns with oil, garlic powder, cumin, onion powder, salt and pepper. Transfer to greased air fryer basket.

Cook at 200°C for 5-6 minutes or until cooked through.

Assemble tortillas filled with prawns, tomatoes, capsicum, avocado, red onion and coriander.

Squeeze over lemon juice and add lemon slices to serve.

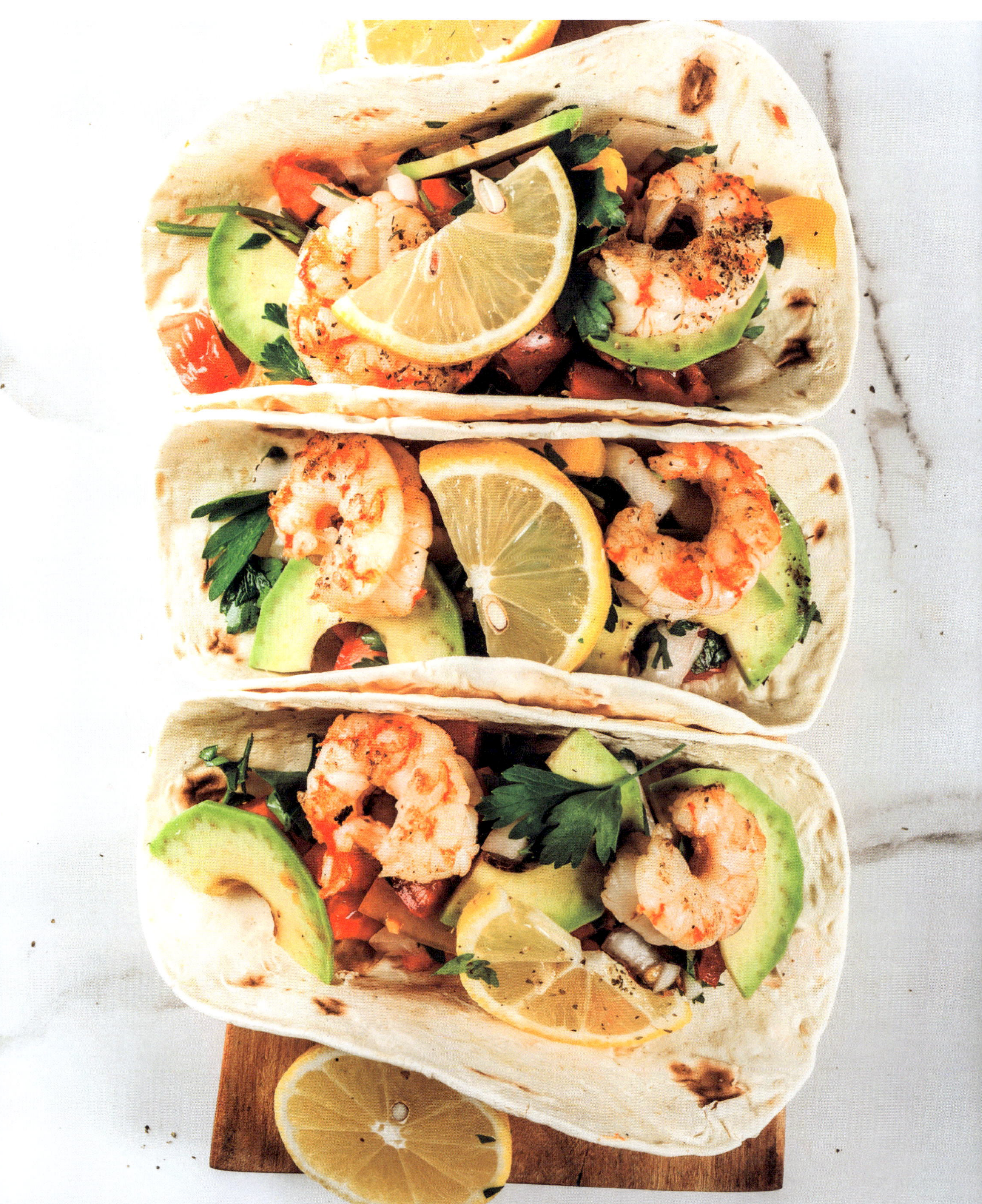

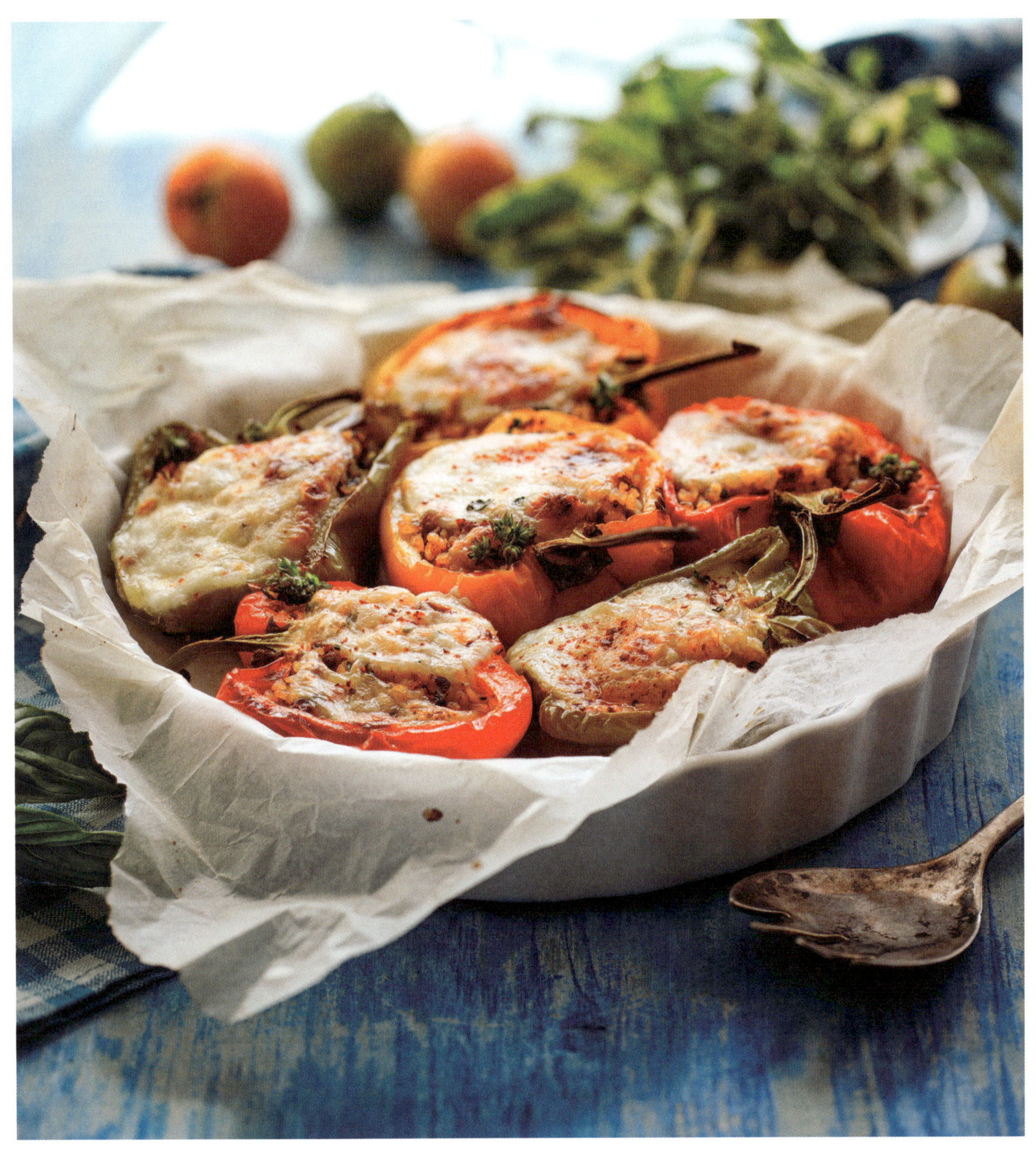

Stuffed Capsicums

SERVES 2

PREP + COOK TIME: 40 MINS

GLUTEN FREE

STUFFED CAPSICUMS

1 tsp olive oil
1 onion, diced
250g beef mince
½ tsp salt
¼ tsp pepper
¼ tsp garlic powder
1 cup (165g) cooked rice
1 cup (225g) passata
2 large or 3 small capsicums, halved lengthways
¾ cup (90g) grated mozzarella cheese

Heat the olive oil in a large pan over medium heat.

Add the onion and cook, stirring, for 3-5 minutes until soft and translucent. Add beef mince, salt, pepper and garlic powder. Cook, stirring occasionally, for about 10 minutes until beef is browned. Stir in rice and passata until well combined. Remove from the heat.

Place capsicum halves into the air fryer basket. Fill each with the beef and rice mixture.

Cook for 15 minutes at 180°C.

Sprinkle over cheese and cook for a further 2 minutes.

Caesar Salad

SERVES 2

PREP + COOK TIME: 25 MINS

1 large chicken breast
1 tbsp olive oil
1 tsp garlic powder
1 tsp onion powder
½ tsp chilli powder
Salt and pepper to taste
1 cos lettuce, leaves washed and dried
½ cup (50g) grated Parmesan cheese
1 cup (30g) croutons
½ cup (120g) Caesar dressing

Brush chicken with olive oil. Season all over with garlic, onion and chilli powders, salt and pepper.

Air fry chicken for 5 minutes at 190°C. Flip chicken and cook for another 5-8 minutes, until cooked through. Rest for 5 minutes then slice.

In a large bowl, combine chicken, lettuce, cheese and croutons. Drizzle with dressing to serve.

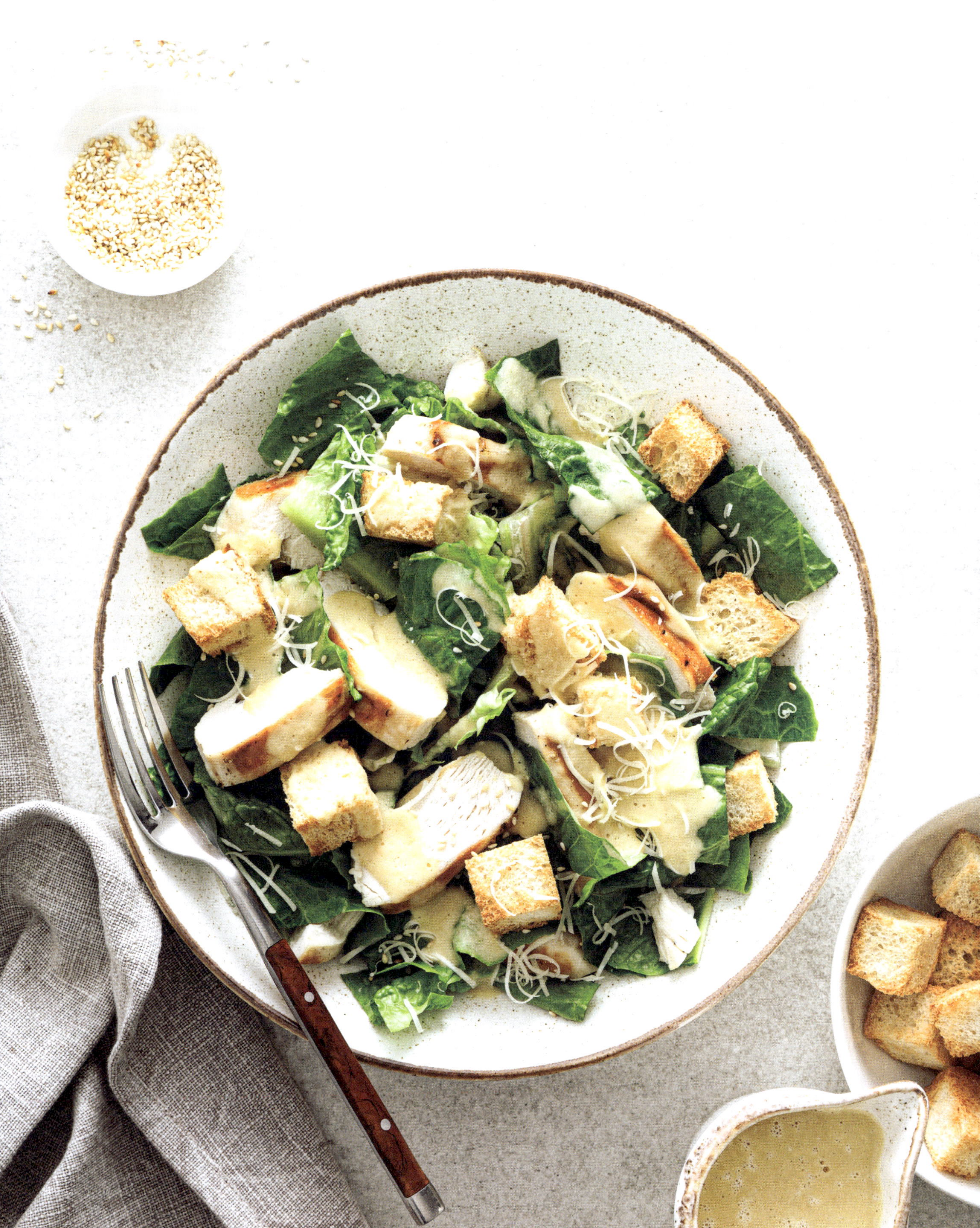

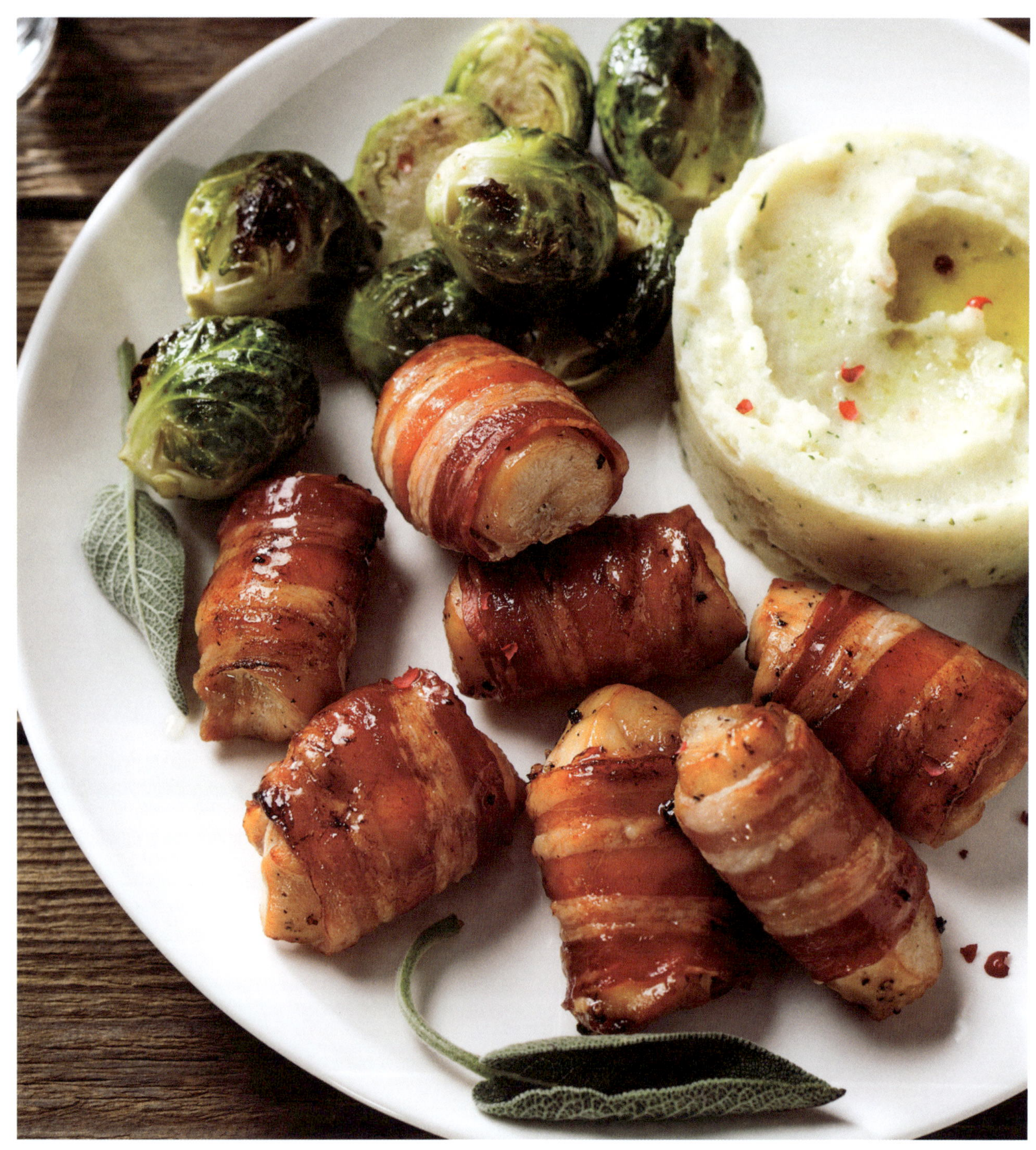

Bacon-Wrapped Chicken Bites

SERVES 2

PREP + COOK TIME: 30 MINS

GLUTEN FREE

BACON-WRAPPED CHICKEN BITES

2 skinless chicken breasts

Salt and pepper to taste

8 sage leaves

4 rashers streaky bacon, cut in half

Cut each of the chicken breasts into four equal pieces and transfer to a large bowl. Season with salt, pepper and toss to coat.

Place a sage leaf on top of each piece of chicken. Wrap half a bacon rasher around the chicken, tucking the ends on the underside of each piece.

Spray air fryer basket with cooking spray then carefully transfer chicken to basket. Make sure bacon is still tucked under firmly.

Cook at 200°C for 15-18 minutes or until chicken is cooked through and internal temperature reaches 74°C.

CHICKPEA SALAD

1 x 400g can chickpeas, drained and rinsed

2 tbsps olive oil

¼ tsp salt

3 tsps ground cumin

2 tsps paprika

150g rocket

1 avocado, sliced

½ cup (100g) cherry tomatoes, halved

1 tbsp lime juice + lime wedges to serve

Place chickpeas, 1 tablespoon olive oil, salt and spices in a bowl. Toss to coat.

Transfer to air fryer and cook at 190°C for 15 minutes, shaking the basket once or twice during cooking.

Add to the salad ingredients in a serving bowl.

Drizzle with lime juice and remaining olive oil and toss to coat.

GARLIC PRAWNS

500g raw king prawns, peeled and deveined

1 tsp garlic powder

¼ tsp dried chilli flakes

1 tbsp olive oil

½ tsp salt

½ tsp pepper

Lemon wedges and fresh coriander leaves to serve

Into a medium-sized bowl, place prawns, garlic powder, chilli flakes, oil, salt and pepper. Toss to coat.

Transfer the prawns to your air fryer. Cook for 10 minutes at 200°C until the prawns are opaque and just cooked through.

Serve with lemon wedges and fresh coriander leaves.

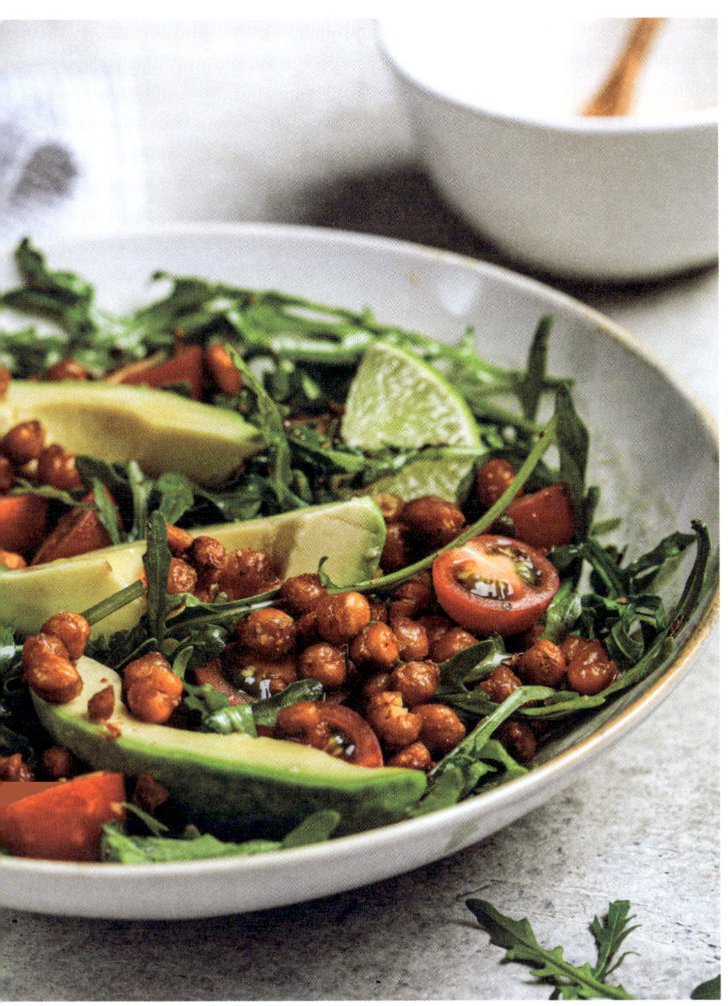

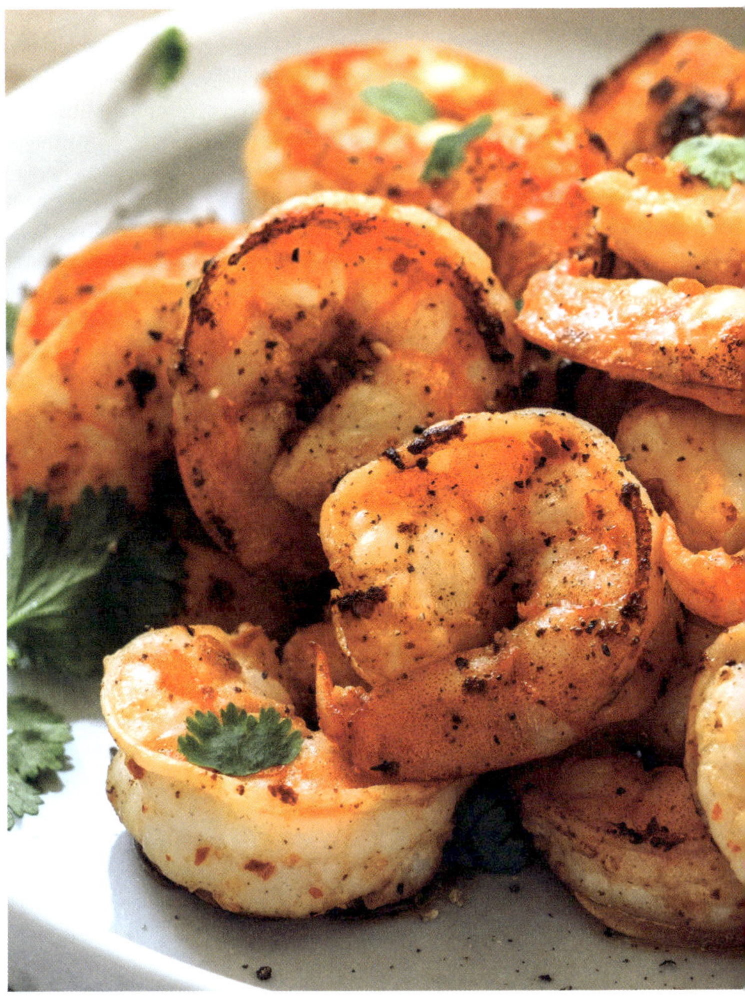

Chickpea Salad

SERVES 2

PREP + COOK TIME: 25 MINS

VEG • GLUTEN FREE

Garlic Prawns

SERVES 4

PREP + COOK TIME: 15 MINS

GLUTEN FREE

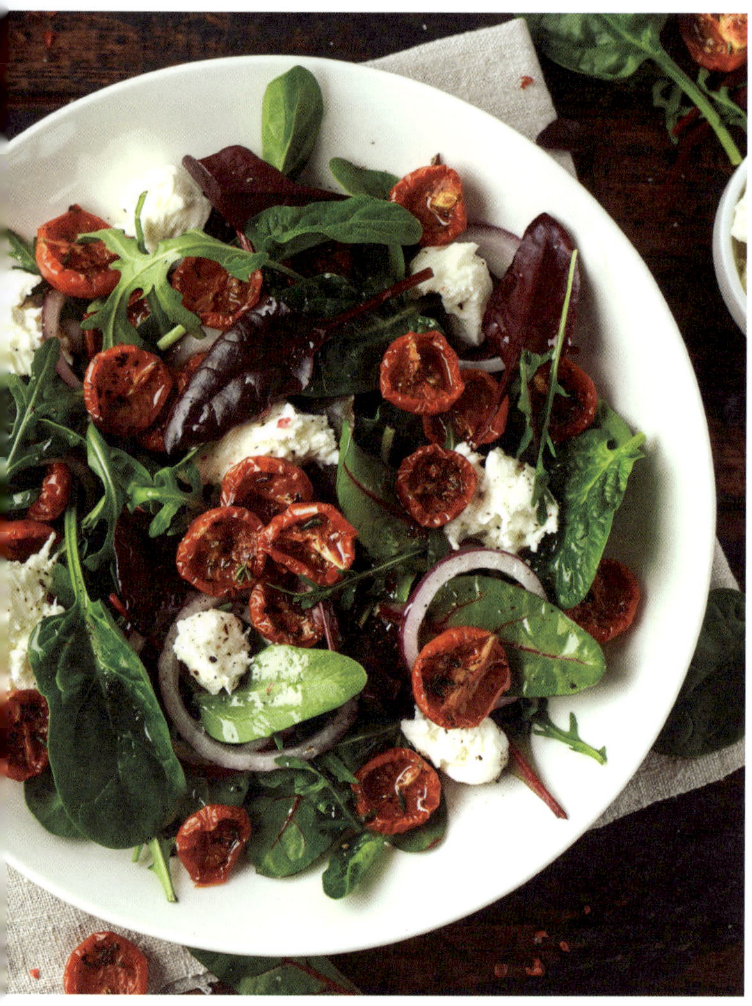

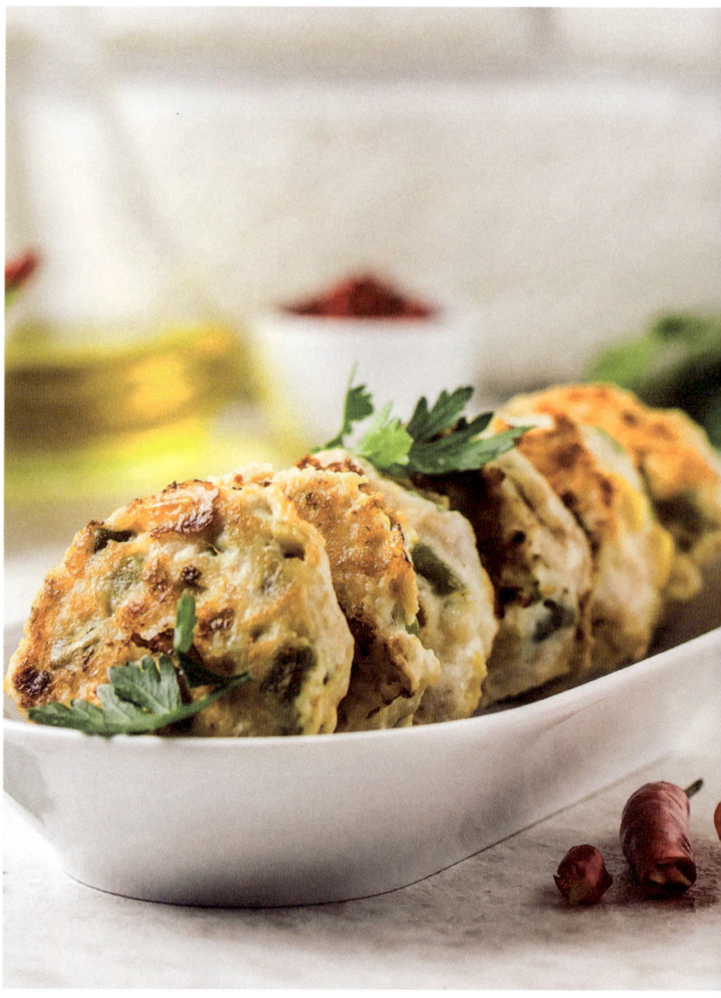

Italian Salad

SERVES 2

PREP + COOK TIME: 30 MINS

VEG • GLUTEN FREE

Chicken & Vegetable Patties

SERVES 4

PREP + COOK TIME: 30 MINS

GLUTEN FREE

ITALIAN SALAD

1 cup (250g) cherry tomatoes, halved
3 tbsps olive oil
Salt and pepper to taste
150g mixed salad leaves
¼ red onion, sliced
150g fresh mozzarella, torn

Drizzle the tomatoes with half the olive oil and season with salt and pepper.

Place in the air fryer basket cut-side up.

Cook for 20-24 minutes at 180°C.

Toss tomatoes with remaining salad ingredients. Drizzle with olive oil and season with salt and pepper.

CHICKEN & VEGETABLE PATTIES

600g chicken mince
1 onion, finely chopped
½ green capsicum, finely chopped
2 tbsps chopped parsley
¼ tsp dried chilli flakes
½ cup (60g) grated Cheddar cheese
½ cup (125ml) thickened cream
½ tsp salt or to taste
½ tsp pepper or to taste

Mix together all the ingredients until well combined.

Using hands, form into four to six evenly sized patties.

Preheat the air fryer to 200°C.

Place the patties in the air fryer and cook for 15 minutes.

Flip the chicken patties and cook for another 5 minutes until golden brown.

Cheese Souffle

SERVES 4
PREP + COOK TIME: 35 MINS
VEG

¼ cup (30g) panko breadcrumbs
30g butter
½ cup (60g) plain flour
1¼ cups (310ml) milk
½ cup (60g) grated Cheddar cheese
¼ cup (30g) grated Parmesan cheese
½ tsp ground nutmeg
4 large eggs, separated
4 ramekins or souffle dishes

Preheat air fryer to 165°C.

Spray four small souffle dishes or ramekins with olive oil spray and sprinkle with breadcrumbs.

Heat butter in a small saucepan, over medium-low heat. When melted add flour and stir until smooth. Add the milk a little at a time, whisking to remove any lumps. Bring to a simmer, stirring constantly until sauce thickens.

Remove sauce from heat and whisk in cheeses and nutmeg. Add egg yolks and beat until smooth.

In a separate bowl, whisk egg whites until stiff peaks form. Use a metal spoon to gradually fold egg whites into the sauce.

Divide mixture between dishes. Use a knife to flatten the tops.

Place dishes in air fryer basket. Cook for 18-20 minutes, until cheese is puffed up and golden brown.

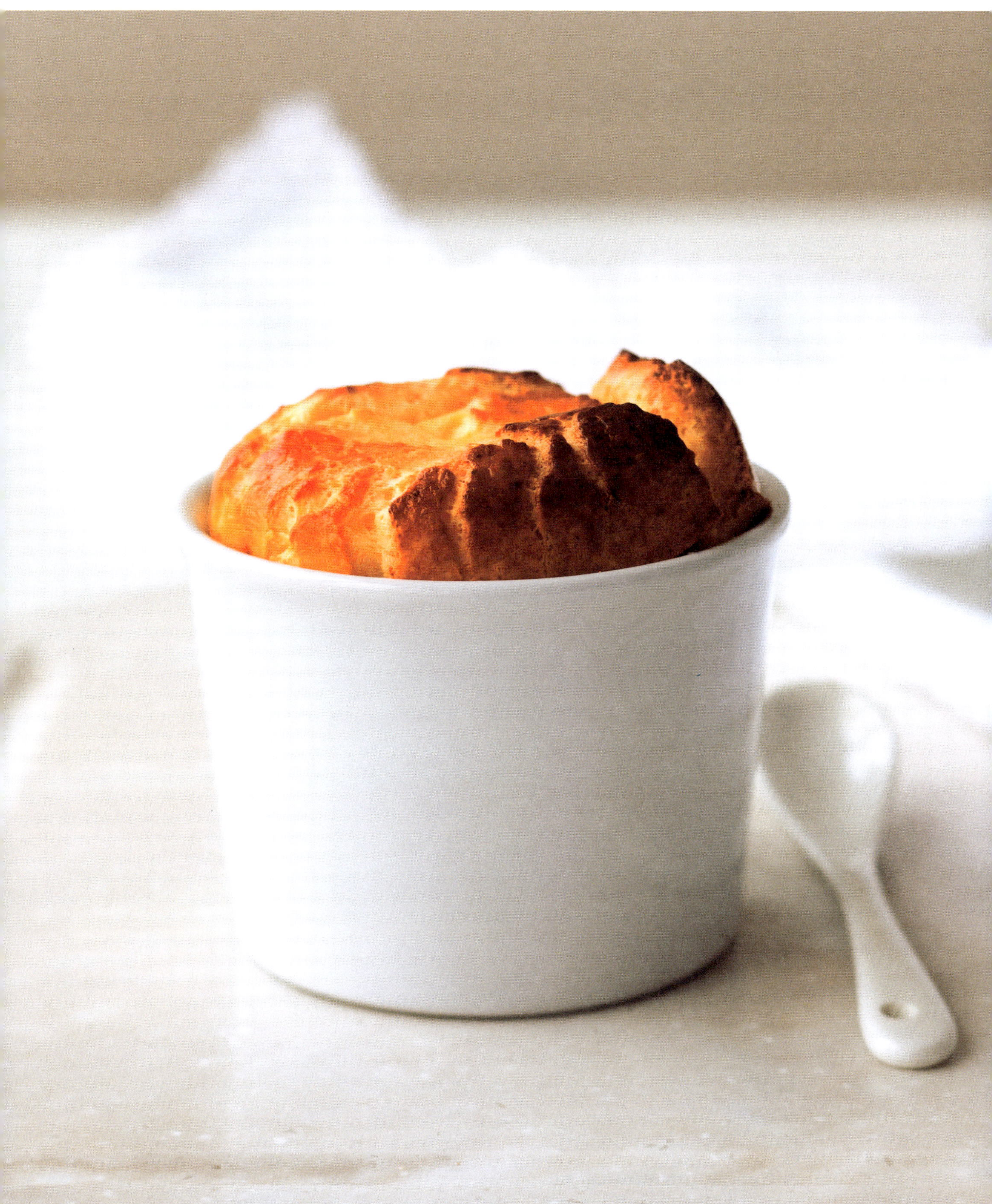

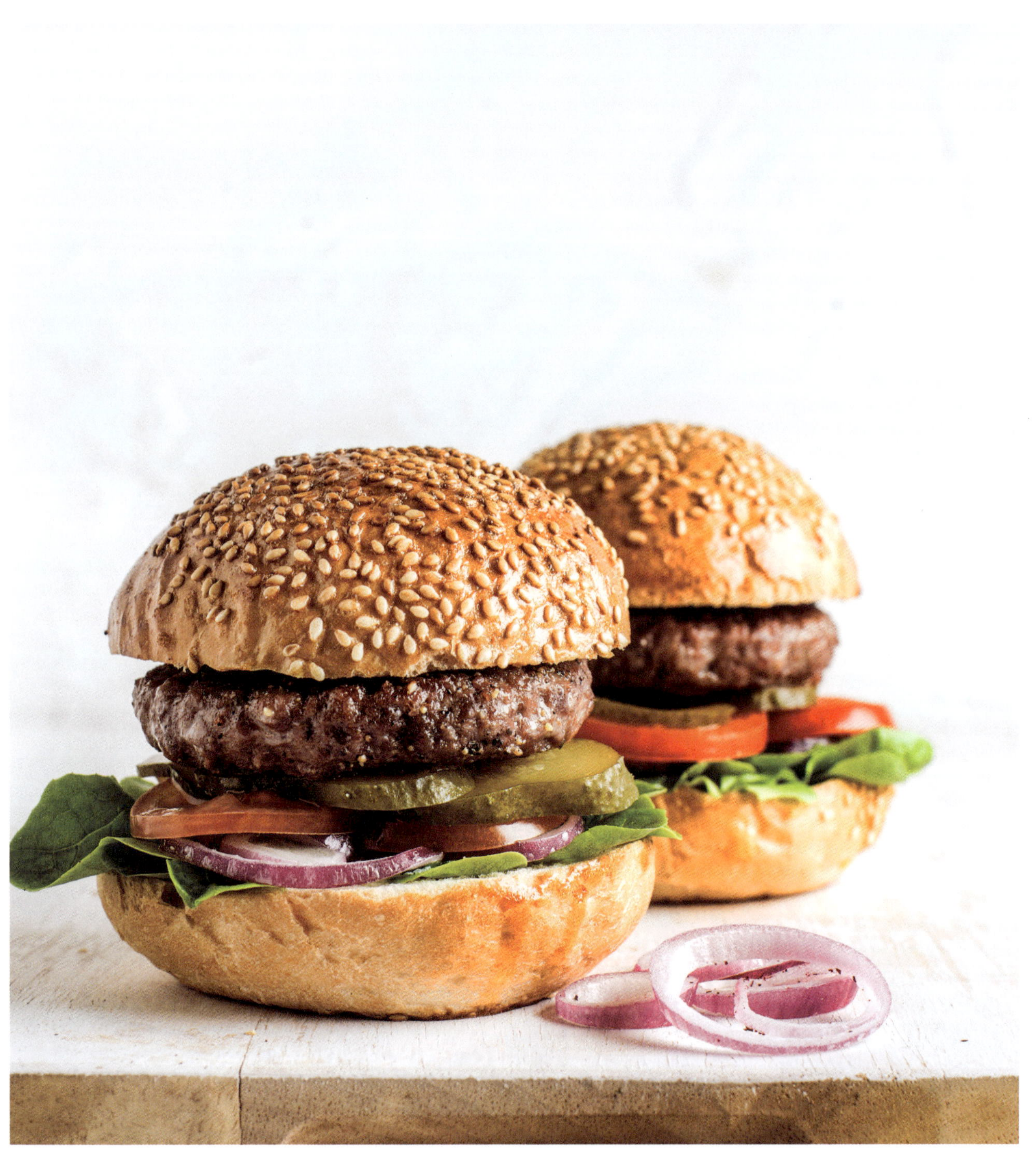

Beef Burgers

SERVES 4

PREP + COOK TIME: 20 MINS

DAIRY FREE

BEEF BURGERS

500g beef mince
1 tbsp Worcestershire sauce
1 tsp barbecue sauce
½ tsp garlic powder
½ tsp onion powder
½ tsp salt
½ tsp pepper
½ tsp dried oregano
4 sesame seed burger buns
2 tbsps mayonnaise
1 tbsp Dijon mustard
4 butter lettuce leaves
½ red onion, cut into rings
2 tomatoes, sliced
2 gherkins, sliced

Preheat the air fryer to 180°C.

Place mince, Worcestershire sauce, barbecue sauce, garlic powder, onion powder, salt, pepper and oregano together in a large mixing bowl and mix well to combine.

Shape the mixture into four burger patty shapes, using your hands.

Spritz the patties on both sides with cooking spray and place into the air fryer basket.

Cook for 10 minutes.

Spread burger bun bases with mayonnaise and mustard. Then layer with lettuce, red onion, tomatoes and gherkins. Top with burger patties and bun lids.

Cheesy Pastries

MAKES 8

PREP + COOK TIME: 1 HOUR

VEG

2 tbsps olive oil
3 onions, sliced
1 tbsp brown sugar
2 tbsps balsamic vinegar
½ tsp salt
½ tsp pepper
2 sheets frozen puff pastry, thawed
50g Brie, finely diced
50g Gorgonzola, finely diced
¼ cup (60ml) milk

Heat oil in a large pan on medium-high heat. Add onions and cook for about 10 minutes until wilted. Add sugar, vinegar, salt and pepper. Reduce heat and cook gently, uncovered, for 20-25 minutes or until caramelised. Add a little water if needed.

Preheat air fryer to 200°C.

Cut each sheet of pastry into four squares. Scoop even amounts of onion onto each pastry square. Top with cubes of Brie and Gorgonzola. Fold the four corners of each pastry square into the centre. Moisten the edges with some water and pinch along the seams to seal. Brush with milk.

Working in batches, transfer pastries to air fryer in a single layer. Bake for 10 minutes until golden brown. Repeat with remaining pastries.

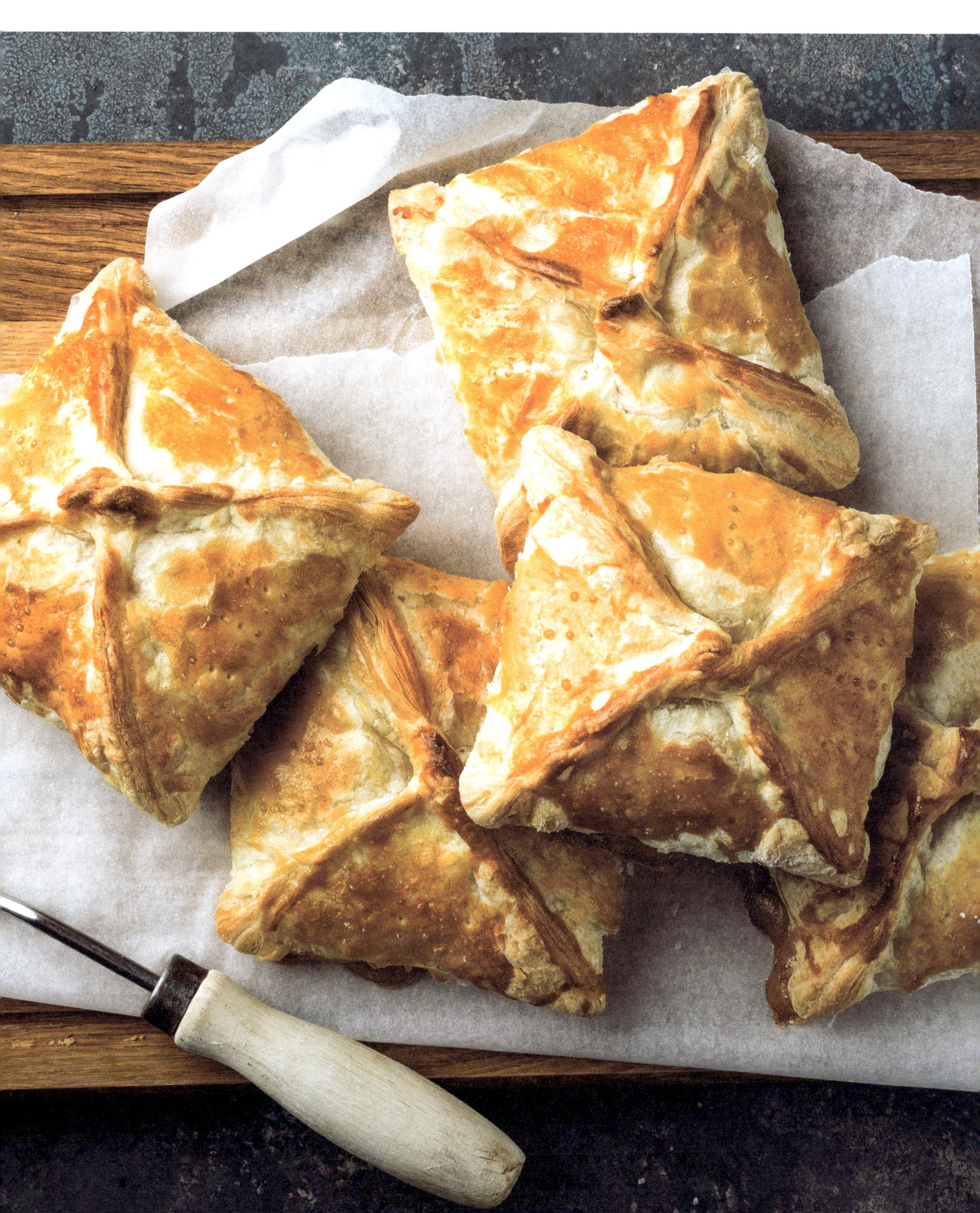

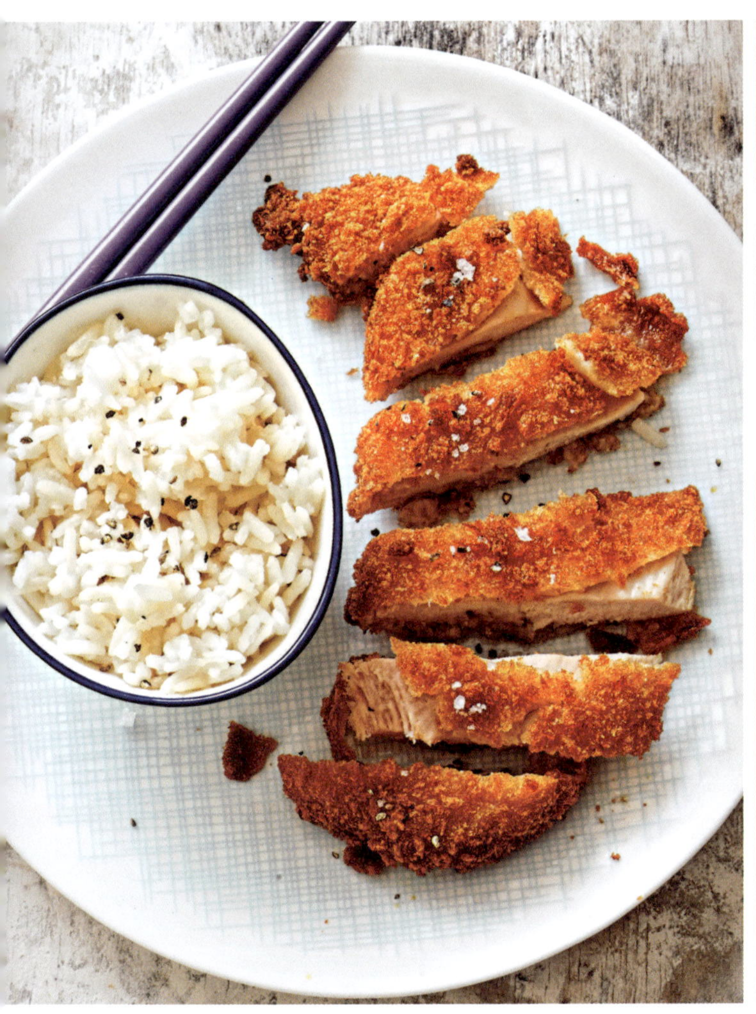

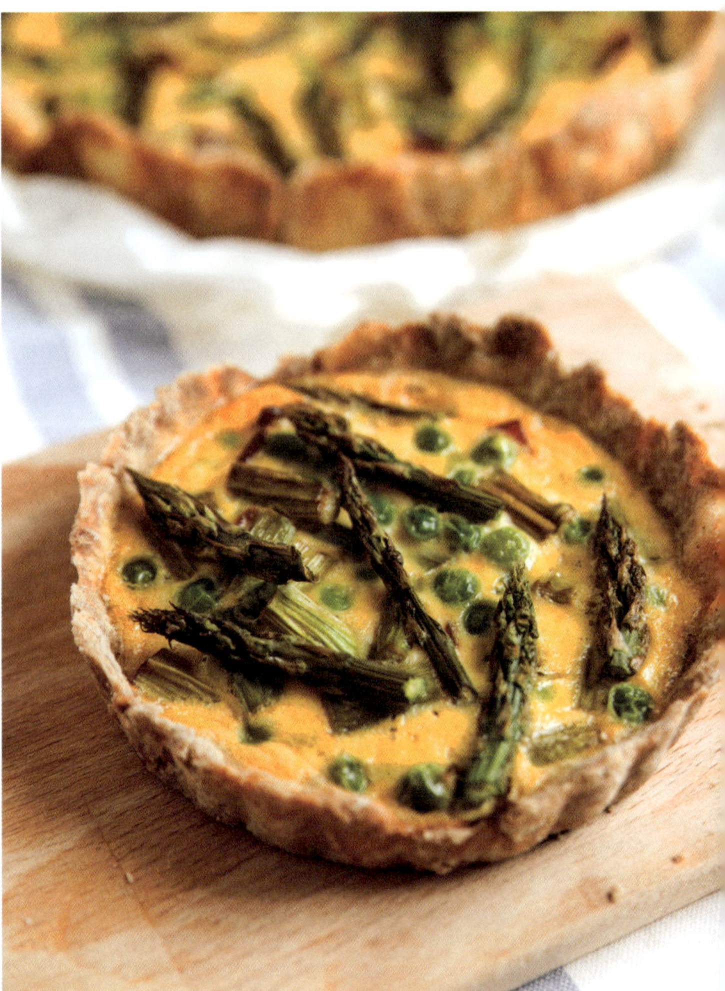

Chicken Katsu

SERVES 4

PREP + COOK TIME: 30 MINS

DAIRY FREE

Asparagus Pea Tarts

SERVES 4

PREP + COOK TIME: 20 MINS

VEG

CHICKEN KATSU

500g boneless, skinless chicken breast, sliced in half horizontally

Salt and pepper to taste

2 large eggs, beaten

1½ cups (185g) panko breadcrumbs

Steamed rice, to serve

Preheat air fryer to 175°C.

Lay chicken pieces on a clean work surface. Season with salt and pepper.

Place beaten eggs in a shallow dish. Pour breadcrumbs into a second shallow dish. Dredge chicken pieces in egg and then in breadcrumbs. Repeat by dredging chicken in egg and then breadcrumbs again, pressing down so that the breadcrumbs stick to the chicken.

Place chicken pieces in the air fryer basket. Spray the tops with cooking spray.

Cook for 10 minutes. Flip chicken pieces over and spray the tops with cooking spray. Cook for 8 minutes more. Transfer chicken to a chopping board and slice. Serve with steamed rice.

ASPARAGUS PEA TARTS

1 sheet frozen puff pastry

4 eggs

¾ cup (200ml) double cream

¼ cup (30g) finely grated Cheddar cheese

Salt and pepper to taste

1 bunch asparagus, cut into 5cm lengths

½ cup (80g) fresh or frozen peas

4 individual quiche dishes or ramekins

Lightly grease the quiche dishes or ramekins.

Lay pastry on a lightly floured work surface.

Cut around the quiche dishes on the pastry to create four pastry rounds. Line the base and sides of the quiche dishes with pastry.

In a medium jug whisk together eggs, cream and cheese. Season with salt and pepper.

Arrange asparagus and peas in the pastry cases and pour over egg mixture. Place quiche dishes in the air fryer and cook at 180°C for 12-15 minutes until the filling is set.

Serve warm or cold.

CRISPY TOFU

½ cup (60g) plain flour
2 eggs, beaten
1 tbsp water
450g semi-firm tofu, dried and cut into 3cm cubes
Salt to taste

Line air fryer basket with greaseproof paper and spray with cooking spray.

Place flour in one bowl, mix eggs and water in another.

Dip each piece of tofu into the flour and then the egg. Then repeat process to dip in the flour and egg once again.

Arrange tofu in air fryer basket. Spray with cooking spray and sprinkle with salt.

Cook at 190°C for 8 minutes, then gently remove the greaseproof paper from beneath the tofu and cook for a further 4 minutes.

CRISPY CHICKEN SALAD

1 egg, beaten
½ cup (60g) plain flour
1 cup (125g) panko breadcrumbs
2 chicken breasts, cut into strips
150g mixed salad leaves
½ cup (50g) shaved Parmesan

DRESSING

½ cup (120g) mayonnaise
½ clove garlic, finely minced
1 anchovy fillet
1 tbsp fresh lemon juice
1 tsp Dijon mustard
1 tsp Worcestershire sauce
¼ cup (25g) grated Parmesan
2 tbsps milk
Salt and pepper to taste

Preheat the air fryer to 200°C.

Place the egg, flour and panko in three separate shallow bowls.

Dredge the chicken strips through the flour mixture, then into the egg, then through the panko, pressing in firmly to ensure they are covered. Spray the chicken lightly with cooking spray.

Place the chicken into the air fryer basket. Cook in batches if needed. Cook for 20 minutes, turning halfway.

Whiz dressing ingredients in a food processor until smooth.

Place chicken and salad leaves in a large bowl. Drizzle with the dressing and top with shaved Parmesan.

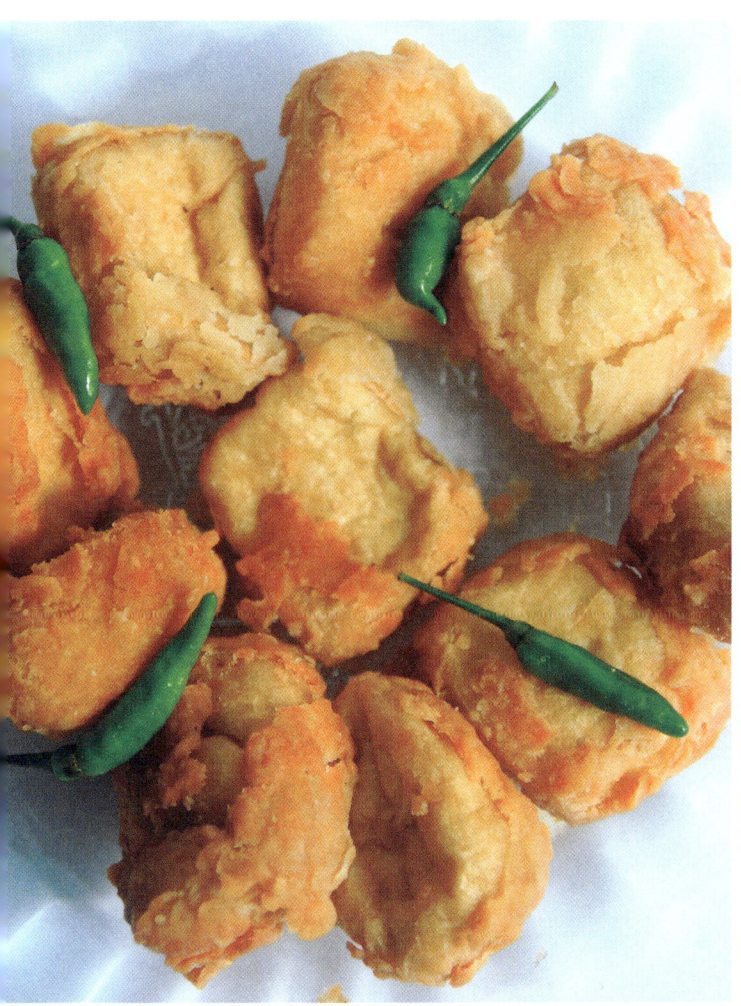

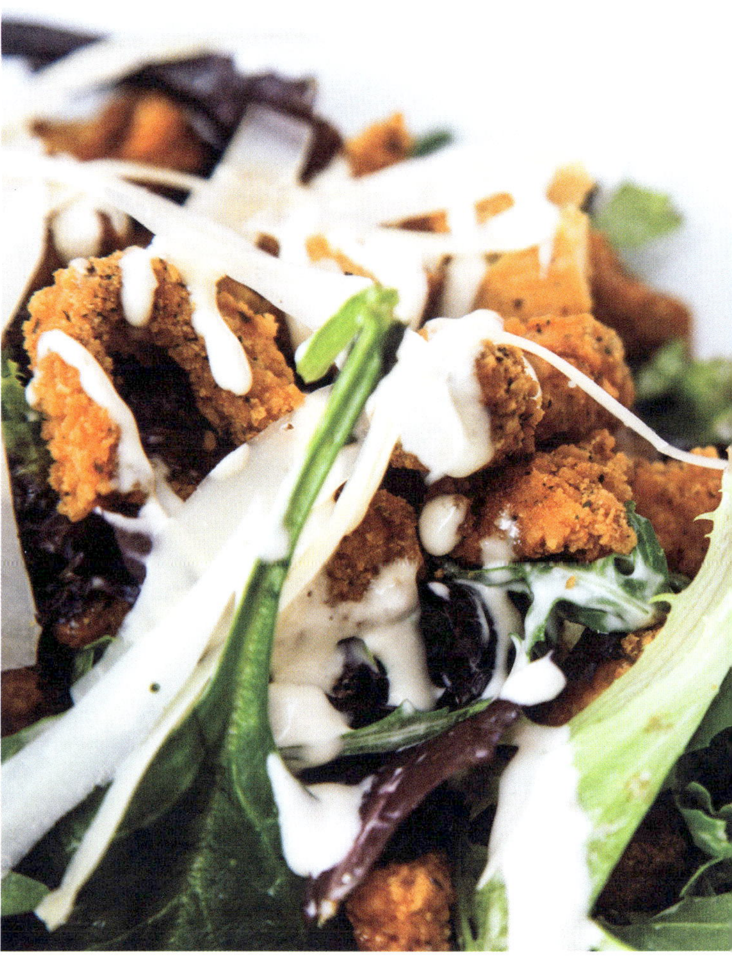

Crispy Tofu

SERVES 2

PREP + COOK TIME: 25 MINS

VEG • DAIRY FREE

Crispy Chicken Salad

SERVES 4

PREP + COOK TIME: 30 MINS

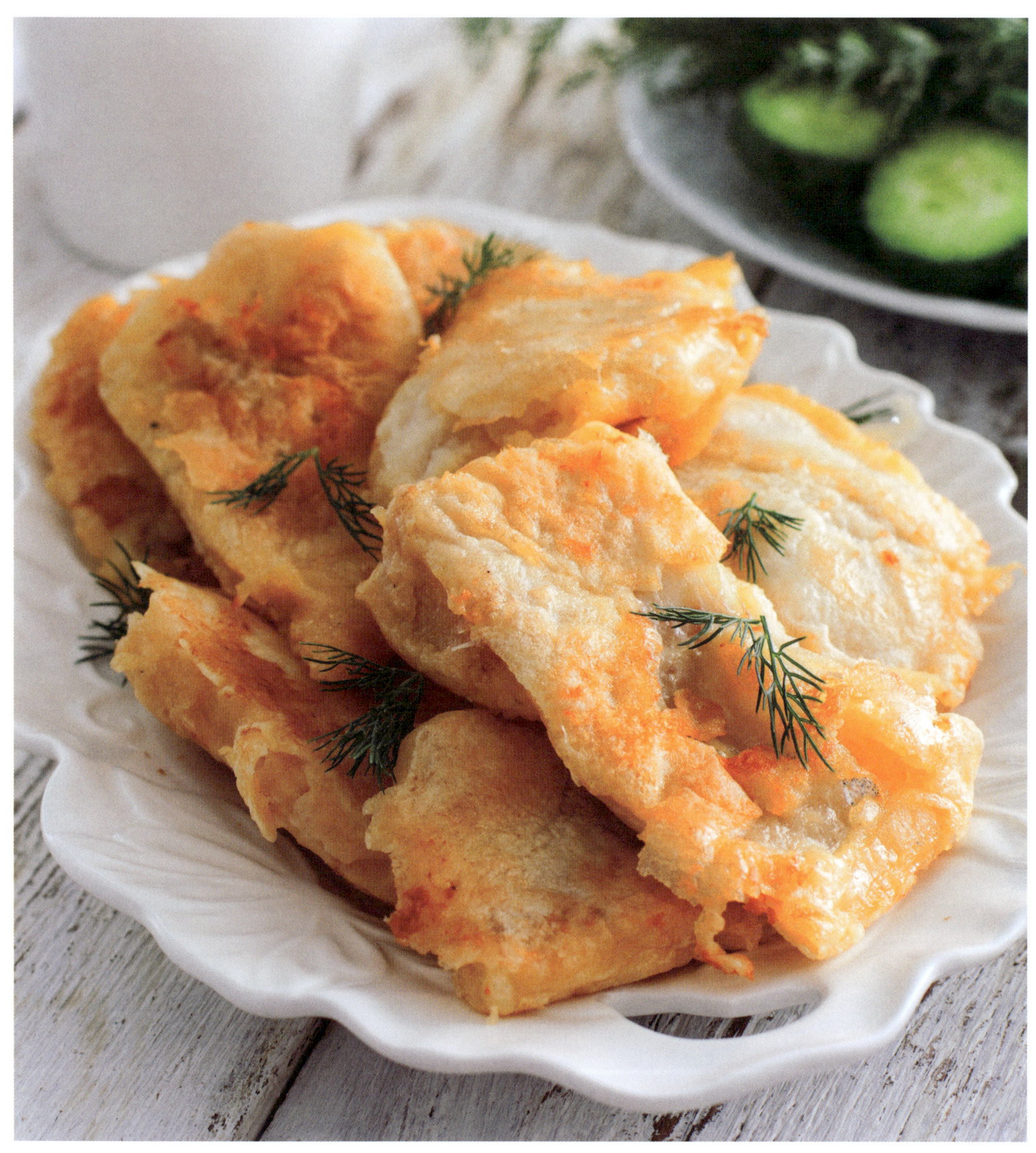

Beer-Battered Fish

SERVES 4

PREP + COOK TIME: 45 MINS

DAIRY FREE

BEER-BATTERED FISH

1¾ cups (215g) plain flour

2 tbsps cornflour

½ tsp bicarbonate of soda

¾ cup (180ml) beer

1 egg, beaten

½ tsp paprika

1 tsp salt

¼ tsp pepper

Pinch of cayenne pepper

700g cod or other firm white fish fillet, at least 3cm thick, cut into 4 pieces

Combine 1 cup flour, cornflour and bicarb in a large bowl. Add the beer and egg and whisk until smooth. Cover the bowl and refrigerate for at least 20 minutes.

Combine the remaining ¾ cup of flour, paprika, salt, pepper and cayenne pepper in a shallow dish.

Pat the fish fillets dry with a paper towel. Dip the fish first into the batter, coating all sides. Let the excess batter drip off and then coat each fillet with the seasoned flour. Sprinkle any leftover flour on the fish fillets and pat gently to coat.

Preheat the air fryer to 200°C.

Generously spray both sides of the fish fillets with cooking spray and place them in the air fryer basket. Air fry for 12 minutes, spraying once more with cooking spray halfway through cooking.

Serve hot.

Chicken Potato Salad

SERVES 2
PREP + COOK TIME: 45 MINS
GLUTEN FREE • DAIRY FREE

2 chicken breasts
4 tsps olive oil
Salt and pepper to taste
½ tsp garlic powder
1 tbsp thyme leaves
250g potatoes, sliced
100g baby spinach

DRESSING

1 tbsp finely diced shallot or white onion
1 tbsp lemon juice
2 tbsps olive oil

Brush the chicken breasts with 2 teaspoons of the olive oil. Sprinkle with salt, pepper, garlic powder and thyme leaves.

Place chicken in the air fryer basket. Cook at 180°C for 8 minutes. Then flip over and cook for another 8-10 minutes until cooked through. Remove from air fryer and wrap in foil to keep warm.

Toss potato slices with remaining olive oil, salt and pepper. Place potatoes in air fryer basket and cook for 12 minutes at 180°C. Shake air fryer basket then cook potatoes at 200°C for 5 minutes.

Slice chicken and serve in bowls with potatoes and spinach. Combine dressing ingredients and pour over chicken to serve.

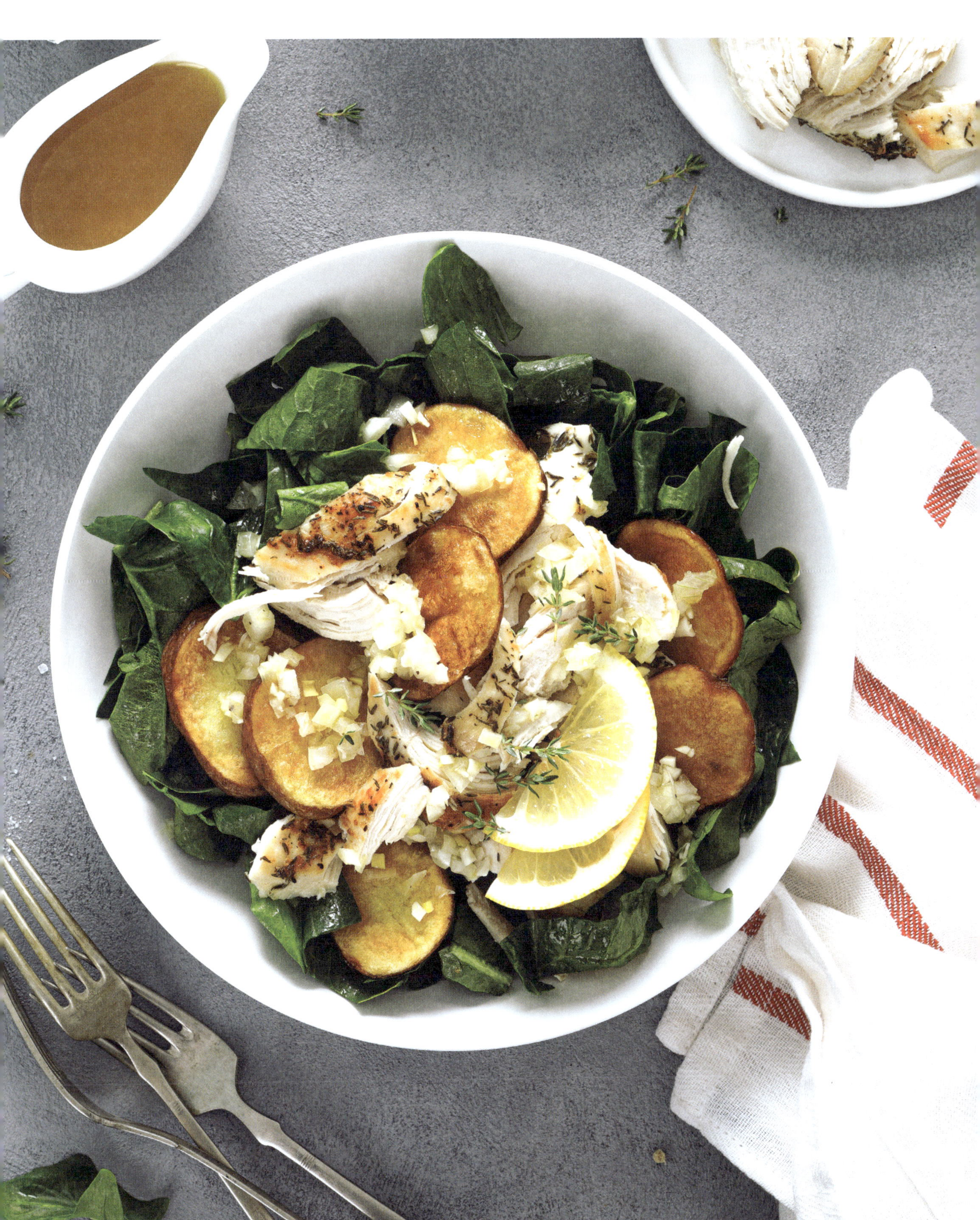

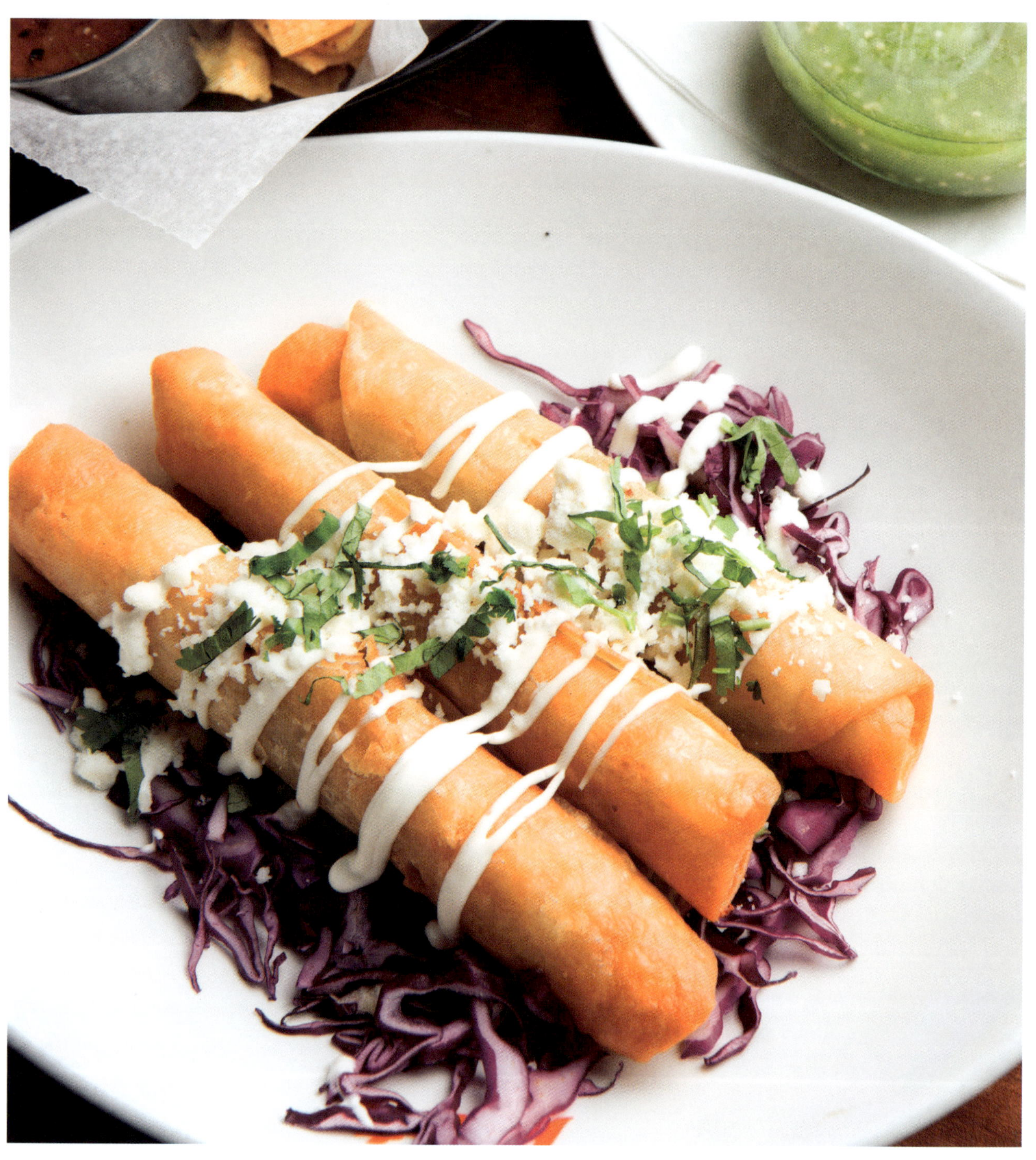

Chicken Taquitos

SERVES 4

PREP + COOK TIME: 35 MINS

GLUTEN FREE

CHICKEN TAQUITOS

1 tbsp olive oil

½ onion, diced

2 cloves garlic, minced

1 tbsp dried oregano

1 tsp ground cumin

½ tsp smoked paprika

600g cooked chicken, shredded

¼ cup (60g) passata

Salt and pepper to taste

12 corn tortillas

½ cup (60g) grated Cheddar cheese

½ cup (25g) red cabbage, finely sliced, to serve

2 tbsps sour cream, to serve

1 tbsp fresh coriander, chopped, to serve

Heat the oil in a large frying pan over medium-high heat. Add the onion and fry for 3-5 minutes until soft and translucent. Add the garlic, oregano, cumin and paprika. Fry for 1 minute until fragrant. Add the chicken and passata. Season with salt and pepper and cook for 2-3 minutes until chicken is heated through.

Spoon small amounts of chicken mix along the centre of the tortillas. Top with cheese and roll into taquitos. Secure with a toothpick. Repeat with the remaining tortillas.

Preheat air fryer to 200°C. Spray the basket with cooking spray.

Place four taquitos at a time into the air fryer basket. Spray with cooking spray. Cook for 5-6 minutes until golden brown and crispy. Repeat with the remaining taquitos.

Remove toothpicks and place cooked taquitos on a bed of shredded cabbage, drizzle with sour cream and sprinkle with chopped coriander to serve.

BEEF KOFTE

1 tbsp oil

500g beef mince

4 tbsps parsley, chopped

2 cloves garlic, minced

1 tbsp all-purpose seasoning

1 tsp salt

Skewer rack

Combine all the ingredients in a large mixing bowl. Cover and transfer to the fridge to chill for 30 minutes (or longer if convenient).

Form the kebabs into sausage shapes using your hands. When roughly done insert a skewer in the centre and then gently roll to reshape if needed.

Place kebabs on the skewer rack and spritz with olive oil.

Preheat the air fryer to 190°C. Cook for 10 minutes or to an internal temperature of 71°C with a thermometer.

BAKED SWEET POTATOES

3 sweet potatoes

1 tbsp olive oil

1 tsp salt

3 tbsps sour cream

1 tbsp fresh chives, chopped

Scrub potatoes and pat dry with paper towels. Prick a few times with a fork. Sprinkle with olive oil and salt, and rub evenly into the potato skin.

Preheat the air fryer to 200°C.

Place potatoes into the air fryer basket. Cook for 40 minutes until tender.

Serve with sour cream and chives on top.

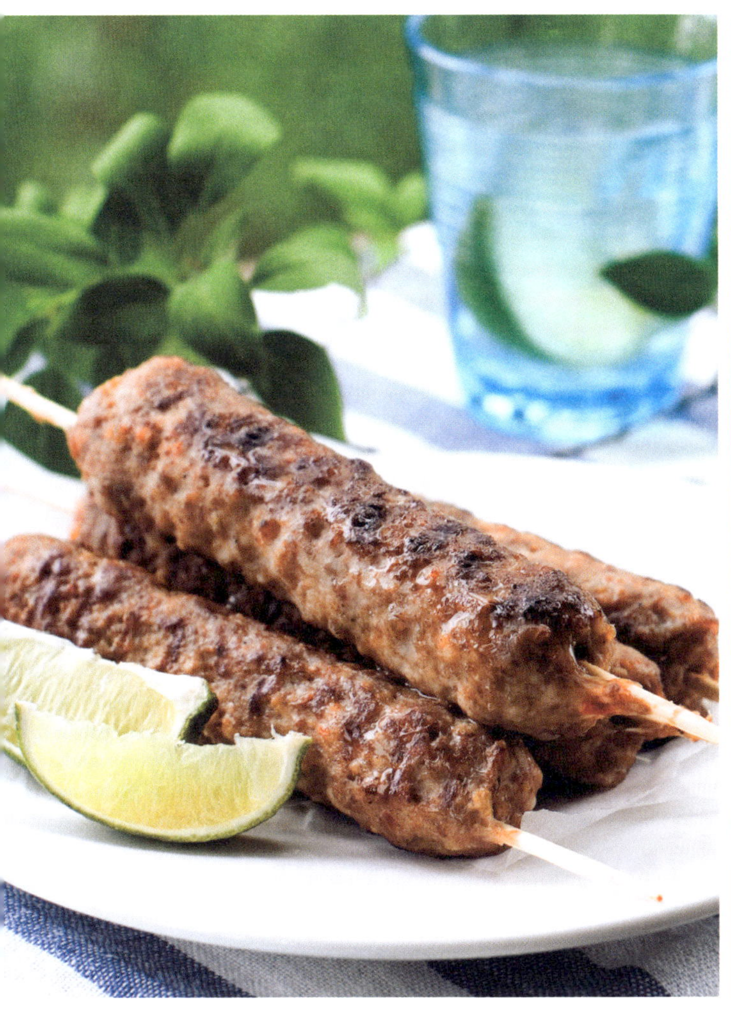

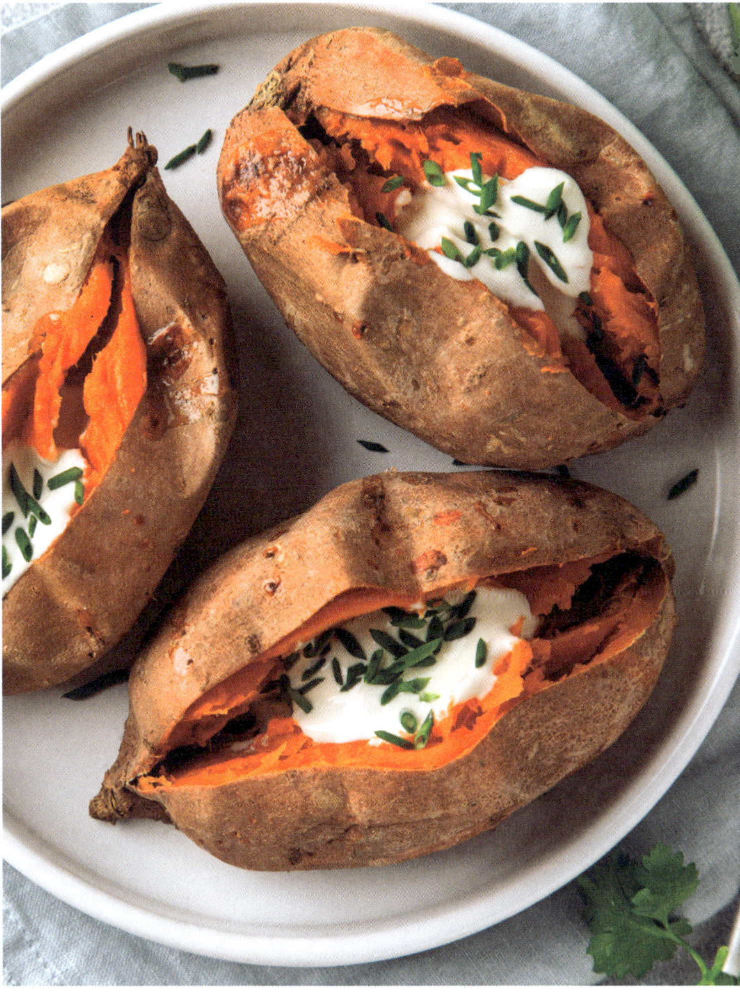

Beef Kofte

SERVES 4

PREP + COOK TIME: 20 MINS + CHILLING

GLUTEN FREE • DAIRY FREE

Baked Sweet Potatoes

SERVES 3

PREP + COOK TIME: 45 MINS

VEG • GLUTEN FREE

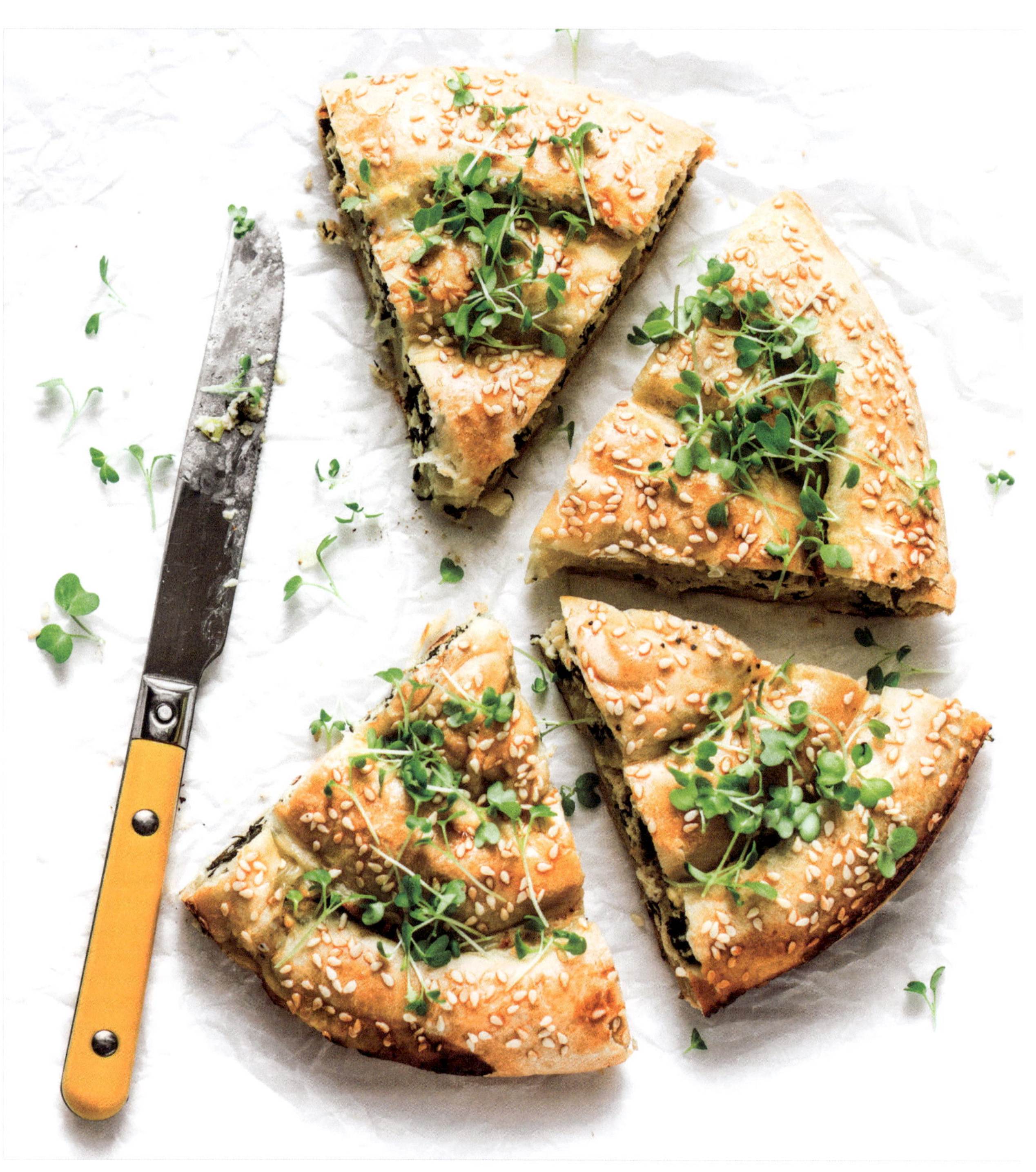

Spanakopita

SERVES 4

PREP + COOK TIME: 50 MINS

VEG

SPANAKOPITA

250g spinach

6 tbsps olive oil

1 small onion, finely chopped

3 spring onions, thinly sliced

2 cloves garlic, thinly sliced

100g cream cheese

1 small egg

Pinch of nutmeg

1 tbsp fresh dill leaves

½ cup (10g) mint leaves, roughly chopped

Zest of ½ lemon zest

Salt and pepper to taste

100g feta

3 sheets filo pastry

1 tsp sesame seeds

Baking tin

Place spinach in a large colander over a sink. Boil a kettle full of water and slowly pour over the spinach. Leave to cool. When cool enough to handle, squeeze out excess moisture. Transfer the spinach to a chopping board and roughly chop.

Heat 2 tablespoons of oil in a large pan over medium heat. Add onion, spring onion and garlic and cook, stirring regularly, for 5-7 minutes, until onion is soft and translucent. Add the spinach and cook for another minute. Remove from the heat and set aside to cool.

In a separate large bowl, mix together cream cheese, egg, nutmeg, dill, mint, lemon zest and salt and pepper. Add the cooled spinach and mix to combine. Crumble in the feta and carefully fold through.

Grease a round baking tin that fits in your air fryer. Preheat air fryer to 160°C.

Remove one sheet of filo pastry and lay it out on a clean work surface with the long end in front of you. Keep the remaining filo sheets rolled up and cover them with a damp tea towel.

Brush your first filo sheet with olive oil. Take a third of the spinach mixture and spread it out along the long end of the filo pastry sheet in a 2cm-thick sausage. Leave 1-2cm at each end with no filling. Roll the filo pastry sheet tightly around the filling and continue rolling until you get to the end. Coil the tube up to make a tight spiral and place it in the middle of your baking tin. This is your first coil which is the start of your spiral. The other coils move out from that first one. Repeat the process with the remaining sheets of filo pastry and spinach filling, working out from your first coil until the dish is full. Brush the top with olive oil and sprinkle with sesame seeds.

Cook for 15-20 minutes until golden brown and crisp.

CHICKEN DRUMSTICKS

1 tsp salt
½ tsp pepper
1 tsp garlic powder
1½ tsps smoked paprika
¼ tsp chilli powder
1 tsp onion powder
8 chicken drumsticks
2 tbsps olive oil
Chopped spring onion, to serve

Preheat air fryer to 200°C.

In a small bowl combine all the spices and herbs, set mixture aside.

Place chicken in a large bowl. Add olive oil and toss to coat.

Add spice mixture to bowl and toss to coat.

Place chicken drumsticks in air fryer basket and cook for 10 minutes.

Flip chicken drumsticks over and cook for an additional 10 minutes until cooked through.

Scatter with spring onion to serve.

SPINACH & CHEESE ROLLS

2 cups (500g) ricotta
¾ cup (75g) finely grated Parmesan cheese
250g feta, broken into small pieces
125g baby spinach, finely chopped
1 tsp nutmeg
Salt and pepper to taste
1 egg
4 sheets filo pastry
2-4 tbsps olive oil

Preheat the air fryer to 180°C.

Place all ingredients except the beaten egg and the pastry into a large bowl and mix until combined.

Cut pastry sheets in half lengthways. Brush one half sheet with olive oil, then add a spoonful of mixture in a line along one of the short edges. Roll up the pastry and brush the outside with olive oil. Repeat process until all the pastry and mixture have been used up.

Place the rolls into the air fryer basket.

Cook for 12 minutes until golden.

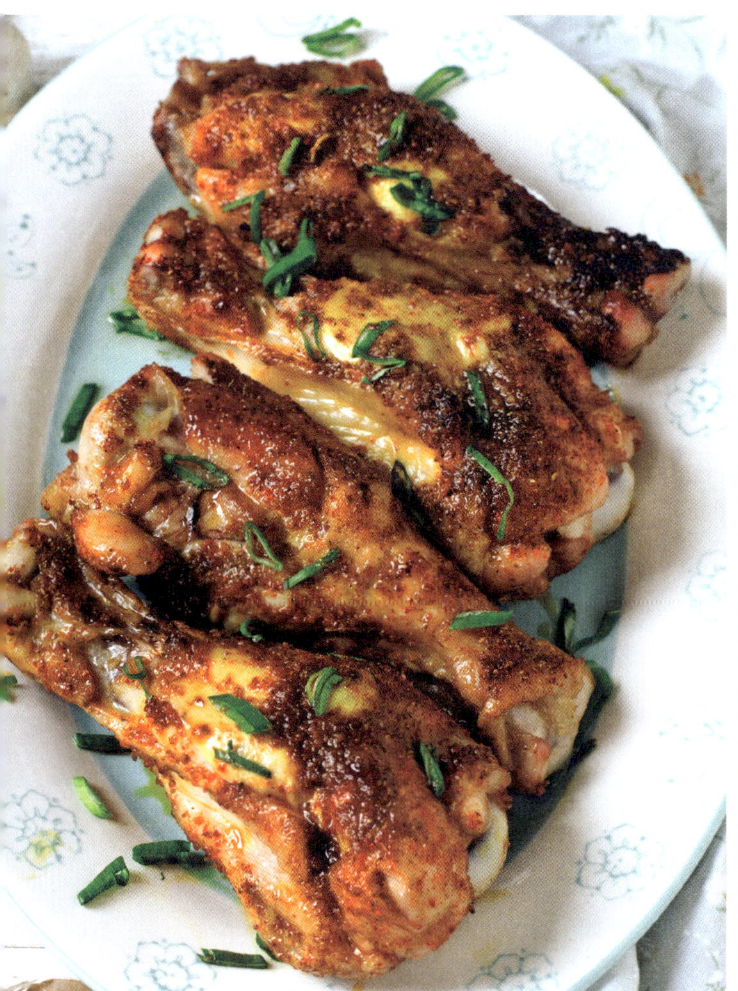

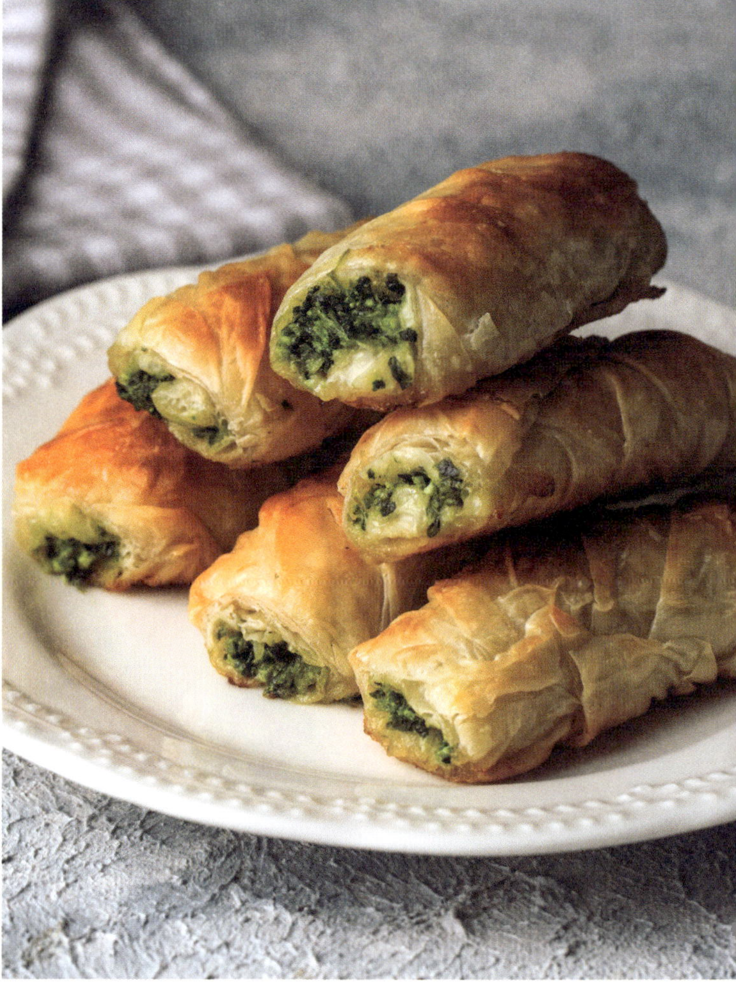

Chicken Drumsticks

SERVES 4

PREP + COOK TIME: 25 MINS

GLUTEN FREE • DAIRY FREE

Spinach & Cheese Rolls

SERVES 4

PREP + COOK TIME: 25 MINS

VEG

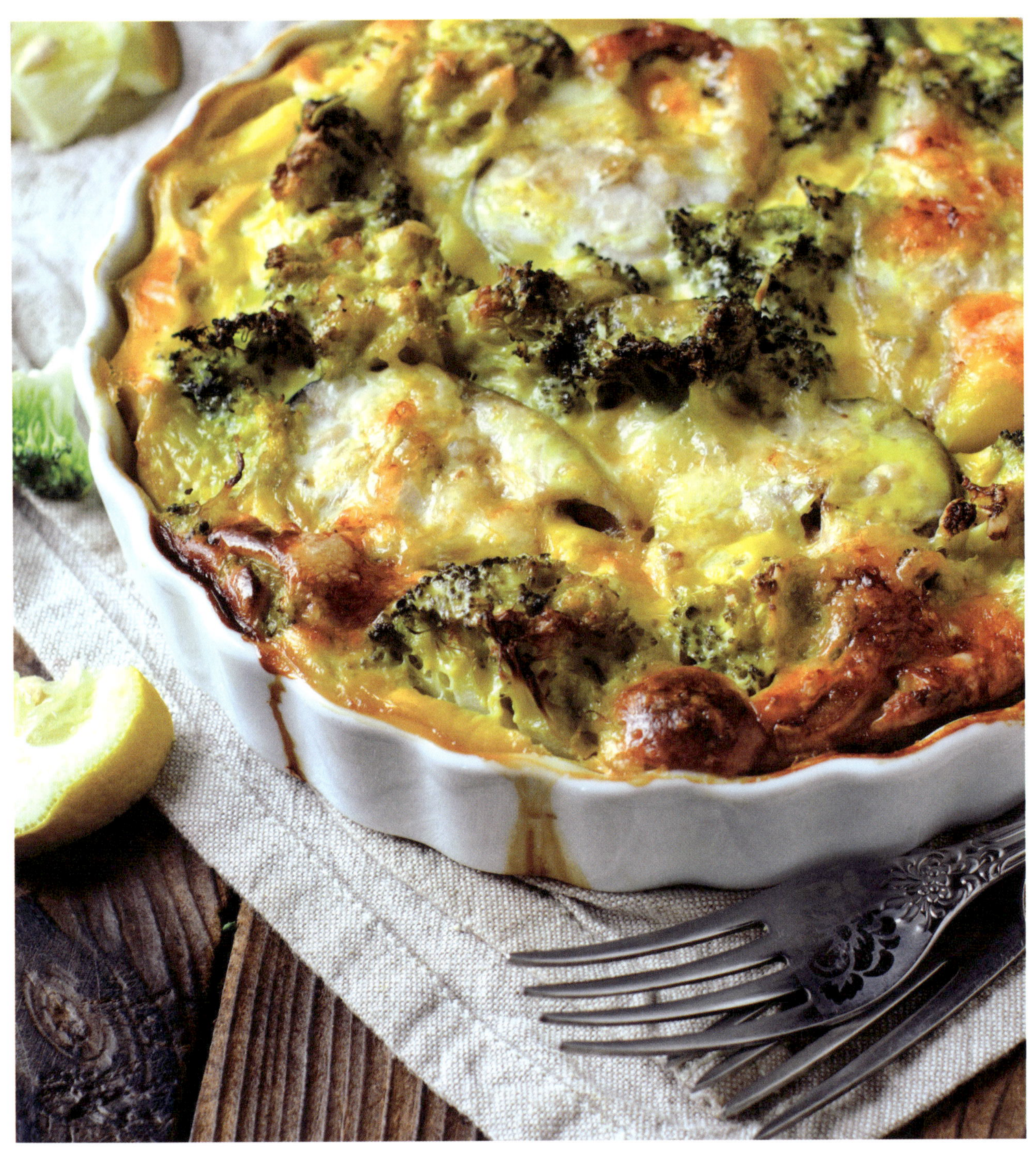

Broccoli & Salmon Casserole

SERVES 4

PREP + COOK TIME: 40 MINS

GLUTEN FREE

BROCCOLI & SALMON CASSEROLE

2 x 150g salmon fillets
2 tsps olive oil
Salt and pepper to taste
450g fresh broccoli florets
¼ cup (60ml) water
250g cream cheese, room temperature
¼ cup (60ml) sour cream
1½ cups (185g) grated Cheddar cheese
Baking dish

Preheat the air fryer to 190°C. Spray the baking dish with cooking spray.

Rub the salmon fillets with olive oil and season with salt and pepper. Add the salmon fillets to the air fryer and cook for 6 minutes until just cooked through. Set aside for 5 minutes, then cut into 2cm chunks.

Add the broccoli and the water to a large microwave-safe bowl. Cover tightly with plastic wrap and microwave for 5 minutes. Let stand, covered, for 3 minutes. Carefully remove the plastic wrap and drain the liquid.

Add the salmon, cream cheese, sour cream and 1 cup Cheddar to the bowl with the broccoli. Season with salt and pepper. Stir gently to combine. Pour broccoli mixture into the prepared baking dish. Cover with foil.

Air fry at 180°C for 10 minutes. Remove the foil and top the casserole with the remaining cheese.

Return the pan to the air fryer and cook, uncovered, for 5 minutes.

Zucchini & Capsicum Pizza

SERVES 2

PREP + COOK TIME: 40 MINS + 1 HOUR PROVING

VEG

2 cups (250g) baker's (or plain) flour
1 x 7g sachet dry active yeast
1 tsp caster sugar
1 tsp salt
¾ cup (200ml) warm water
1 tbsp olive oil

TOPPING

2 tbsps olive oil
2 cloves garlic, minced
¾ cup (175g) passata
2 tsps dried oregano
Salt and pepper to taste
1 zucchini, thinly sliced
1 orange capsicum, cut into chunks
½ red onion, sliced
150g fresh mozzarella, sliced
1 tbsp fresh rosemary leaves
1 tsp dried parsley
½ tsp dried chilli flakes

Sift flour into a large bowl. Stir in yeast, sugar and salt. Make a well in the centre and pour in water and oil. Bring the dough together with your hands, then turn out onto a lightly floured surface. Knead for 5 minutes until the dough is smooth. Place the dough in a lightly greased bowl. Cover and set aside in a warm place to prove for 1 hour, until doubled in size.

Meanwhile heat 1 tablespoon oil in a small pan over medium heat. Add garlic and cook for 1 minute until fragrant. Add passata and 1 teaspoon dried oregano. Season with salt and pepper. Simmer for 10 minutes until thick. Set aside.

Knock back the dough by punching it to remove air and divide into two balls.

Preheat air fryer to 190°C. Spray air fryer basket with cooking spray.

Roll out one ball of pizza dough. Carefully transfer to air fryer and brush with olive oil. Spread with sauce. Top with half the zucchini, capsicum, red onion and mozzarella. Scatter with half the remaining oregano, rosemary, parsley and chilli flakes.

Air fry for 7 minutes until crust is crispy and cheese is melted. Season with salt and pepper.

Repeat with remaining ball of pizza dough.

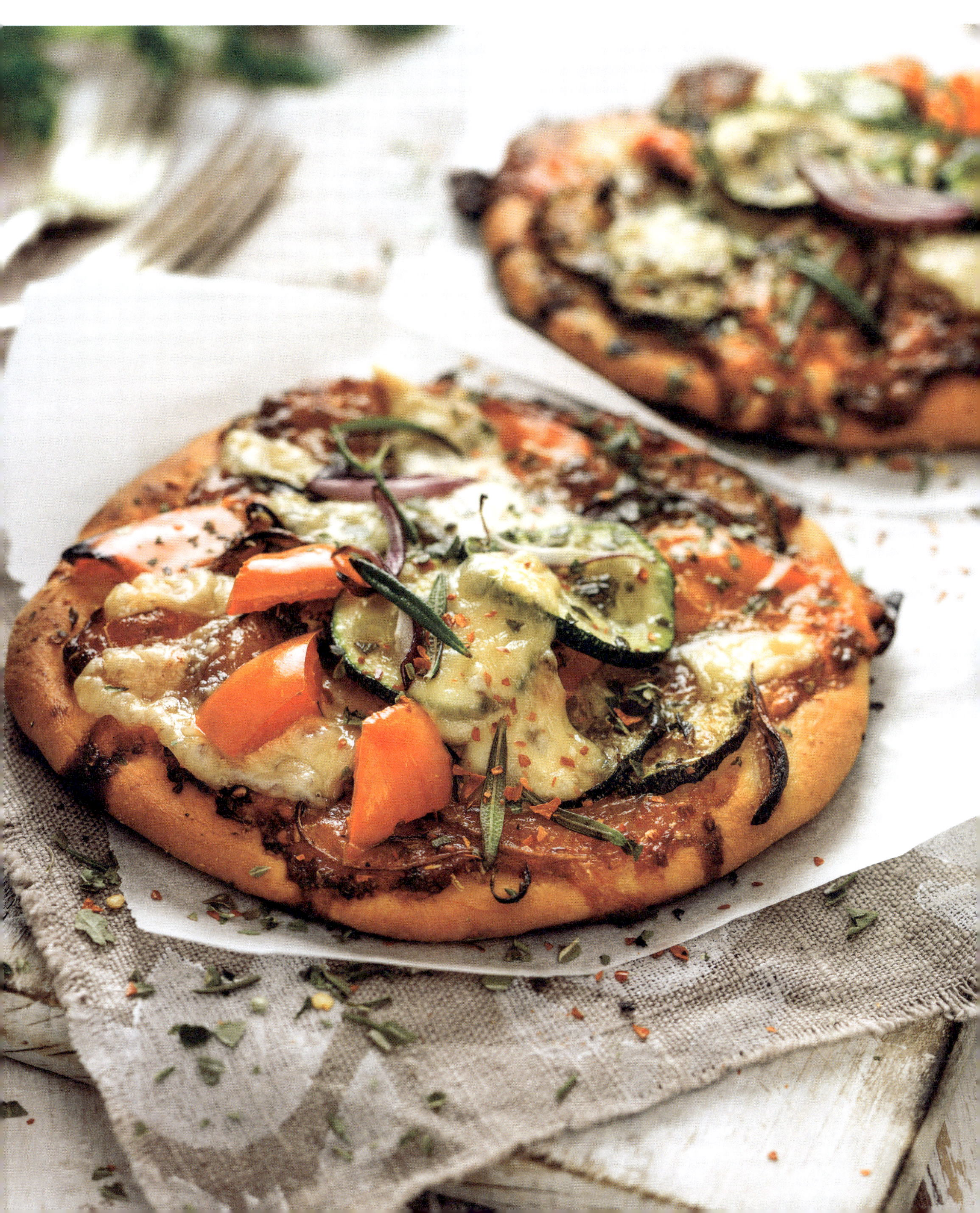

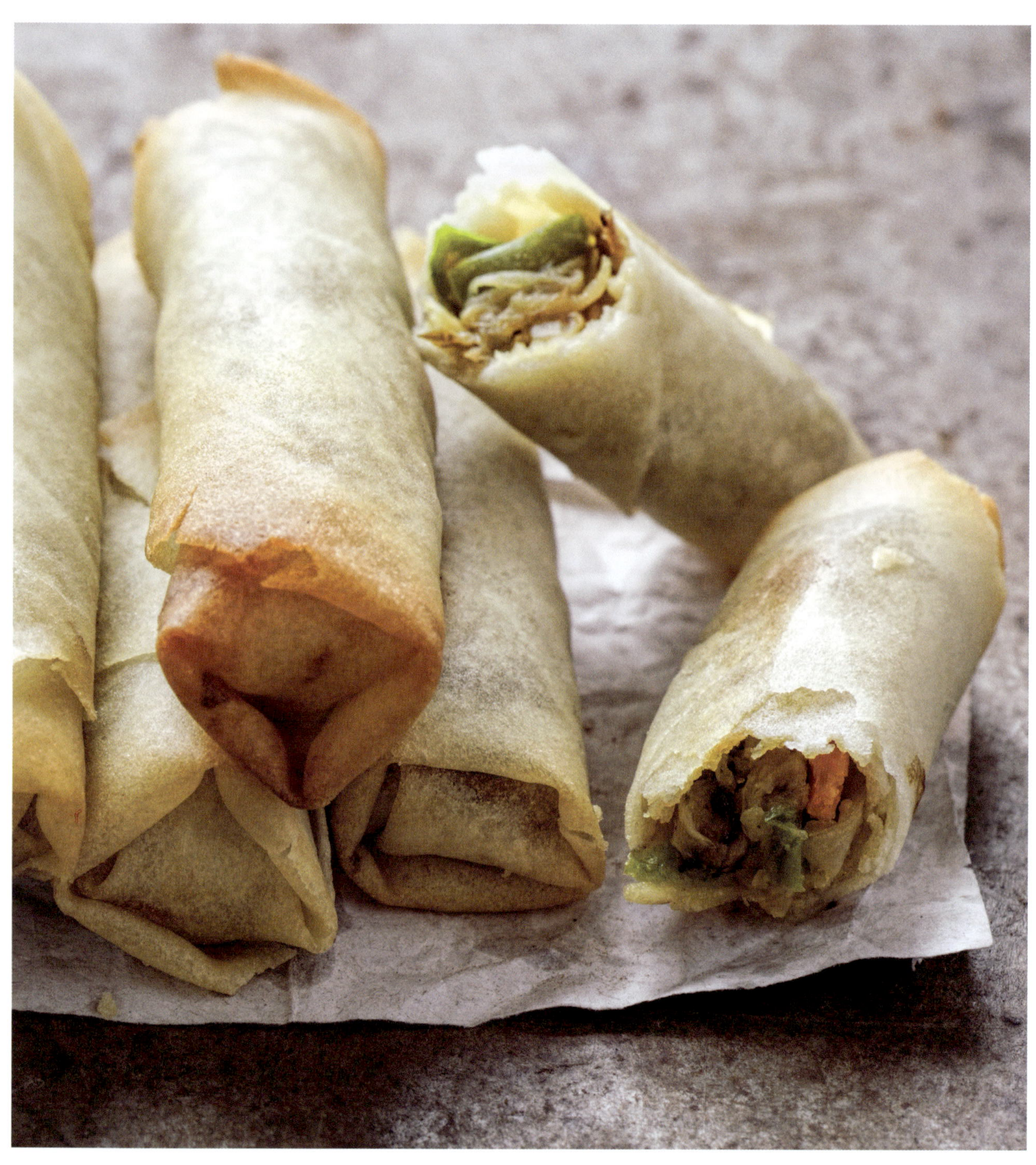

Spring Rolls

SERVES 12

PREP + COOK TIME: 30 MINS

SPRING ROLLS

2 tbsps sesame oil

1 clove garlic, minced

250g pork mince

2 cups (200g) shredded cabbage

2 carrots, cut into matchsticks

½ cup (75g) thinly sliced bamboo shoots

1 tbsp fresh lime juice

3 tsps fish sauce

2 tsps soy sauce

12 square spring roll wrappers

Preheat air fryer to 200°C.

Heat sesame oil in a frying pan over medium-high heat and cook garlic for 30 seconds until fragrant. Add pork and cook for 2-3 minutes until browned. Add cabbage, carrots and bamboo shoots and cook, stirring, for 5 minutes until tender. Remove pan from heat and stir in lime juice, fish sauce and soy sauce.

Place some of the vegetable mixture in one corner of one wrapper, just below the centre. Fold the bottom point over the filling and tuck under. Fold in both sides and roll up tightly. Use water to seal the wrapper. Repeat with remaining vegetable mixture and wrappers.

Spray air fryer basket with cooking spray. Place spring rolls into the basket, working in batches as needed, and spray rolls with cooking spray.

Cook spring rolls in air fryer for 5 minutes; turn over and cook for a further 5 minutes, until evenly browned.

Eggplant Schnitzel

SERVES 2

PREP + COOK TIME: 30 MINS + DRAINING

VEG

1 eggplant

1 tsp salt

1 cup (125g) breadcrumbs

1 tsp Italian herbs

¼ cup (60ml) olive oil

2 eggs

½ cup (60g) plain flour

Slices the eggplant lengthwise into four or five even slices. Place the eggplant in a colander over a bowl and sprinkle with the salt. Allow to drain for 45 minutes. Discard water in the bowl.

Combine the breadcrumbs, herbs and olive oil together in a shallow bowl.

Beat the eggs in a shallow bowl.

Place the flour in a shallow bowl.

Dip the eggplant slices first in the flour and then in the egg mixture, shaking off any excess.

Then dip into the breadcrumb mixture, pressing in to ensure they are evenly covered.

Preheat the air fryer to 200°C.

Place a single layer of breaded eggplant into the basket of the air fryer and cook for 14 minutes, turning halfway during cooking.

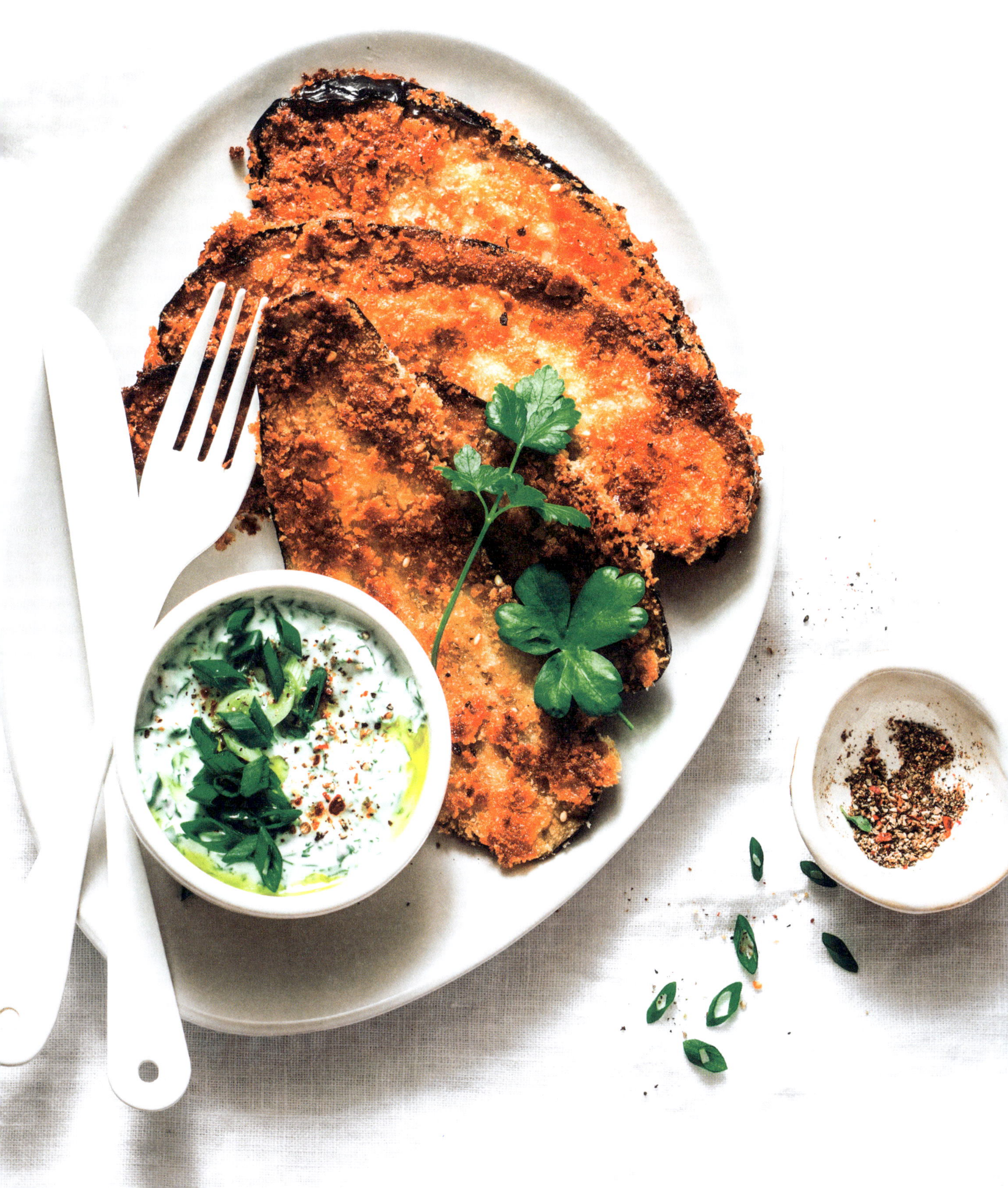

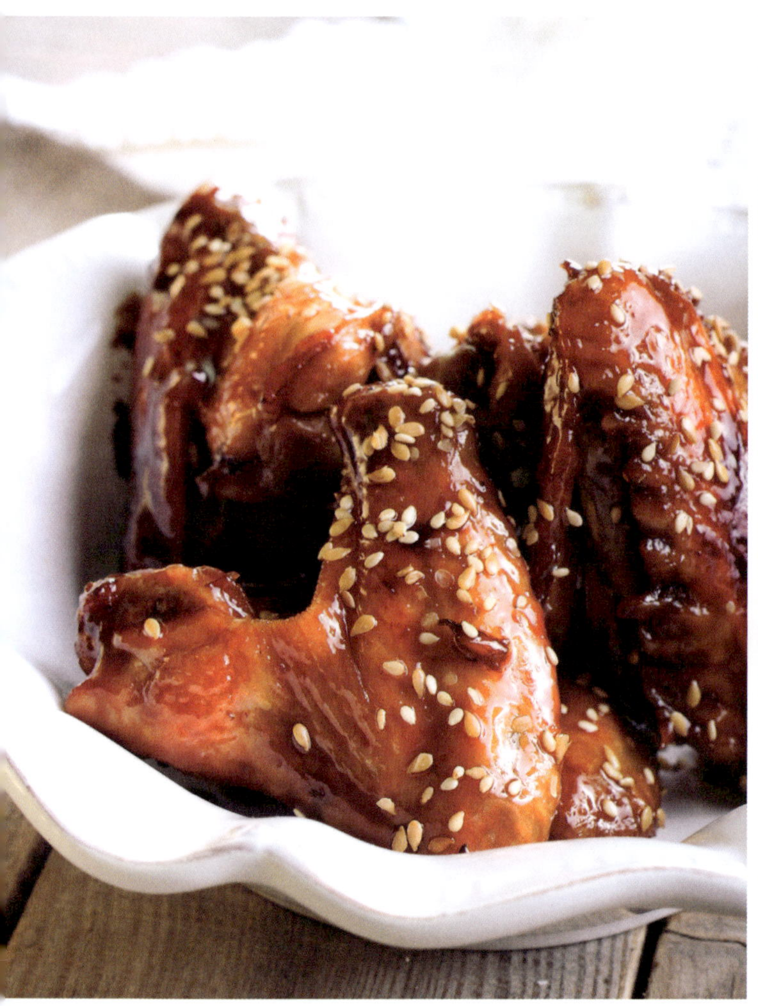

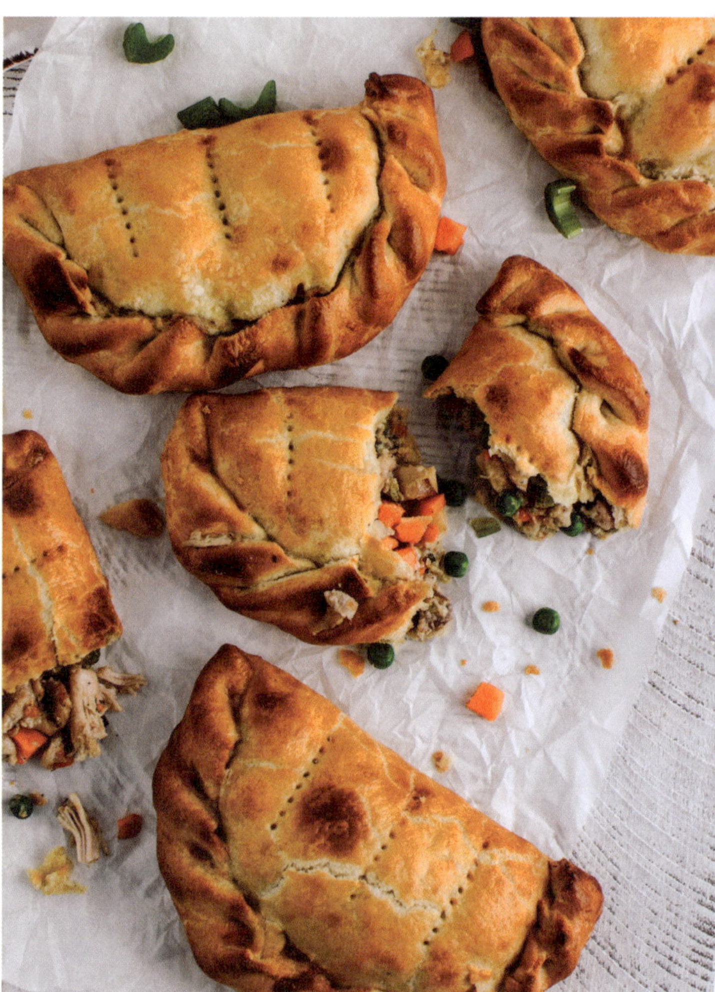

Sticky Wings

SERVES 2

PREP + COOK TIME: 25 MINS + 30 MINS MARINATING

GLUTEN FREE

Chicken & Vegetable Pies

SERVES 4

PREP + COOK TIME: 25 MINS

STICKY WINGS

2 cloves garlic, chopped

Small piece ginger, minced

2 tbsps honey

1 tbsp tamari

1 tbsp rice wine vinegar

2 tsps sesame oil

1 tsp Sriracha

6 chicken wings

1 tbsp toasted sesame seeds

Combine first seven ingredients in a large bowl and stir.

Add the chicken and toss to coat. Cover and place in the fridge for at least 30 minutes.

Air fry the wings at 190°C for 20 minutes, turning every 5 minutes.

Sprinkle over sesame seeds to serve.

CHICKEN & VEGETABLE PIES

1 tbsp olive oil

1 onion, finely chopped

2 stalks celery, finely chopped

1 carrot, finely diced

2 cloves garlic, minced

1½ cups (190g) diced cooked chicken

1 cup (170g) frozen peas

2 tsps Dijon mustard

½ cup (125ml) sour cream

¼ cup (30g) grated Cheddar cheese

4 sheets frozen shortcrust pastry, thawed

1 egg, beaten lightly

Heat oil in a large frying pan over medium-high heat. Add onion, celery and carrot and cook, stirring, for 3-5 minutes until the onion is soft and translucent. Add garlic and cook for 1 minute until fragrant. Add chicken, peas, mustard, sour cream and cheese and stir until heated through.

Cut one 22cm circle from each pastry sheet. Spoon a quarter of the filling in the centre of each circle. Brush the edge of the pastry with beaten egg. Fold the pastry over to enclose the filling, then fold the curved edges back and crimp and press with your thumb to seal. Brush pasties with remaining egg and prick a few holes in the top with a fork.

Preheat air fryer to 190°C.

Place pasties in air fryer basket and cook for 10 minutes until golden brown and crisp.

NACHOS

1 ripe avocado

½ clove garlic, crushed

Pinch of salt

Juice of ½ lime

2 cups (55g) corn chips

1 cup (245g) chilli con carne, warmed (see recipe page 233)

1 cup (125g) grated Cheddar cheese

½ red chilli, sliced

2 tbsps fresh coriander leaves

Use a fork to mash avocado in a small bowl with garlic, salt and lime juice. Mix well and set aside.

Line base and two sides of air fryer basket with aluminium foil. Preheat air fryer to 190°C.

Place corn chips in basket, spoon over chilli con carne and sprinkle with cheese. Cook for 1-2 minutes, until cheese is just melted.

Remove nachos from the air fryer and top with avocado, chilli slices and fresh coriander. Serve immediately.

ASPARAGUS PARCELS

1 bunch asparagus (about 450g), ends trimmed

1 tbsp olive oil

Salt and pepper to taste

3 sheets frozen puff pastry, thawed

250g soft goat's cheese, sliced into 3mm slices

1 egg, beaten

Toss asparagus in olive oil and season with salt and pepper.

Cut each sheet of pastry into four squares.

Place two or three stalks of asparagus diagonally across each pastry square. Top the asparagus with slices of goat's cheese.

Lift two opposite corners of the puff pastry squares and wrap them around the asparagus and press to seal.

Brush pastry with beaten egg.

Air fry in batches at 160°C for 8-10 minutes.

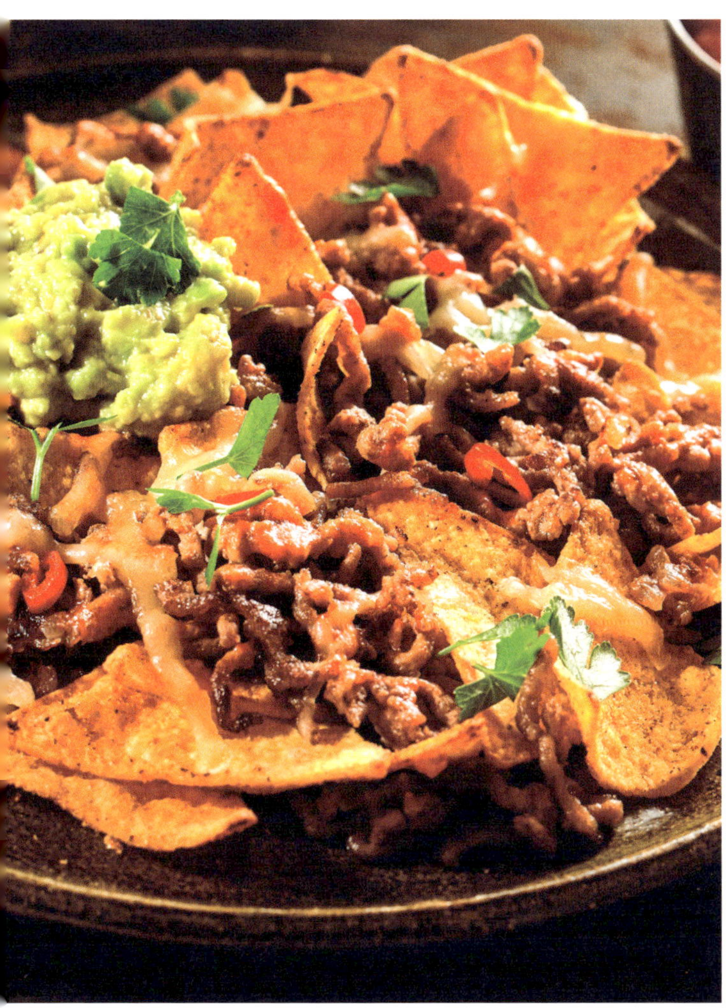

Nachos

SERVES 4

PREP + COOK TIME: 10 MINS

GLUTEN FREE

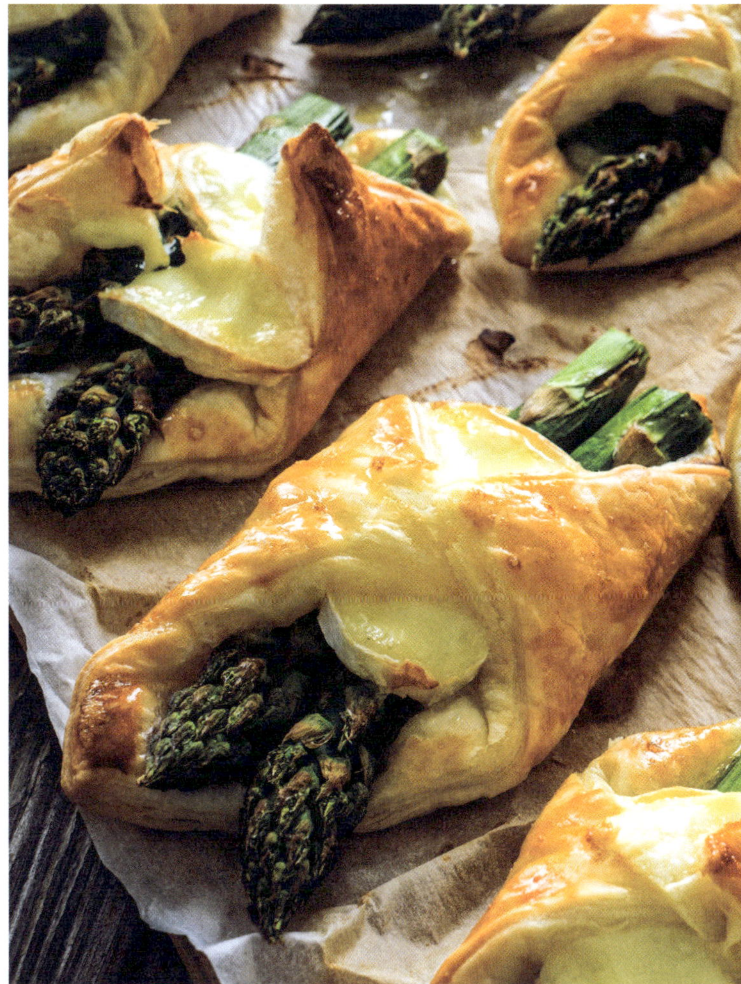

Asparagus Parcels

SERVES 12

PREP + COOK TIME: 20 MINS

VEG

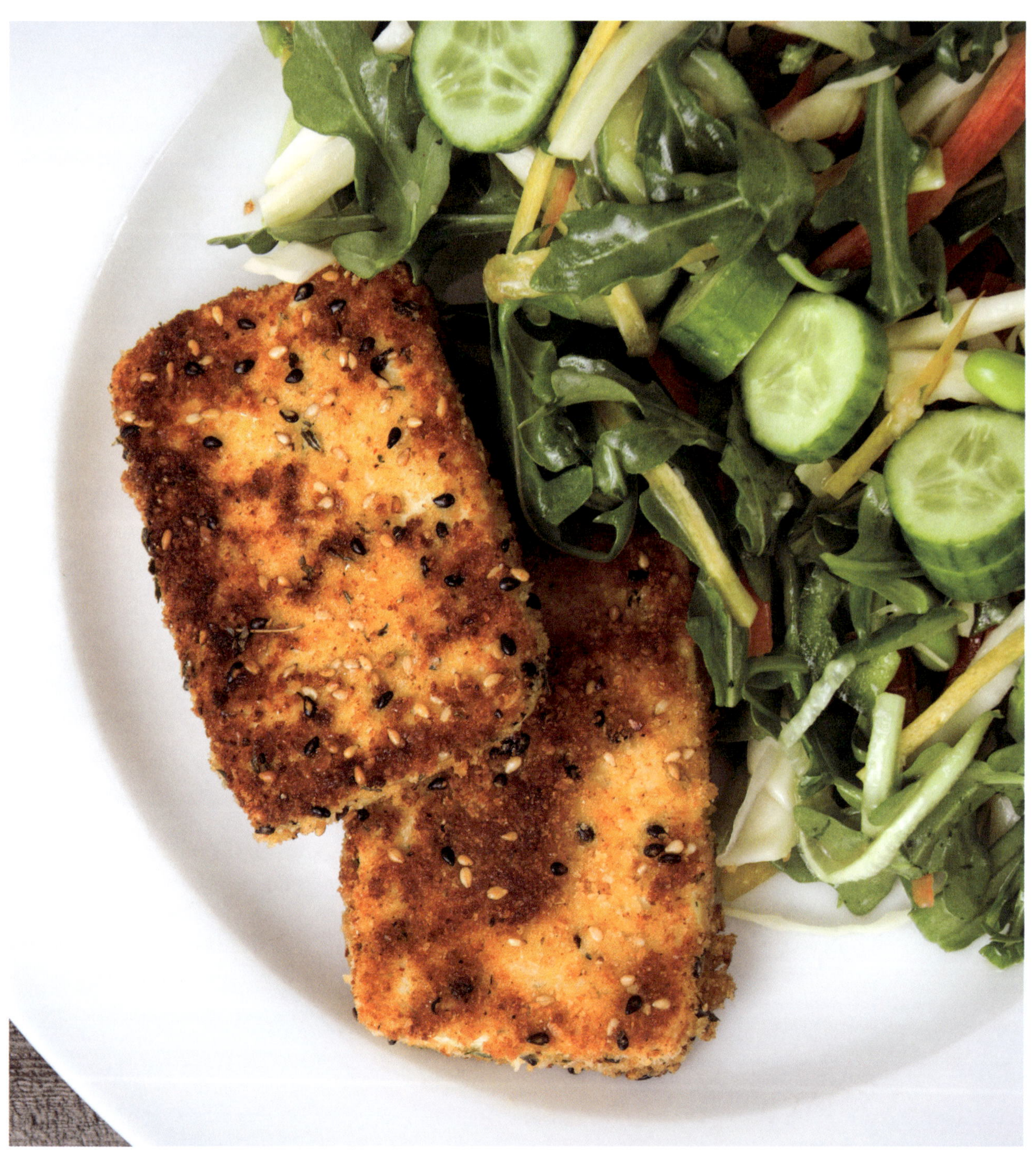

Crumbed Tofu

SERVES 2

PREP + COOK TIME: 30 MINS

VEG • GLUTEN FREE

CRUMBED TOFU

¾ cup (90g) gluten-free breadcrumbs

1 tbsp black and white sesame seeds

2 tsps garlic powder

½ tsp salt

225g firm tofu

Green salad to serve (optional)

Preheat air fryer to 180°C.

Combine breadcrumbs, sesame seeds, garlic powder and salt in a shallow dish. Slice tofu into rectangular pieces approximately 1cm in thickness. Dip each piece of tofu into the crumb mix, pressing down so the crumb sticks. Turn to coat all sides.

Lightly spray the tofu with cooking spray and place in a single layer in the air fryer basket. Work in batches or use a double-layer accessory if needed.

Cook for 12-13 minutes until tops are golden brown. Flip the tofu and spray once more with cooking spray. Cook for a further 7-8 minutes until golden brown.

Serve with green salad, if desired.

Parmesan Chicken Wings

SERVES 4
PREP + COOK TIME: 35 MINS
GLUTEN FREE

1kg chicken wings

2 tbsps olive oil

Salt and pepper to taste

2 tsps garlic powder

¼ tsp dried chilli flakes

¼ cup (10g) chopped parsley

½ cup (60g) finely grated Parmesan cheese

Ranch or other dipping sauce to serve (optional)

In a large bowl, drizzle wings with oil, then season generously with salt and pepper. Add garlic powder, chilli flakes, parsley and half the Parmesan cheese and toss to coat.

Arrange chicken wings in air fryer basket and cook at 190°C for 22-26 minutes, or until wings are cooked through. Toss the wings every 5 minutes throughout the cooking process to ensure even cooking.

Remove wings from air fryer and sprinkle with remaining Parmesan cheese. Serve immediately, with ranch dip if desired.

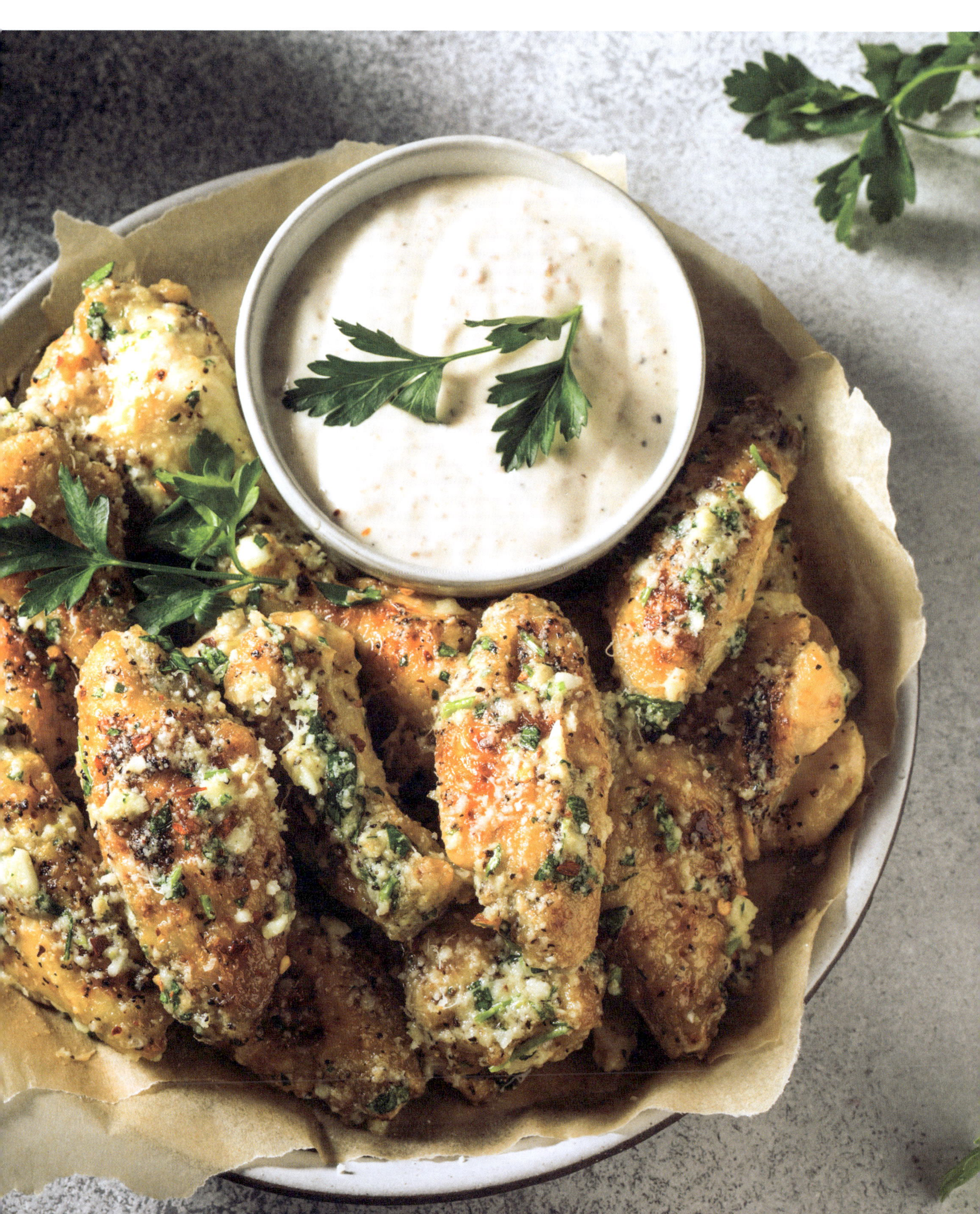

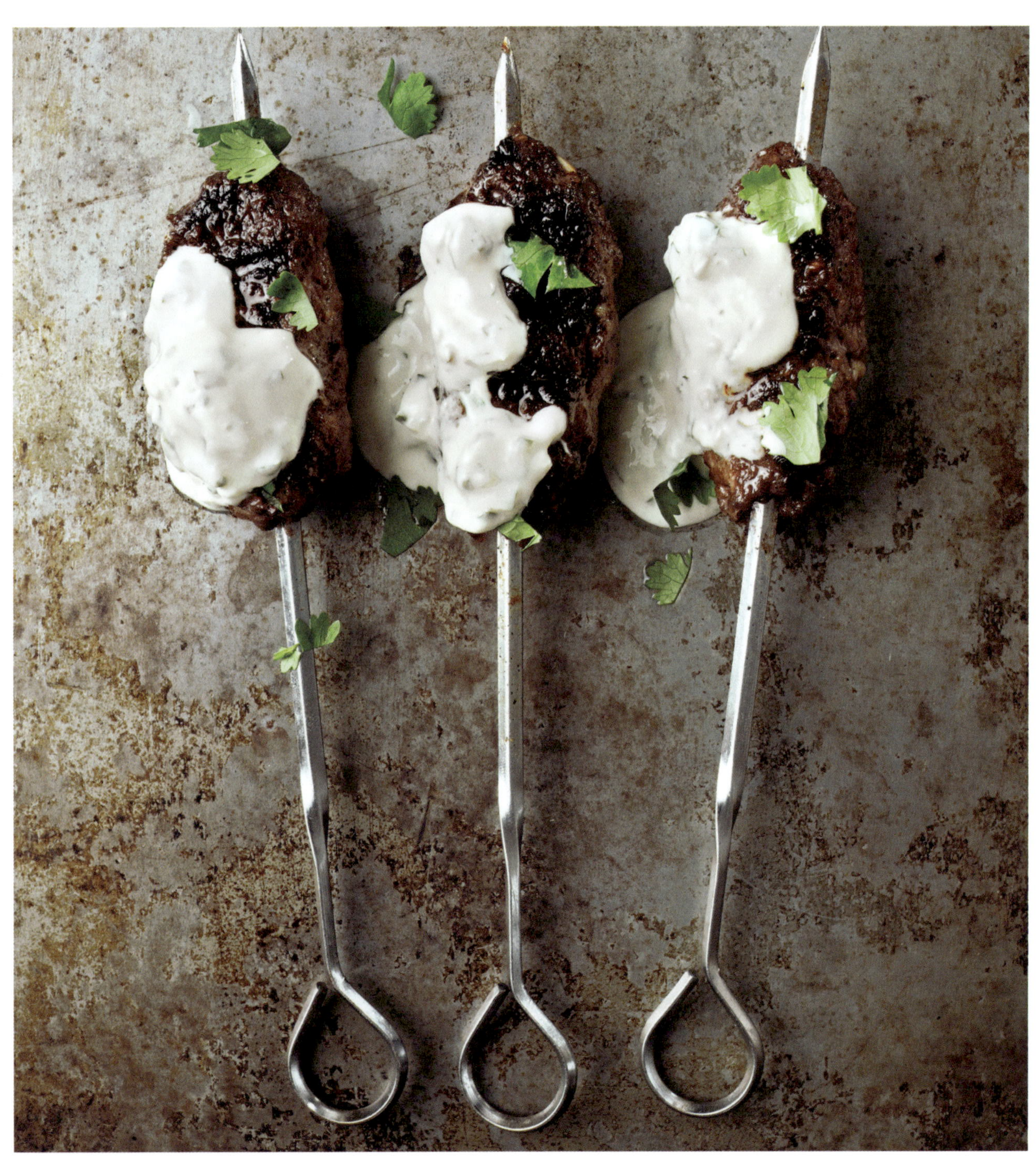

Lamb Koftes with Yoghurt Sauce

SERVES 4

PREP + COOK TIME: 30 MINS + CHILLING

VEG • GLUTEN FREE • DAIRY FREE

LAMB KOFTES WITH YOGHURT SAUCE

500g lamb mince

½ onion, grated

2 cloves garlic, crushed

2 tbsps fresh coriander, chopped

2 tsps cumin

2 tsps coriander

2 tsps paprika

½ tsp ground cinnamon

1 tsp salt

½ tsp pepper

1 tsp cayenne pepper (optional)

Skewer rack

YOGHURT SAUCE

1 cup (250ml) Greek yoghurt

1 tbsp olive oil

1 clove garlic, crushed

1 tsp cumin

1 tbsp chopped fresh coriander

1 tbsp lemon juice

¼ tsp salt

¼ tsp pepper

Combine the ingredients for the yoghurt sauce in a small bowl. Mix well to combine and refrigerate for at least 30 minutes or overnight.

Place the lamb mince in a large bowl with the grated onion, garlic, fresh coriander, spices and salt and pepper.

Mix well with hands then divide into eight equal portions. Push and shape the meat onto eight skewers. Spray with olive oil cooking spray.

Place the skewers in the air fryer basket, ensuring there is space between each skewer. Cook in batches or use a double layer accessory if necessary.

Cook at 190°C for 10-12 minutes, turning halfway through.

Remove from air fryer and serve with prepared yoghurt sauce.

AUTUMN SALAD

1 medium sweet potato, cut into 2cm chunks

1 cup (135g) butternut pumpkin, cut into 2cm chunks

1 medium beetroot, cut into 2cm slices

1 medium carrot, thickly sliced

100g mushrooms, sliced

1 zucchini, cut into 1cm-thick half moons

3 tbsps olive oil (or avocado oil)

1 tsp salt

1 tsp garlic powder

150g mixed salad leaves

Chopped dill, to garnish

Place sweet potato, pumpkin, beetroot and carrot in a bowl of cold water to soak for at least 10 minutes.

Preheat air fryer to 180°C.

Drain the soaked vegetables and pat dry.

Mix olive oil, salt and garlic powder in a large bowl. Add the drained vegetables and toss to coat. Transfer to air fryer basket and cook for 5 minutes.

Shake basket then add mushrooms and zucchini.

Air fry for 10-15 minutes, shaking the basket every 5 minutes until the vegetables are tender and golden brown.

Add vegetables to a large bowl with salad leaves. Top with dill to serve.

FALAFEL

2 x 400g cans chickpeas, drained and rinsed

¼ cup (10g) fresh parsley, chopped

¼ cup (10g) fresh coriander, chopped

2 tsps ground cumin

1 tsp paprika

2 cloves garlic, minced

1 small onion, finely diced

3 tbsps plain flour

1 tbsp lemon juice

1 tsp salt

6 pitta breads

Rocket, grated carrot, cucumber, tomato and red onion to serve

TAHINI SAUCE

1¼ cups (310ml) Greek yoghurt

¼ cup (60g) tahini

2 tbsps fresh lemon juice

Combine chickpeas, herbs, spices, garlic, onion, flour, lemon juice and salt in a food processor. Blend into a rough paste.

Shape mixture into tablespoon-sized balls.

Preheat air fryer to 175°C. Spray air fryer basket with cooking spray.

Cooking in batches, arrange falafel in air fryer basket and spray with cooking spray. Cook for 8 minutes then flip over and cook for another 6 minutes until golden brown and crispy. Repeat with remaining falafel.

Combine ingredients for sauce in a small bowl. Mix well. Serve falafel hot in pitta bread with salad and tahini sauce.

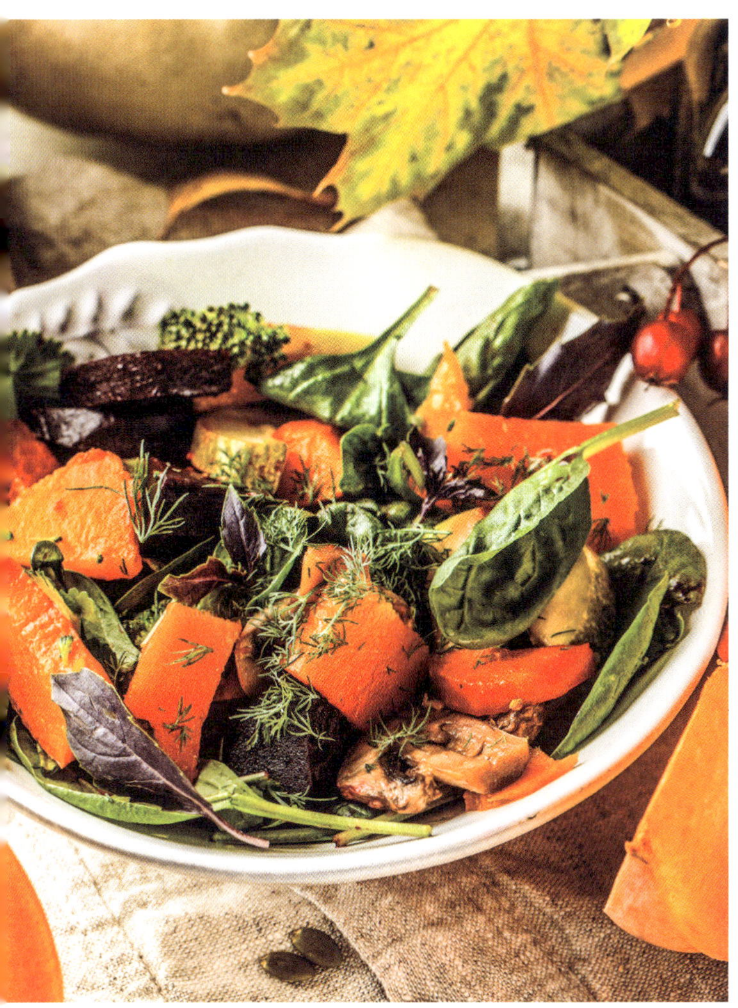

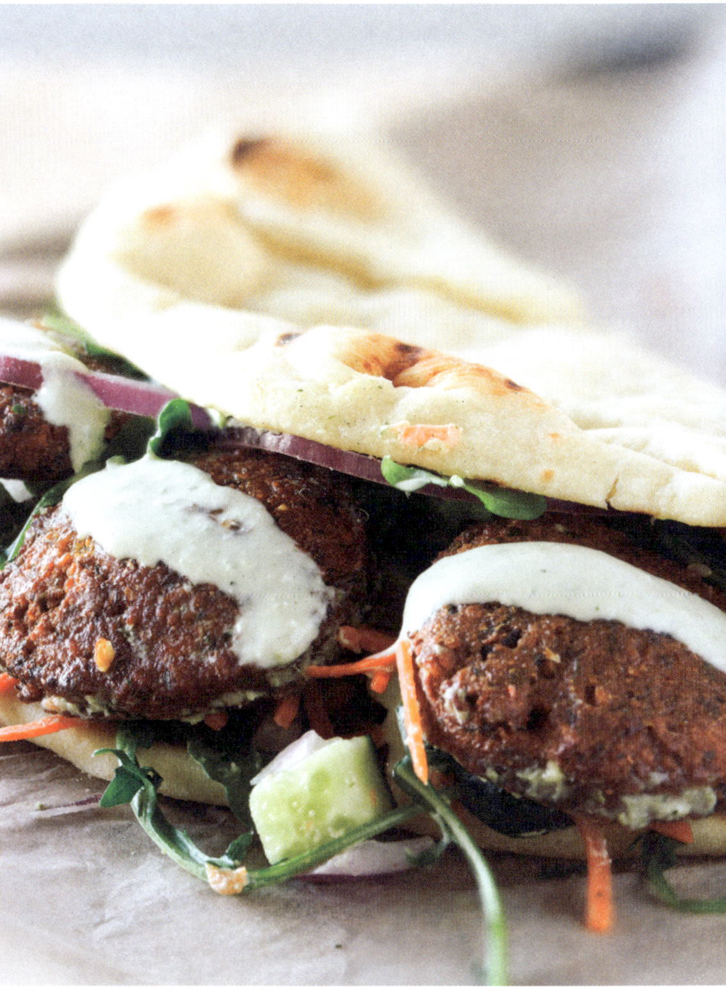

Autumn Salad

SERVES 4

PREP + COOK TIME: 35 MINS

VEG • GLUTEN FREE • DAIRY FREE

Falafel

SERVES 6

PREP + COOK TIME: 20 MINS

VEG

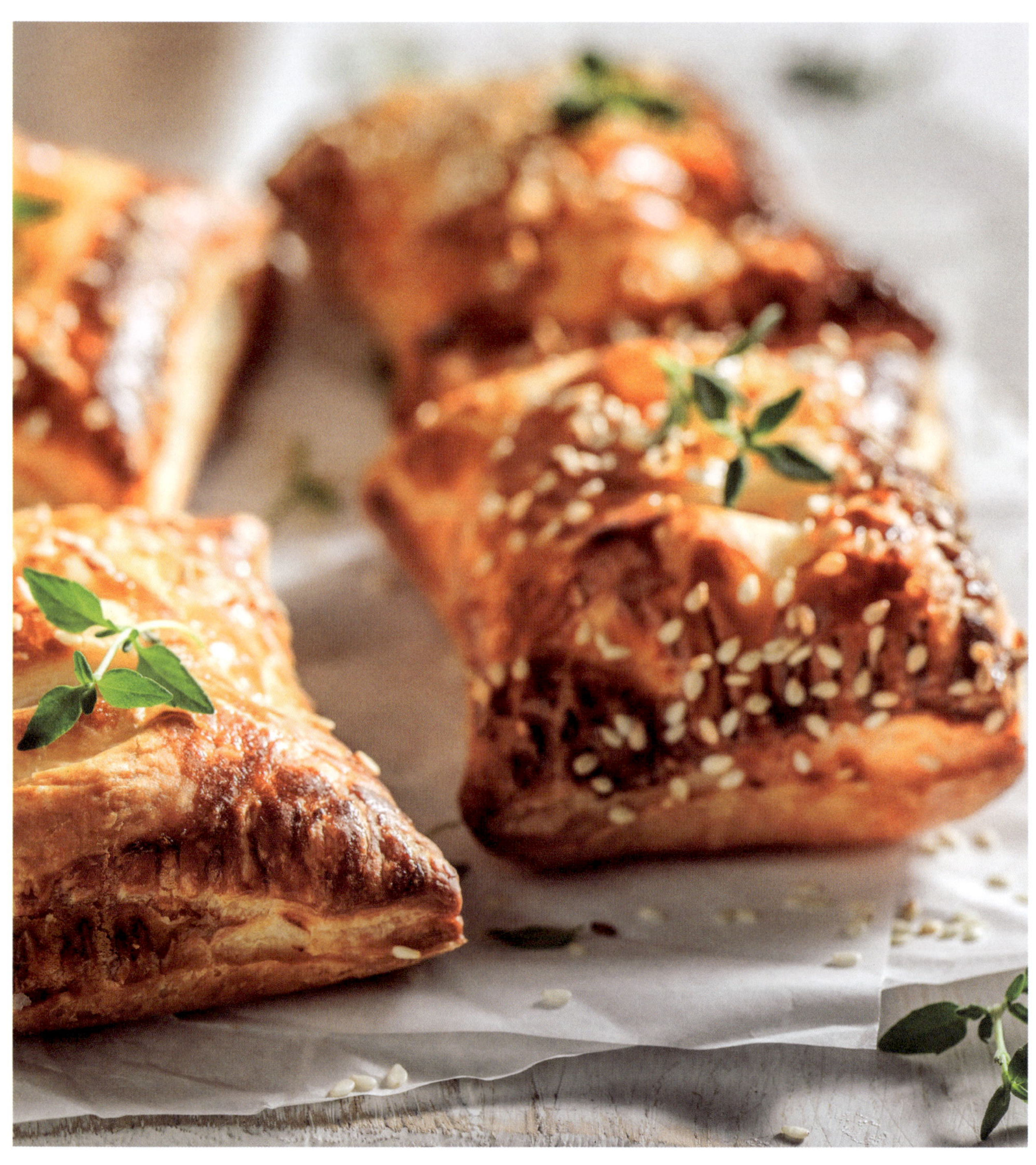

Mushroom Pastry Parcels

SERVES 4

PREP + COOK TIME: 45 MINS

VEG

MUSHROOM PASTRY PARCELS

1 tbsp olive oil
1 onion, finely chopped
4 cloves garlic, minced
350g mushrooms, finely chopped
1 tsp fresh thyme leaves
½ tsp dried chilli flakes
Salt and pepper to taste
2 sheets frozen puff pastry, thawed
1-2 tbsps milk
1 tbsp sesame seeds

Heat the oil in a large frying pan over medium heat. Add the onion and cook for 3-5 minutes until soft and translucent. Add garlic and cook for 1 minute until fragrant. Add mushrooms, thyme and chilli flakes. Season with salt and pepper and cook for 5 minutes until tender. Set aside to cool for about 10 minutes.

Cut the pastry sheets in half to make four rectangles.

Spread the mushroom mixture over one half of each of the pastry rectangles, leaving a 1cm border around the edge. Brush the edges with milk, then fold the pastry sheets in half, covering the mixture, and press the edges with a fork. Brush pastry parcels with milk, cut two or three slits in the top of each parcel with a sharp knife and scatter with sesame seeds.

Spray air fryer basket with cooking spray.

Place the mushroom parcels into the air fryer basket. Air fry for 8-10 minutes at 165°C until golden brown. Allow to cool slightly before serving.

Chapter Four

Everyday Dinners

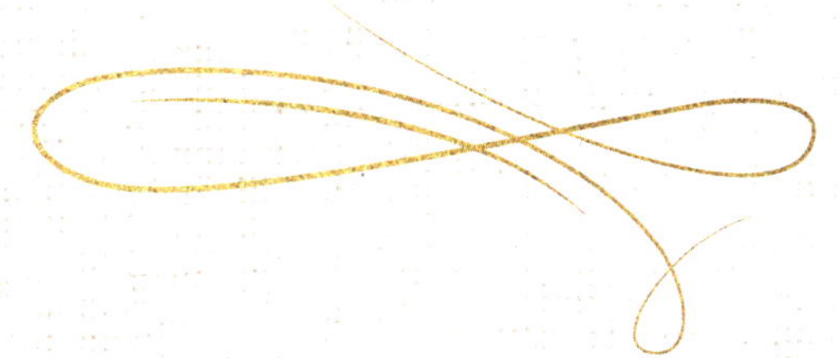

Air Fryer Pot Roast

SERVES 4-6

PREP + COOK TIME: 40 MINS + 8 HOURS MARINATING

GLUTEN FREE • DAIRY FREE

1 tbsp rosemary, chopped
½ onion, finely chopped
3 tbsps olive oil
1 tbsp balsamic vinegar
1 tsp salt
½ tsp pepper
1.2kg beef chuck roast

Place the rosemary, onion, olive oil, vinegar, salt and pepper in a small bowl and whisk to combine.

Pour the mixture over the roast, cover and transfer to the fridge to marinate for 8 hours.

Preheat the air fryer to 200°C.

Place roast in the air fryer basket.

Cook for 30 minutes, flipping roast halfway through.

Allow to rest for at least 5 minutes.

Slice into thick cuts to serve.

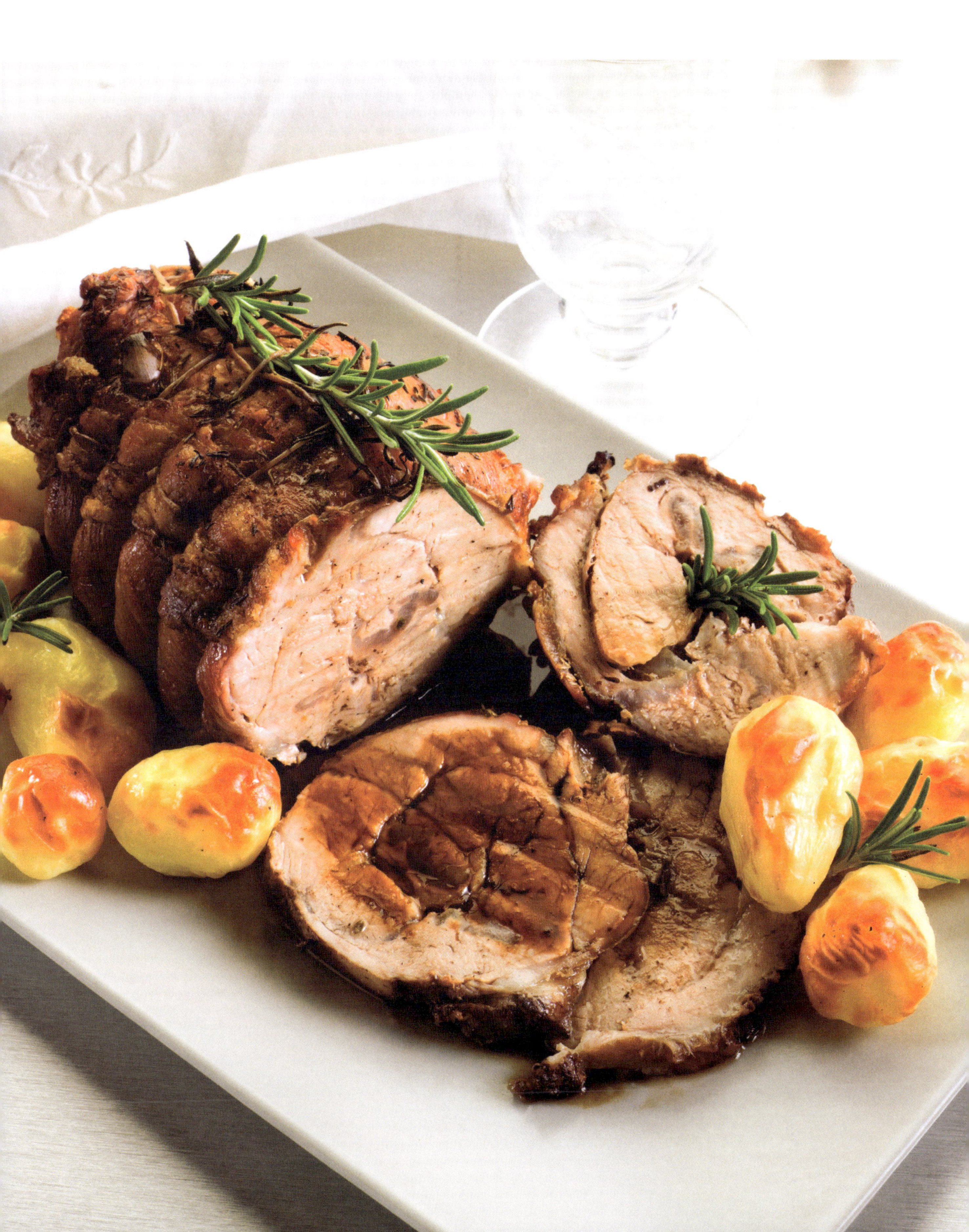

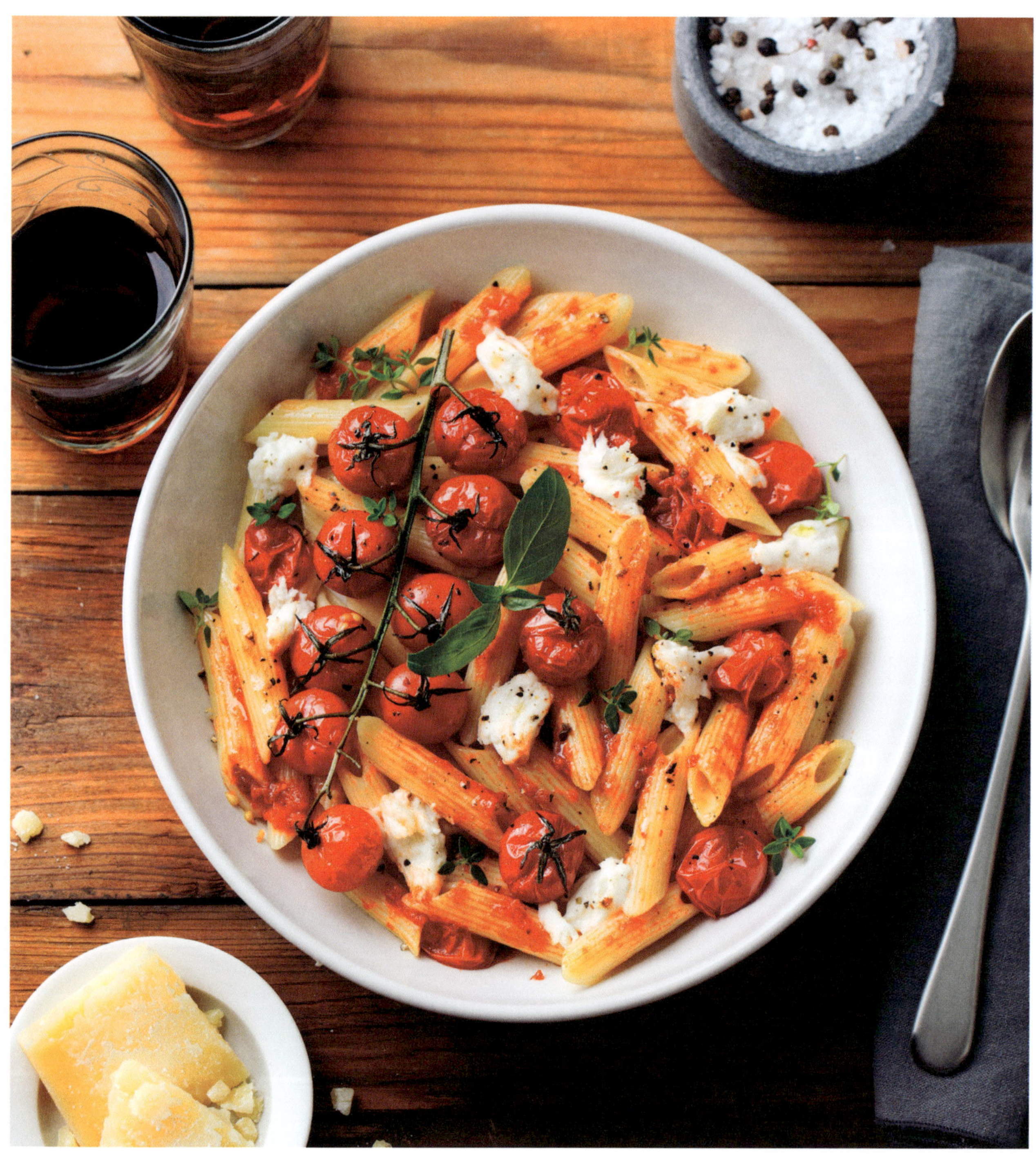

Tomato & Feta Pasta

SERVES 2

PREP + COOK TIME: 25 MINS

VEG

TOMATO & FETA PASTA

500g cherry tomatoes on the vine
2 tbsps olive oil
1 tbsp white wine vinegar
1 clove garlic, minced
1 tsp Italian herbs
1 tbsp fresh basil, chopped
Salt and pepper, to taste
250g penne pasta, cooked
Soft feta, to serve

Preheat the air fryer to 200°C.

Place the tomatoes, olive oil, vinegar, garlic, Italian herbs and basil in a large mixing bowl. Season with salt and pepper and toss to combine.

Transfer the ingredients to basket of the air fryer.

Cook for 20 minutes. During cooking remove from the air fryer a few times to stir with a wooden spoon, crushing some of the tomatoes to create the sauce.

When cooked, toss the cooked pasta with the tomato sauce.

Pour over any liquid from the bottom drawer of the air fryer that has leaked through the basket.

Sprinkle with soft feta to serve.

Tomato & Mozzarella Pizza

SERVES 2
PREP + COOK TIME: 40 MINS + 1 HOUR PROVING
VEG

DOUGH

2 cups (250g) baker's (or plain) flour
1 x 7g sachet dry active yeast
1 tsp caster sugar
1 tsp salt
¾ cup (200ml) warm water
1 tbsp olive oil + extra to grease

TOPPING

1 tbsp olive oil
¼ cup (60g) pizza sauce
150g fresh buffalo mozzarella, cubed
1 tomato, cut into eighths
1 tsp dried oregano
½ red onion, sliced
Mint leaves to garnish
Salt and pepper to taste

Sift flour into a large bowl. Stir in yeast, sugar and salt. Make a well in the centre and pour in water and oil. Bring the dough together with your hands, then turn out onto a lightly floured surface. Clean the bowl for reuse.

Knead for 5 minutes until the dough is smooth.

Lightly grease the bowl with oil, then add dough and cover with a tea towel or plastic wrap. Set aside in a warm place to prove for 1 hour, until doubled in size.

Knock back the dough by punching it to remove air and divide into two balls.

Preheat air fryer to 190°C. Spray air fryer basket with cooking spray.

Roll out one ball of pizza dough to the size of air fryer basket. Carefully transfer to air fryer and brush with olive oil.

Spread with pizza sauce. Top with mozzarella, tomatoes, oregano and onion.

Bake for 7 minutes until crust is crispy and cheese is melted. Top with mint leaves and season with salt and pepper.

Repeat with second ball of pizza dough.

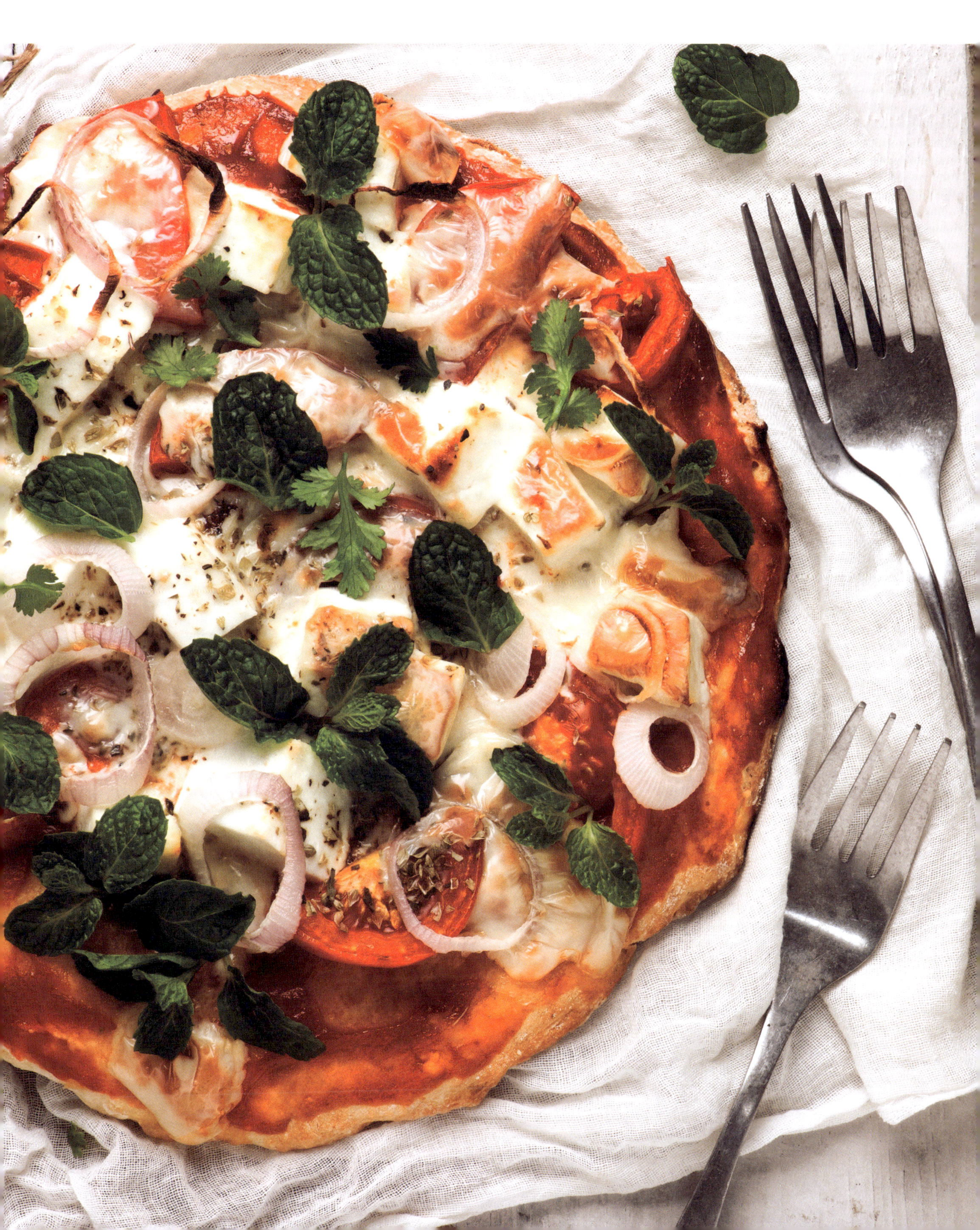

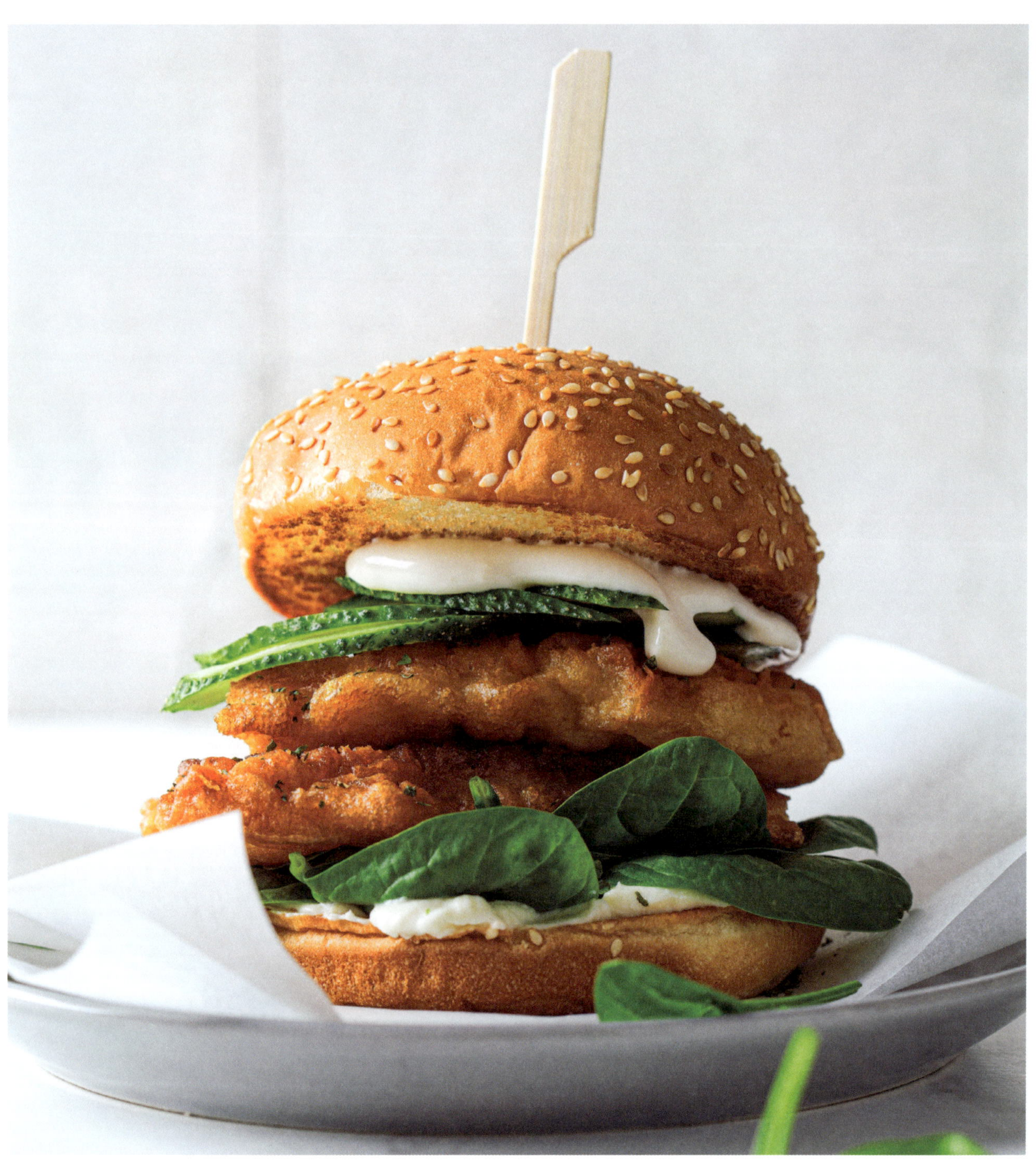

Fish Burgers

SERVES 4

PREP + COOK TIME: 30 MINS

FISH BURGERS

- 1¾ cups (215g) plain flour
- 2 tbsps cornflour
- ½ tsp bicarbonate of soda
- ¾ cup (180ml) soda water
- 1 egg, beaten
- ½ tsp paprika
- 1 tsp salt
- ¼ tsp pepper
- Pinch of cayenne pepper
- 500g cod fillet, cut into roughly 10cm pieces
- 4 toasted burger buns
- 1 cup (30g) baby spinach
- ½ cup (120g) mayonnaise
- ½ cup (120g) tartare sauce
- ½ cup (75g) sliced gherkins

Combine 1 cup flour, cornflour and bicarb in a large bowl. Add the soda water and egg and whisk until smooth. Cover the bowl and refrigerate for at least 20 minutes.

Combine the remaining ¾ cup of flour, paprika, salt, pepper and cayenne pepper in a shallow dish.

Pat the fish fillets dry with a paper towel. Dip the fish first into the batter, coating all sides. Let the excess batter drip off and then coat each fillet with the seasoned flour. Sprinkle any leftover flour on the fish fillets and pat gently to coat.

Preheat the air fryer to 200°C.

Generously spray both sides of the fish fillets with cooking spray and place them in the air fryer basket. Air fry for 12 minutes, spraying once more with cooking spray halfway through cooking.

Fill burger buns with fish pieces, baby spinach, mayonnaise, tartare sauce and sliced gherkins.

Pizza Quesadilla

SERVES 1

PREP + COOK TIME: 10 MINS

1 tbsp pizza sauce

2 large flour tortillas

10 slices pepperoni

½ tsp Italian seasoning

1 cup (125g) shredded mozzarella cheese

½ tbsp butter, melted

Tomato dipping sauce to serve

Preheat the air fryer to 200°C.

Spread pizza sauce over one tortilla. Arrange the pepperoni slices over the pizza sauce, and scatter with Italian seasoning. Cover with mozzarella cheese and top with the second tortilla. Press down on the quesadilla to secure the top tortilla in place. Brush the top of the quesadilla with melted butter.

Using a large spatula, place the pizza quesadilla into the air fryer basket and cook for 5 minutes until golden brown. Be sure to check it halfway through.

Remove the pizza quesadilla from the air fryer. Let cool. Cut into quarters and serve with tomato dipping sauce, if desired.

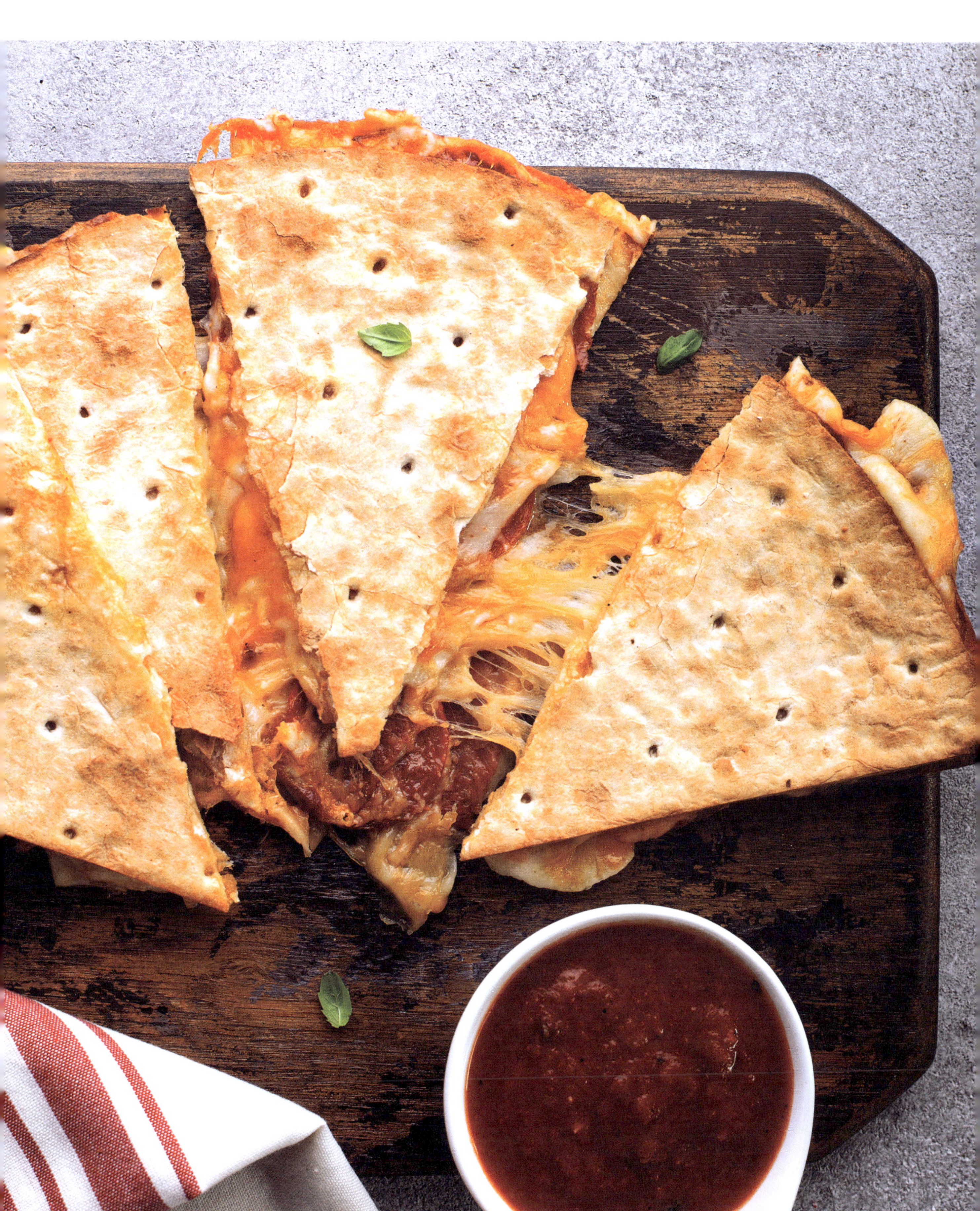

LAMB CHOPS WITH ANCHOVIES & CAPERS

6 small lamb chops
Salt and pepper to taste
3 tbsps olive oil
3 anchovy fillets
½ lemon, thickly sliced
3 tbsps capers, drained
2 cloves garlic, minced
1 tbsp parsley, chopped
Baking pan

Season lamb chops with salt and pepper.

Place olive oil, anchovies, lemon and capers in a pan and place in the air fryer.

Cook for 8-10 minutes at 200°C, stirring every few minutes, until the anchovies break down.

Remove dish from air fryer and stir in garlic and parsley.

Baste lamb chops with anchovy mixture.

Place lamb chops in air fryer.

Cook for 12 minutes at 200°C, turning and basting halfway through cooking.

Rest for 5 minutes before serving.

SALMON & QUINOA PATTIES

2 cups (370g) cooked quinoa
350g cooked salmon, flaked apart
1 spring onion, sliced
2 tbsps fresh parsley, chopped
¼ cup (60g) mayonnaise
2 tsps Dijon mustard
1 egg, beaten
2 tsps fresh lime juice + extra for serving
Salt and pepper to taste

Combine quinoa, salmon, spring onions, parsley, mayonnaise, mustard, egg and lime juice. Season to taste with salt and pepper. Form into eight patties.

Preheat air fryer to 180°C. Spray basket and patties with cooking spray. Cook patties for 6-8 minutes, flipping halfway through, until crisp and golden brown.

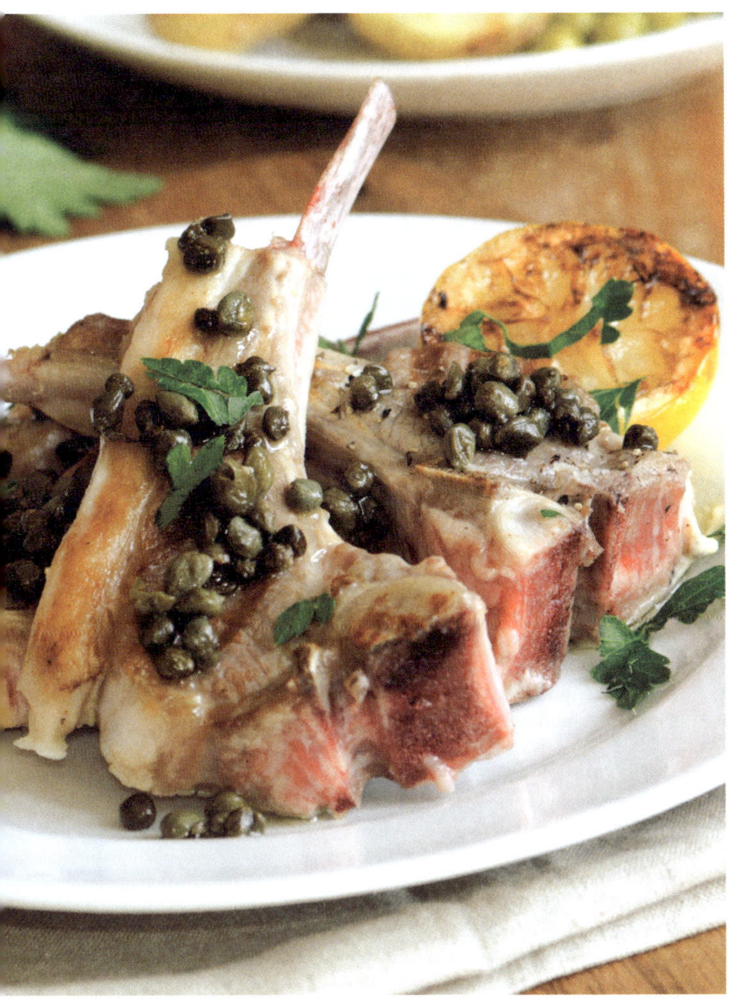

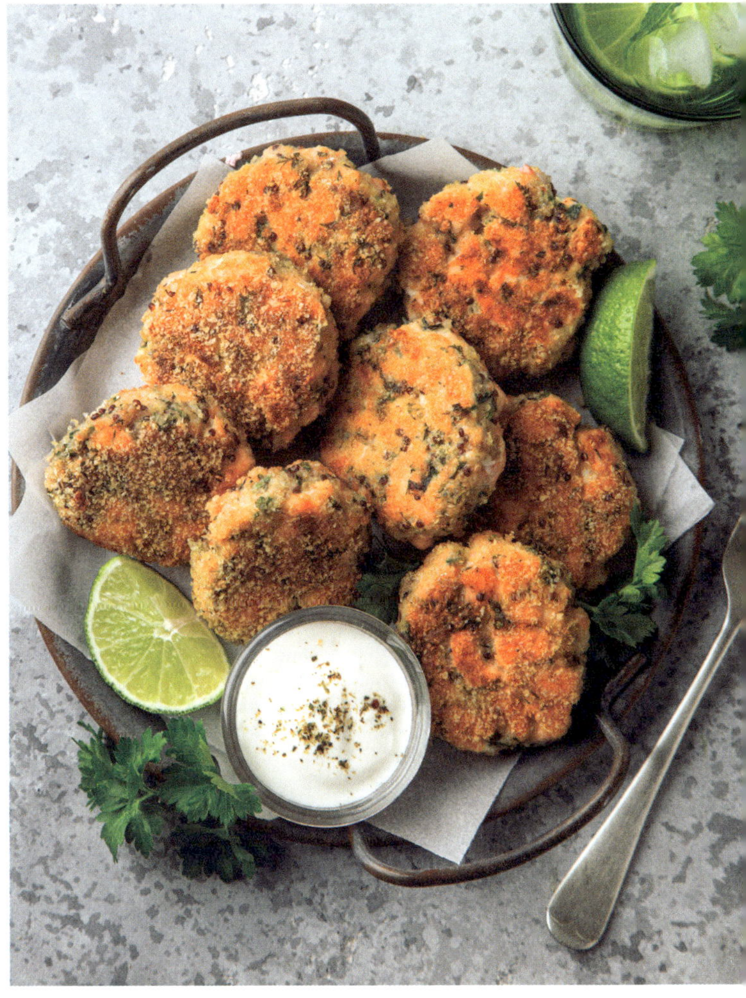

Lamb Chops with Anchovies & Capers

SERVES 2

PREP + COOK TIME: 40 MINS

GLUTEN FREE • DAIRY FREE

Salmon & Quinoa Patties

SERVES 4

PREP + COOK TIME: 15 MINS

GLUTEN FREE • DAIRY FREE

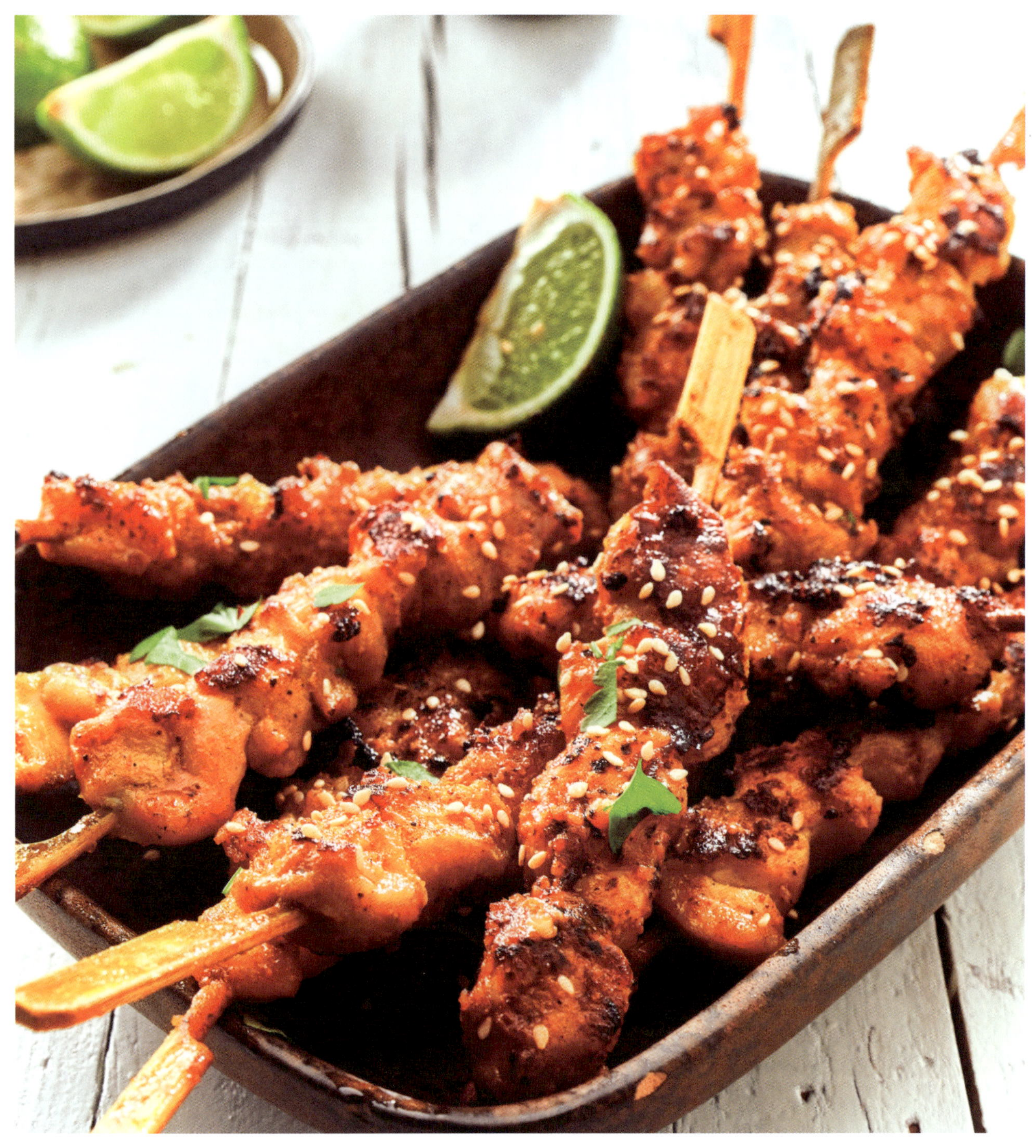

Pork Satay with Peanut Sauce

SERVES 3

PREP + COOK TIME: 20 MINS + 30 MINS MARINATING

DAIRY FREE

PORK SATAY WITH PEANUT SAUCE

2 tbsps garlic, crushed

1 tbsp fresh ginger, minced

2 tsps hot chilli sauce

2 tbsps kecap manis

2 tbsps vegetable oil

400g lean pork chops, cut into cubes

1 spring onion, finely chopped

1 tsp ground coriander

¾ cup (200ml) coconut milk

⅓ cup (100g) unsalted peanut butter

1 tbsp soy sauce

Skewer rack

Whisk together the garlic, ginger, 1 teaspoon hot chilli sauce, kecap manis and 1 tablespoon of the oil in a large bowl. Add the meat and stir to combine. Cover and place in the fridge to marinate for 30 minutes.

Thread the pork cubes onto skewers. Place the kebabs on the skewer rack and spritz with oil.

Preheat the air fryer to 190°C. Spritz the air fryer basket with cooking spray.

Place the skewer rack in the air fryer. Cook for 12 minutes until golden and cooked through, turning halfway during cooking.

To make the peanut sauce, heat 1 tablespoon of the oil in a saucepan. Add the spring onion and coriander and stir-fry for 1 minute. Pour in the coconut milk, peanut butter, soy sauce and remaining chilli sauce and bring to the boil. Cook for 5 minutes, stirring constantly. Add a little water if the sauce is too thick. Serve sauce on the side as an accompaniment to the satay.

Note:

You can easily substitute store-bought satay marinade to make this recipe super quick and easy.

Shepherd's Pie

SERVES 6
PREP + COOK TIME: 1 HOUR
GLUTEN FREE

500g potatoes, peeled and quartered
½ cup (125ml) milk
2 tbsps butter
1 onion, diced
2 carrots, diced
1 tsp melted ghee or olive oil
500g lamb mince
250g mushrooms, diced
2 cloves garlic, minced
2 tbsps tomato paste
1 tbsp Worcestershire sauce
1⅔ cups (400ml) lamb or chicken stock
½ cup (60g) grated Cheddar cheese
Baking pan
6 ramekins

Preheat air fryer to 180°C.

Bring potatoes to a boil in a pan of salted water over medium-high heat. Cook for 15-20 minutes or until soft.

Drain the cooked potatoes and add milk and butter. Mash until smooth. Set aside.

Meanwhile, place onion and carrot in baking pan. Drizzle with ghee or oil and toss to coat. Place pan in air fryer and cook for 5 minutes, stirring halfway through cooking.

Add mince, mushrooms and garlic to the pan. Break up mince with a fork. Cook for 5 minutes to brown the meat.

In a medium bowl or jug, mix together tomato paste, Worcestershire sauce and stock. Add stock mixture to the air fryer pan. Stir well. Cook for 30-35 minutes, stirring about every 5 minutes.

Spoon meat and veggie mix into six ramekins. Divide mashed potato between the dishes, spreading over the top, and top each with a little grated cheese.

Place each dish into the air fryer basket and cook for 8 minutes, or until cheese is melted and golden.

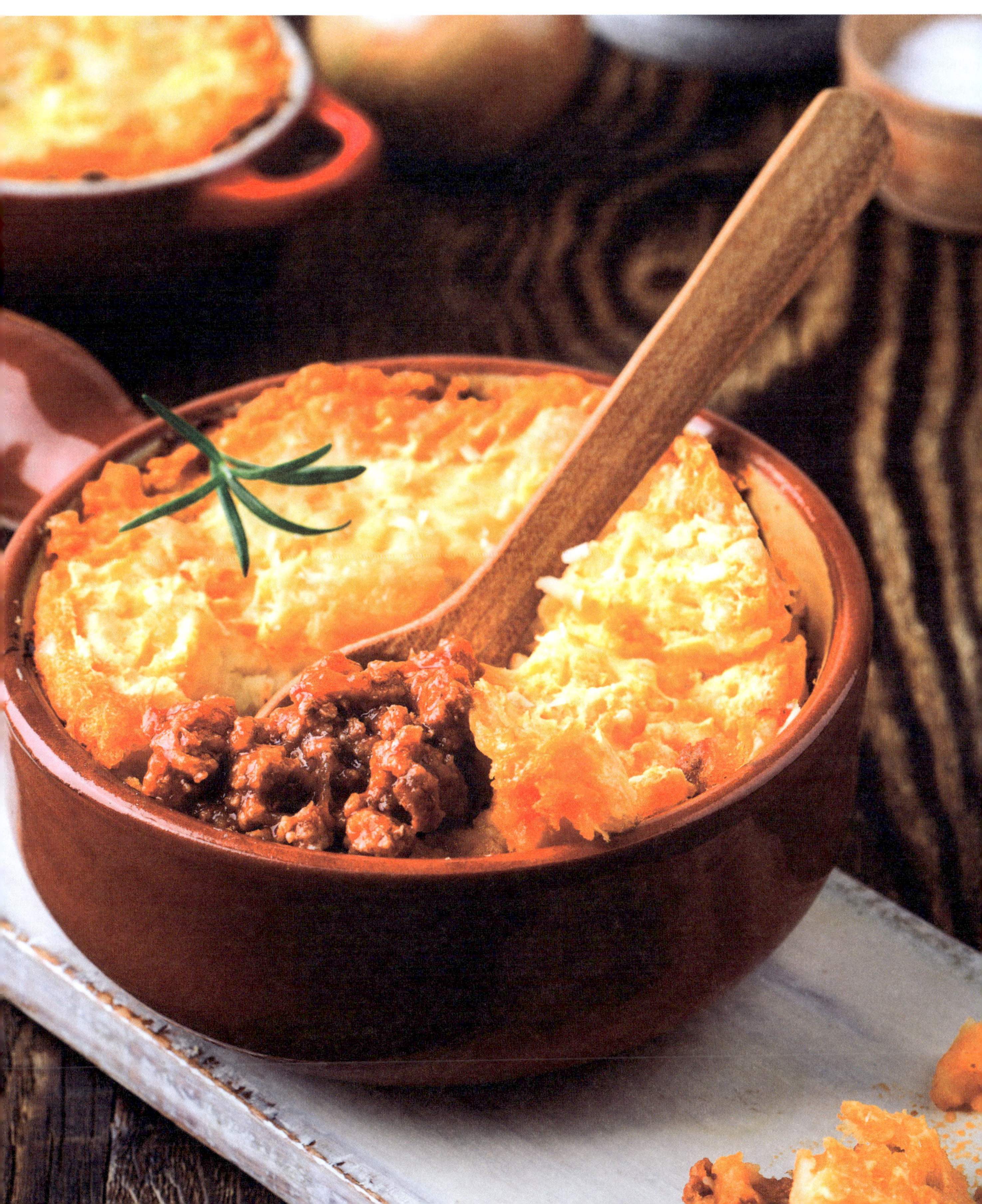

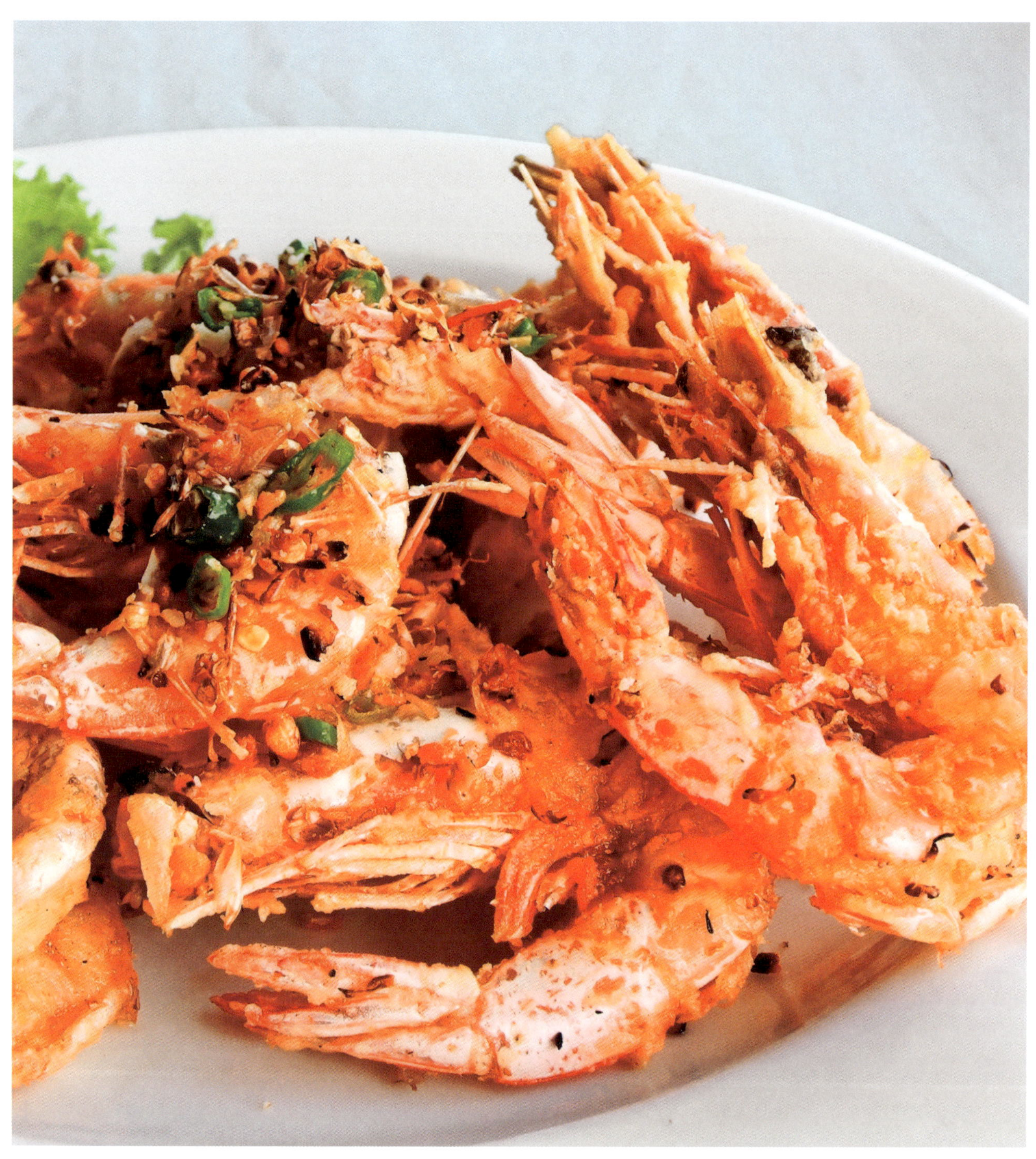

Salt & Pepper Prawns

SERVES 2

PREP + COOK TIME: 15 MINS

GLUTEN FREE • DAIRY FREE

SALT & PEPPER PRAWNS

½ tsp white pepper
½ tsp sugar
¼ tsp salt
2 tsps cornflour
500g shell-on prawns
1½ tsps + 1 tbsp peanut or other neutral oil
1 long red chilli, chopped
5 cloves garlic, chopped
1 spring onion, chopped

Preheat air fryer to 230°C.

In a medium bowl, stir together white pepper, sugar, salt and cornflour. Add prawns and rub in the seasonings. Drizzle on 1½ teaspoons oil and toss to coat.

Cook in air fryer for 2 minutes on each side.

Heat remaining oil in a frying pan over medium-high heat. Add chilli and garlic and cook for 30 seconds, until fragrant. Add prawns, toss to coat and cook for 1 minute. Sprinkle with spring onion to serve.

PORK BELLY

750g pork belly

1½ tsps salt

¼ tsp five-spice powder

2 tsps olive oil

Place pork belly in a pan of boiling water and simmer for 15 minutes. Drain.

When cool enough to handle, pat dry and refrigerate uncovered for 6-8 hours to dry out.

Rub the base of the pork belly with ½ teaspoon salt and the five-spice powder. Rub the top rind with remaining salt and olive oil.

Air fry for 30 minutes at 200°C.

Reduce temperature to 185°C and cook for another 30 minutes.

Allow to rest for 10 minutes.

VEGETARIAN QUESADILLA

4 large flour tortillas

1 cup (125g) grated Cheddar cheese

1 red capsicum, sliced

1 tomato, chopped

1 cup (175g) corn kernels

1 x 400g can black beans, drained and rinsed

2 tbsps coriander, chopped

Preheat air fryer to 200°C.

Place tortillas on a work surface. Sprinkle 2 tablespoons grated cheese over half of each tortilla. Top cheese with capsicum slices, tomato, corn, black beans and coriander. Sprinkle evenly with remaining cheese.

Fold tortillas over to form half-moon shaped quesadillas.

Lightly coat quesadillas with cooking spray and secure with toothpicks.

Spray air fryer basket with cooking spray.

Carefully place two quesadillas in the basket and cook for 10 minutes, turning halfway through, until cheese is melted and vegetables are tender. Repeat with remaining quesadillas.

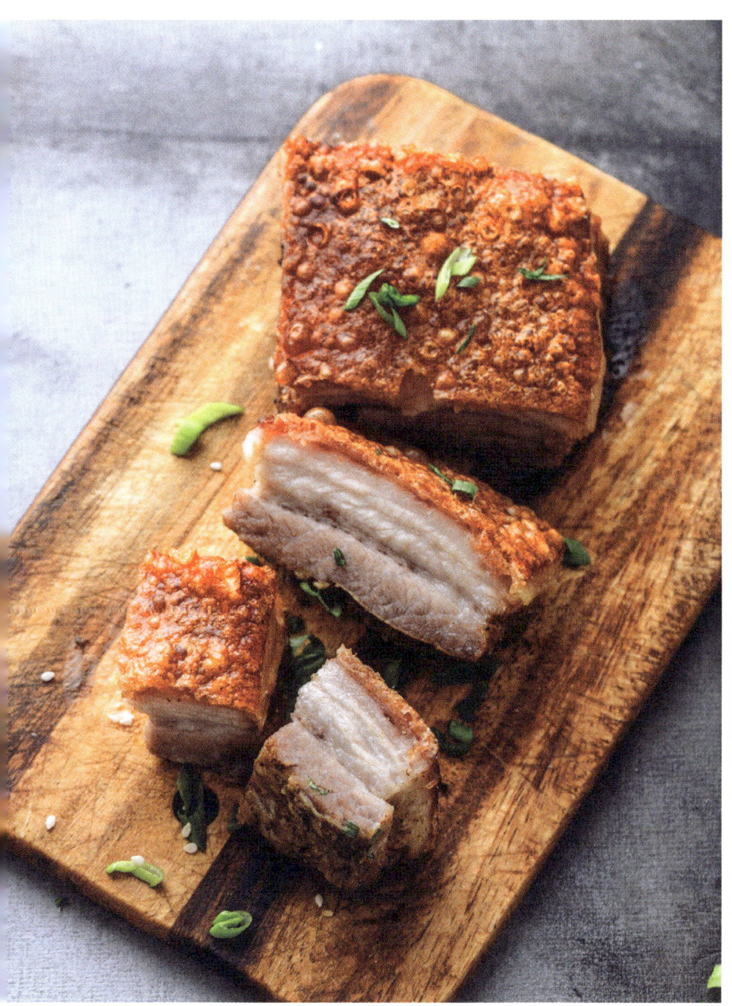

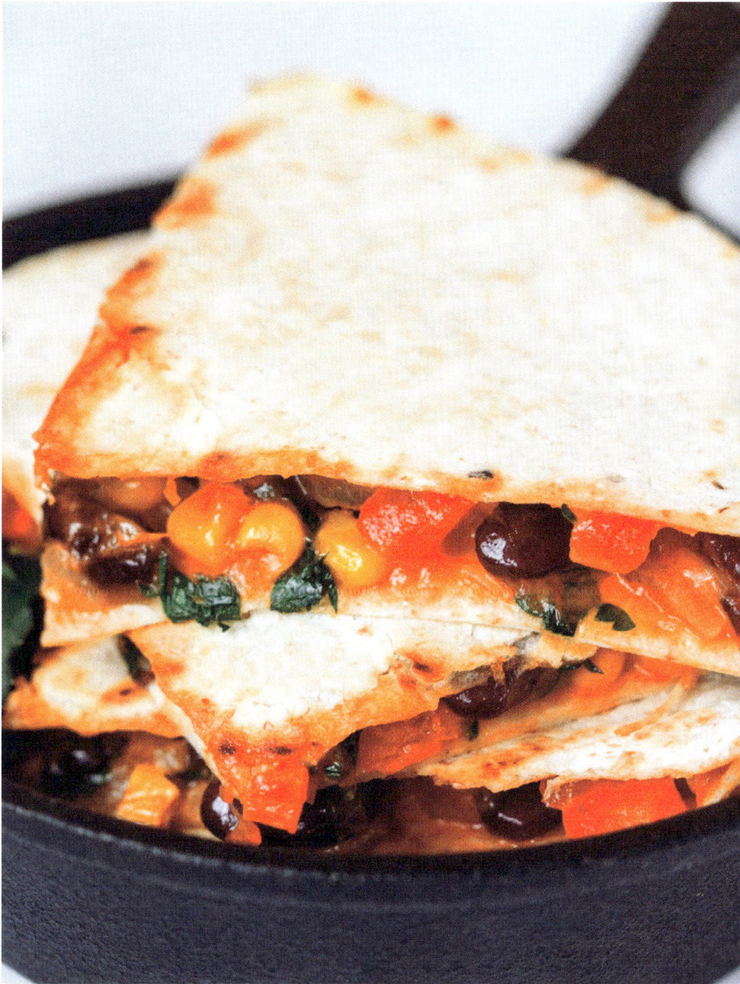

Pork Belly

SERVES 4

PREP + COOK TIME: 1 HOUR 20 MINS + 6 HOURS DRYING

GLUTEN FREE • DAIRY FREE

Vegetarian Quesadilla

SERVES 4

PREP + COOK TIME: 30 MINS

VEG

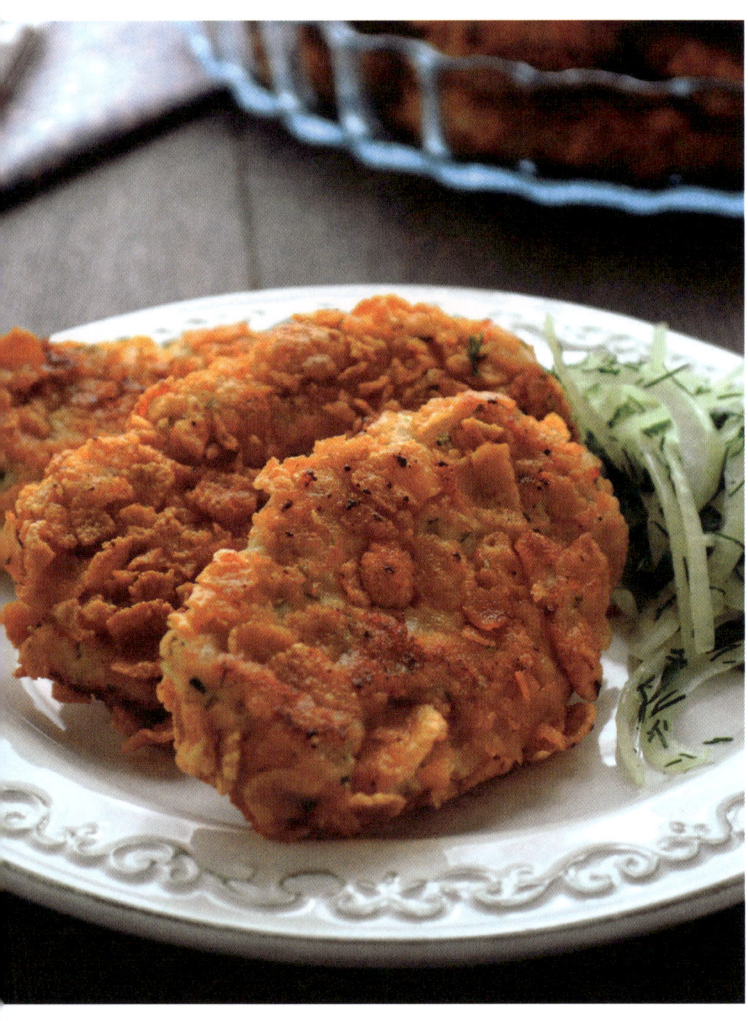

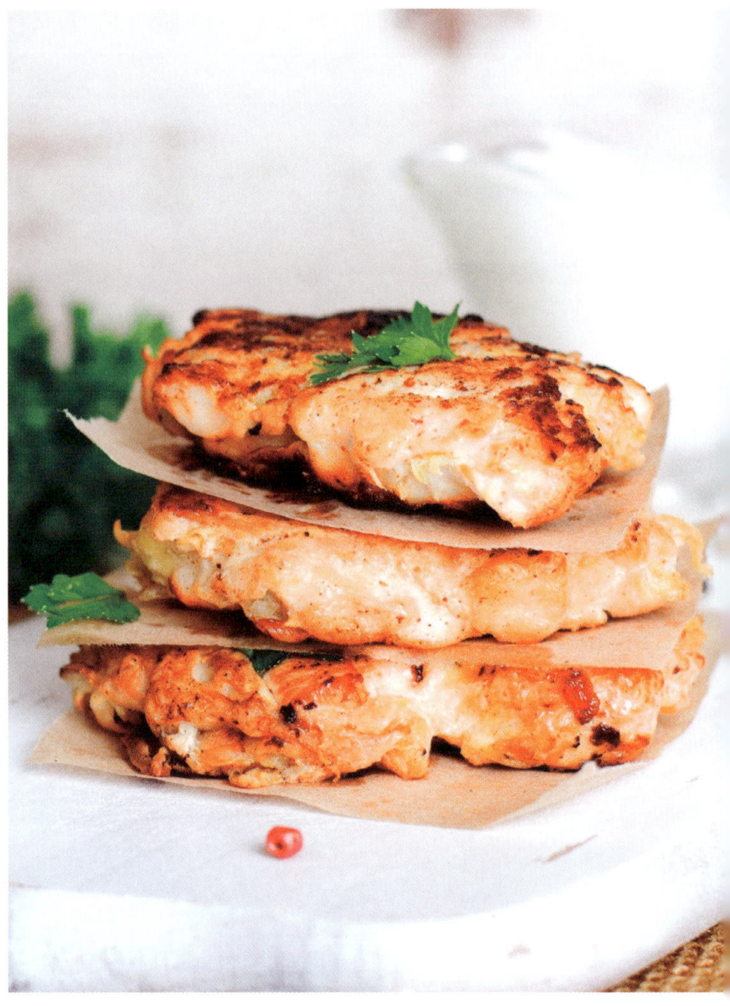

Cornflake Chicken Cutlets

SERVES 4

PREP + COOK TIME: 25 MINS

Fish Cutlets

SERVES 3

PREP + COOK TIME: 20 MINS + 30 MINS CHILLING

VEG • DAIRY FREE

CORNFLAKE CHICKEN CUTLETS

750g chicken tenders or quartered chicken breasts

Salt and pepper to taste

½ cup (125ml) milk

2 eggs

4 cups (120g) cornflakes

1 tsp smoked paprika

¼ tsp onion powder

Season the chicken pieces with salt and pepper.

Place the milk and eggs in a bowl and whisk to combine.

Place cornflakes, paprika, onion powder, salt and pepper in another bowl and mix. Dip each chicken piece into the milk mixture, then roll in the cornflakes.

Spray air fryer basket and chicken with cooking spray.

Arrange chicken in one layer and cook for 15 minutes at 200°C, turning halfway, until chicken is cooked.

FISH CUTLETS

400g skinless white fish fillet

1 tbsp capers, rinsed

1 tbsp parsley, chopped

Zest of 1 lemon

2 tbsps plain flour

Salt and pepper to taste

Finely chop the fish or place in a food processor and pulse until chopped but still chunky.

Add capers, parsley, lemon zest, flour and seasoning. Squeeze the mixture well in your hands to drain any excess liquid, then shape into three cutlets. Refrigerate for 30 minutes.

Preheat air fryer to 180°C.

Spray cutlets and air fryer basket with cooking spray. Place cutlets in air fryer. Cook for 8-10 minutes, until cooked through, turning halfway.

Cauliflower Steaks

SERVES 5

PREP + COOK TIME: 25 MINS+ MARINATING

VEG • GLUTEN FREE • DAIRY FREE

1 head cauliflower

1 tbsp olive oil

½ tsp ground turmeric

1 clove garlic, minced

½ tsp salt

1 tbsp lime juice

¼ cup (30g) toasted hazelnuts

2 tbsps sunflower seeds

¼ cup (10g) chopped fresh coriander

DRESSING

¼ cup (60g) tahini

2 tbsps olive oil

Juice of 1 lime

Salt and pepper to taste

First cut through the centre of the cauliflower head then cut into 3cm-thick slices.

In a bowl mix together the oil, turmeric, garlic, salt and lime juice. Mix well. Spread the mixture on the cauliflower steaks and let them sit for up to an hour.

Preheat air fryer to 175°C.

Place the steaks in a single layer in air fryer basket, working in batches if needed.

Cook for 15 minutes, flipping halfway through cooking.

Combine dressing ingredients in a small bowl. Stir to combine.

Drizzle cauliflower steaks with dressing and scatter with hazelnuts, sunflower seeds and coriander.

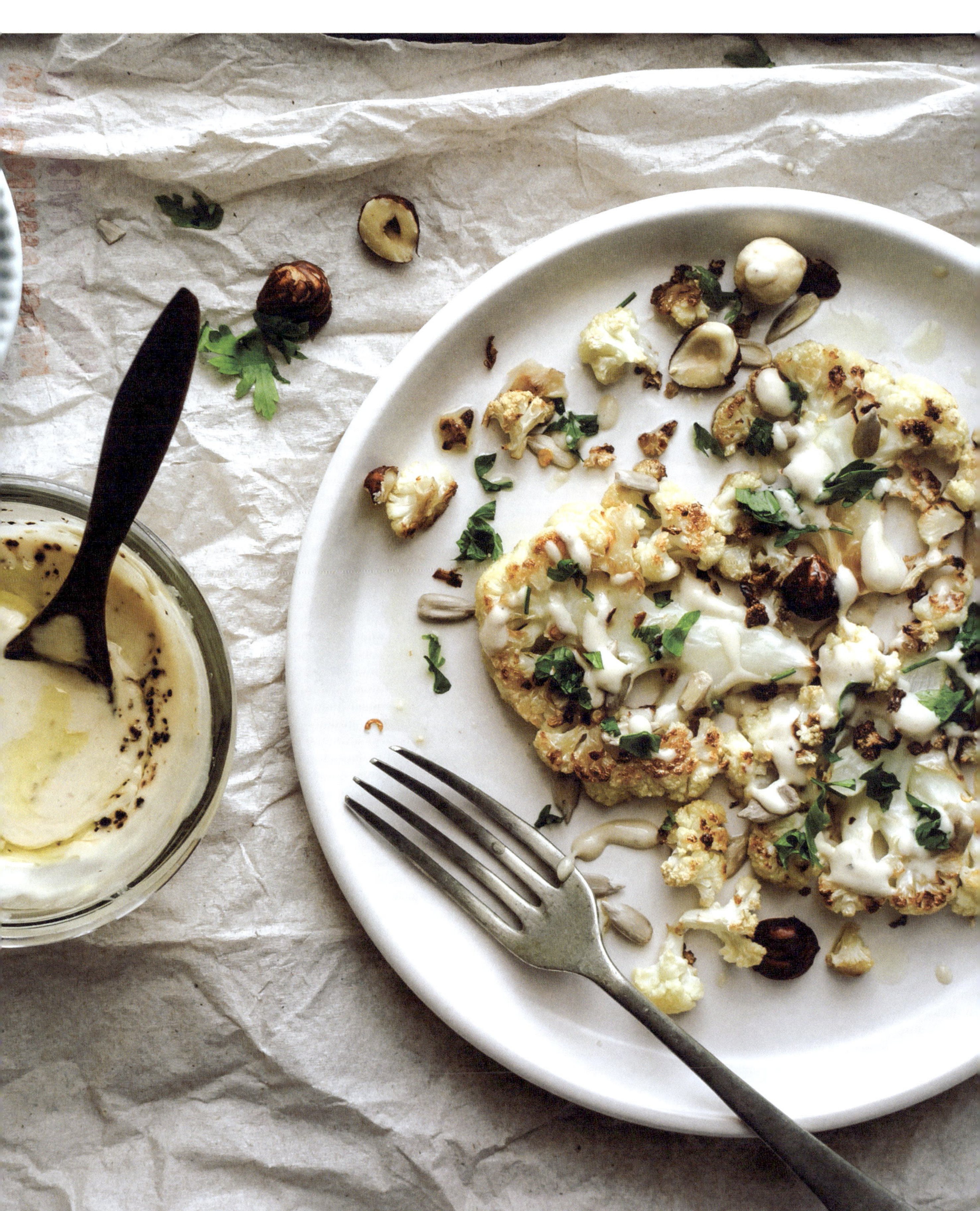

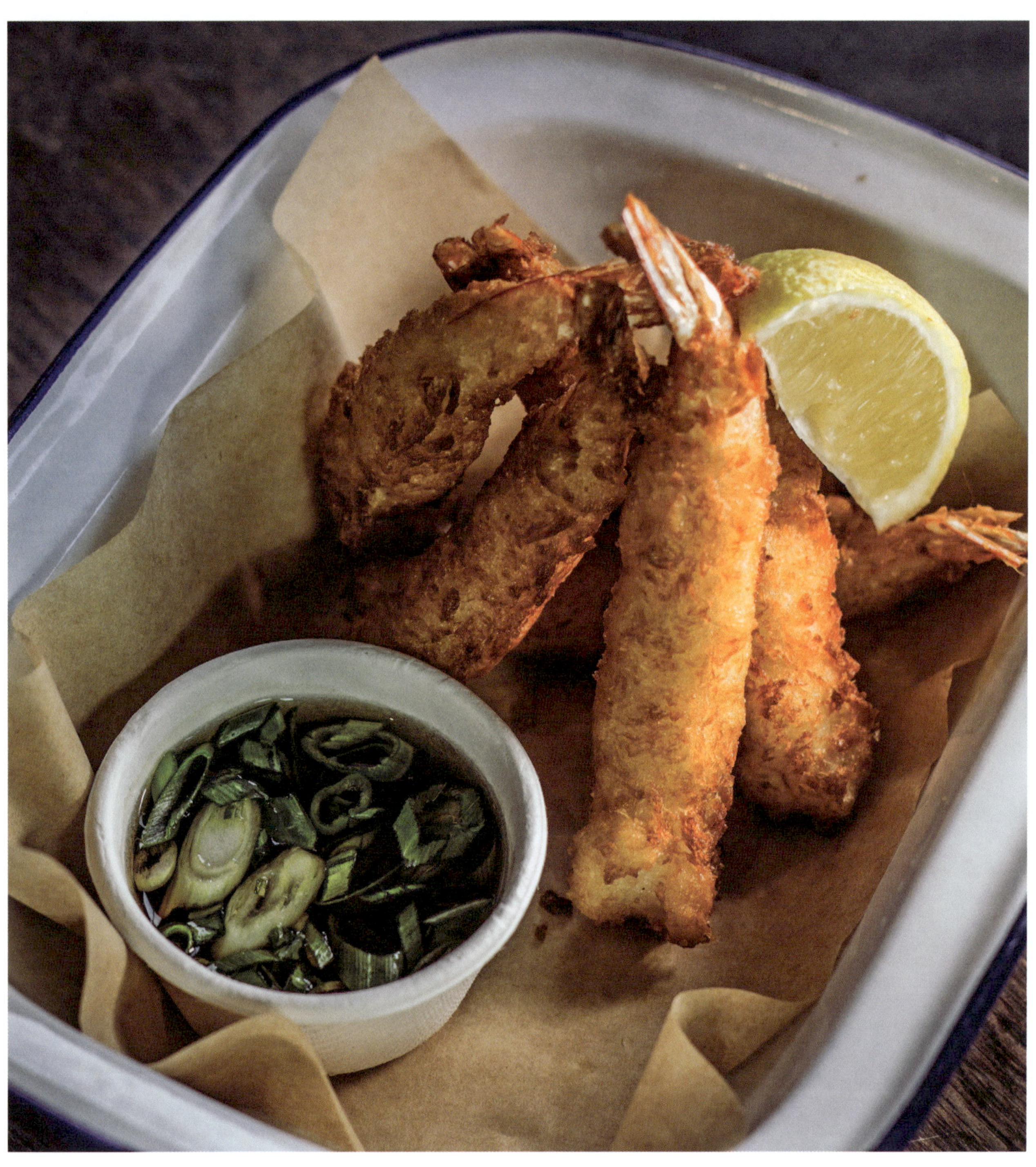

Crispy Prawns

SERVES 2

PREP + COOK TIME: 30 MINS

DAIRY FREE

CRISPY PRAWNS

4 tbsps plain flour

2 eggs

1⅓ tbsps water

1¼ cups (160g) panko breadcrumbs

12 tiger prawns, shelled and deveined, tails intact

Lemon wedges, to serve

DIPPING SAUCE

2 tbsps soy sauce

2 tbsps rice wine vinegar

1 tbsp sweet chilli sauce

3 tsps toasted (dark) sesame oil

1 spring onion, finely sliced

Place flour in a shallow bowl. Beat the eggs and water in another shallow bowl. Place panko breadcrumbs in a third bowl.

Dip the prawns first into the flour, then into the eggs, shaking off any excess. Next press into the panko breadcrumbs, being sure to fully coat each prawn.

Preheat the air fryer to 200°C.

Spray the air fryer basket with cooking spray. Spray the prawns generously with cooking spray.

Working in batches, cook prawns for 6 minutes, turning halfway through cooking.

Combine dipping sauce ingredients in a bowl and stir to combine.

Serve prawns with dipping sauce and lemon wedges.

CHEESY VEGETABLE TART

1 savoury pie crust, chilled (see note)
2 eggs
¼ cup (60ml) milk
Pinch of salt and pepper
½ cup (90g) zucchini, chopped
½ cup (75g) onion, chopped
¼ cup (50g) tomato, chopped
2 button mushrooms, sliced
¼ cup (30g) grated mozzarella cheese
¼ cup (30g) grated Cheddar cheese
Tart pan

Preheat the air fryer to 180°C.

Line the tart pan with the crust and trim off any excess. Prick the base a few times with a fork.

Beat the eggs with an electric mixer until they are pale and fluffy. Add milk, salt and pepper, zucchini, onion, tomato, mushroom and mozzarella cheese. Stir well to combine.

Transfer the mixture into the prepared crust. Don't fill it quite to the top, so there is room for the tart to rise.

Place the tart into the basket of the air fryer. Cook for 15 minutes then remove and sprinkle the top of the tart with the Cheddar cheese. Return to the air fryer to cook for a further 4 minutes until golden and cheese has melted.

Note:

Purchase a pre-made pie crust or make your own. The crust should be big enough to line a 16cm tart pan.

TRADITIONAL SOUTHERN FRIED CHICKEN

1kg chicken pieces
¼ cup (60ml) buttermilk
¾ cup (90g) plain flour
1 packet (75g) coating mix for southern fried chicken
Salt and pepper to taste

Place the chicken in a large bowl. Drizzle over the buttermilk and toss to coat. Cover and transfer to the fridge for 1 hour minimum (longer is better).

When you are ready to cook the chicken, begin by combining the flour, chicken coating mix, salt and pepper in a large, shallow bowl. Stir and mix well.

Dredge the chicken in seasoning mix, ensuring that both sides are fully coated.

Spritz the air fryer basket with cooking spray.

Preheat the air fryer to 200°C.

Place the chicken in the air fryer, being careful not to overcrowd the basket. Cook in batches if necessary.

Cook for a total of 20 minutes on 190°C, flipping the chicken every 5 minutes.

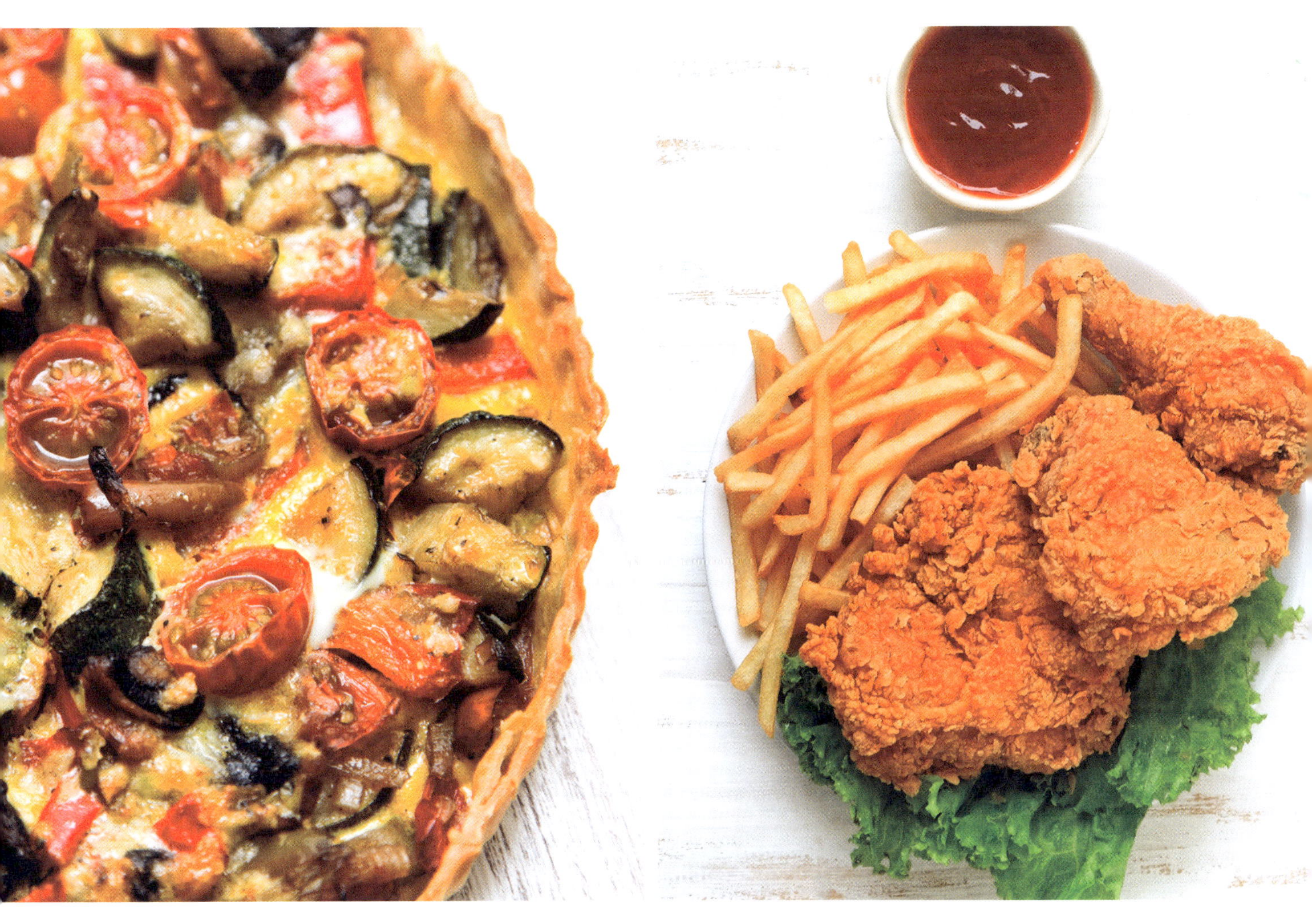

Cheesy Vegetable Tart

SERVES 4

PREP + COOK TIME: 30 MINS

VEG

Traditional Southern Fried Chicken

SERVES 4

PREP + COOK TIME: 30 MINS + 1 HOUR MARINATING

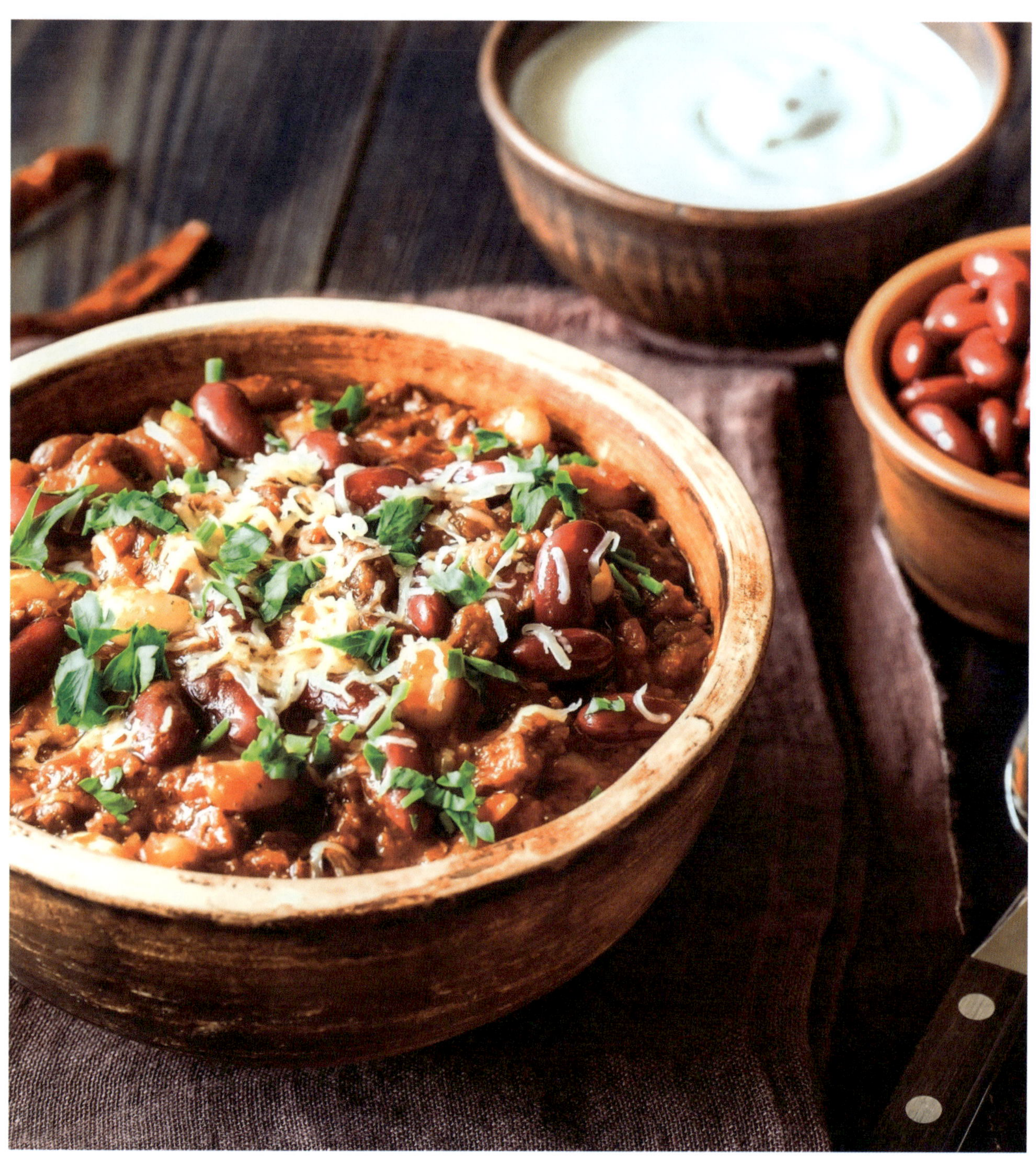

Chilli Con Carne

SERVES 4

PREP + COOK TIME: 1 HOUR

GLUTEN FREE

CHILLI CON CARNE

1 onion, thinly sliced

1 red capsicum, finely diced

1 red chilli, deseeded and finely chopped

1 tbsp olive oil

500g beef mince

2 cloves garlic, minced

2 tsps chilli powder, or to taste

1 tsp ground coriander

1 tsp ground cumin

2 tbsps tomato paste

1⅔ cups (400ml) hot beef stock

1 x 400g can chopped tomatoes

Salt and pepper to taste

1 x 400g can kidney beans, drained and rinsed

1 x 400g can cannellini beans, drained and rinsed

2 tsps cacao powder (optional)

Chopped coriander and grated cheese, to serve

Baking pan

Preheat air fryer to 180°C.

Place the onion, capsicum and chilli in a baking pan, drizzle evenly with oil and place in air fryer. Cook for 5 minutes.

Add the mince and garlic to the pan. Break up the mince with a fork. Cook for 5 minutes to brown the meat.

In a medium bowl or jug, mix together the spices with the tomato paste. Pour in half of the stock and stir to combine. Add the stock mixture and canned tomatoes to the air fryer pan. Stir well and season to taste. Cook for 25 minutes, stirring about every 5 minutes.

Add the canned beans, the remaining stock and cacao if using. Cook for a further 5-10 minutes, stirring halfway through.

Spoon into bowls and top with chopped coriander and grated cheese to serve.

Turmeric Fish Burgers

SERVES 4

PREP + COOK TIME: 25 MINS + 30 MINS MARINATING

DAIRY FREE

TURMERIC FISH BURGERS

4 small white fish fillets (such as flathead)

1 tbsp olive oil

½ tsp salt

1 tsp ground turmeric

4 brioche burger buns, toasted

¼ cup (60g) mayonnaise

1 cup (30g) rocket

1 beef tomato, sliced

1 tbsp olive oil

¼ white onion, very thinly sliced

¼ cup (15g) microgreens

½ red chilli, chopped (optional)

Juice of 1 lime

Pat fish dry using a paper towel.

Rub olive oil into the fillets. Next rub the salt and turmeric into the flesh. Cover and transfer to the fridge to marinate for 30 minutes.

Preheat the air fryer to 180°C.

Place the fish in an even layer in the air fryer basket. Cook for 5 minutes. Increase the temperature of the air fryer to 200°C and cook for a further 7 minutes.

Spread brioche bun bases with mayonnaise, then cover with rocket, tomato slices and a drizzle of olive oil.

Sit the fish fillets on top and scatter with onion, microgreens and chilli. Squeeze over lime juice and finish with burger bun lids.

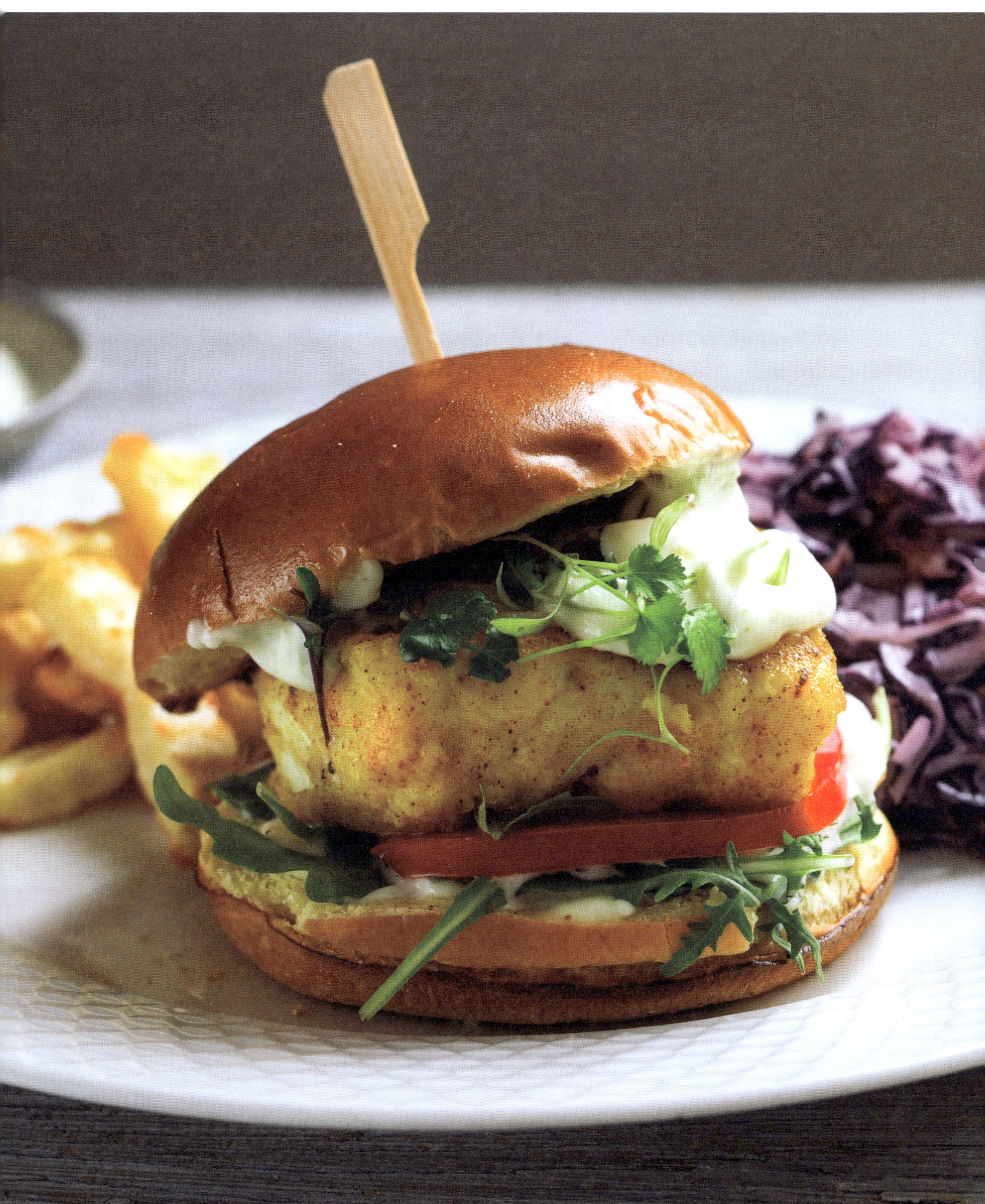

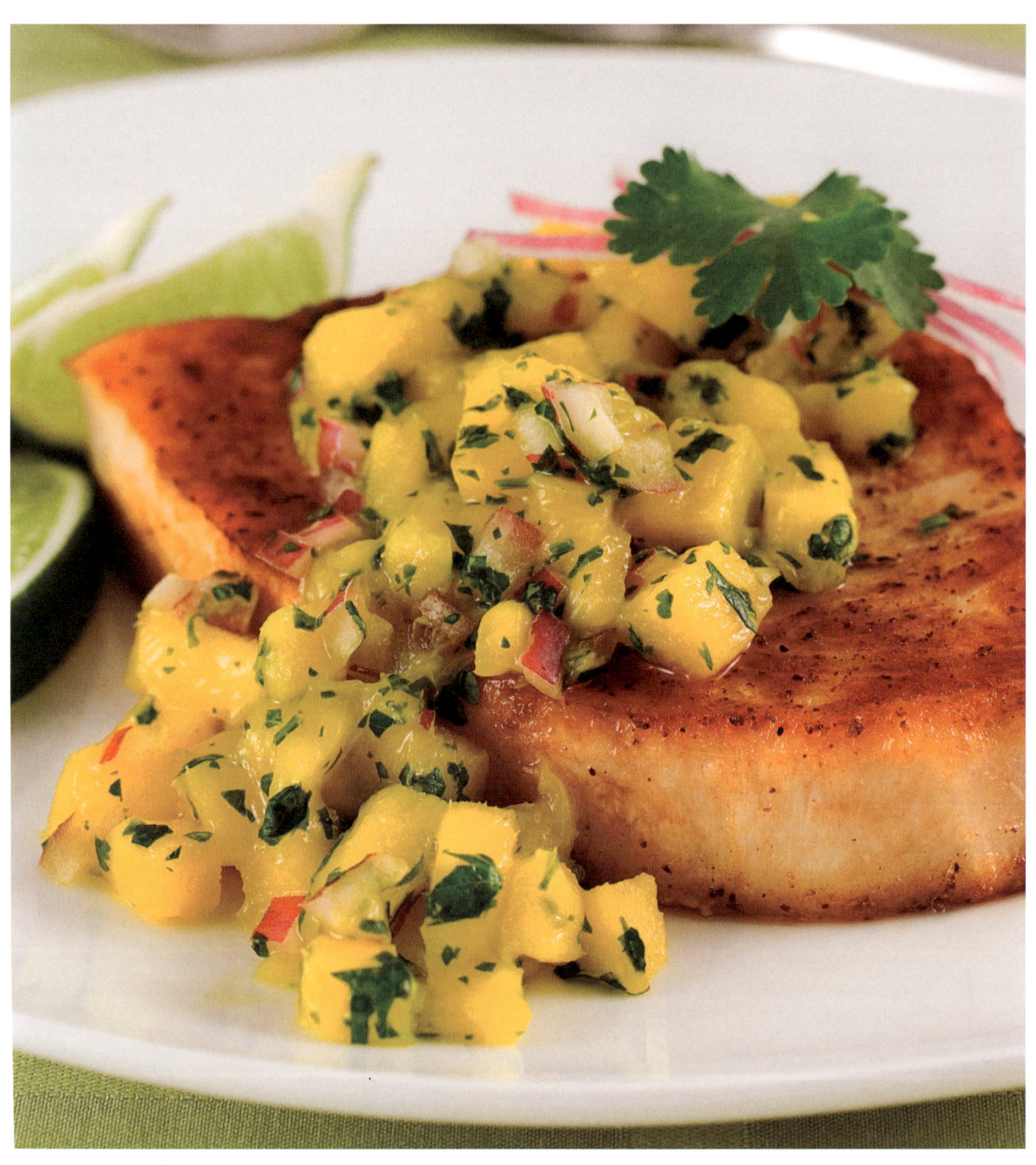

Swordfish with Mango Salsa

SERVES 4

PREP + COOK TIME: 20 MINS

GLUTEN FREE • DAIRY FREE

SWORDFISH WITH MANGO SALSA

4 swordfish steaks
Salt and pepper to taste

MANGO SALSA

2 mangoes, diced
1 red onion, finely diced
1 jalapeno, finely chopped
½ cup (20g) fresh coriander, chopped
2 tbsps lime juice

Preheat air fryer to 200°C.

Season swordfish steaks with salt and pepper. Spray all over with avocado cooking spray.

Place steaks in air fryer basket and cook for 10-12 minutes, flipping halfway through.

Combine salsa ingredients in a bowl. Stir gently. Spoon salsa over swordfish steaks to serve.

Honey Chicken Kebabs

SERVES 2

PREP + COOK TIME: 20 MINS + 1 HOUR MARINATING

DAIRY FREE

2 chicken breasts, diced

Pinch of salt and pepper

⅓ cup (115g) honey

⅓ cup (80ml) soy sauce

1 small zucchini, sliced into rounds

1 red capsicum, deseeded and cut into chunks

Skewer rack

Spray the chicken breasts with oil and season with salt and pepper.

Put the honey and soy sauce in a small bowl and whisk to combine.

Thread the chicken, zucchini and capsicum onto the skewers.

Coat kebabs with the sauce and transfer to the fridge for a minimum of 1 hour.

Preheat the air fryer to 170°C.

Place the kebabs on the skewer rack and place in the air fryer. Cook for 15 minutes.

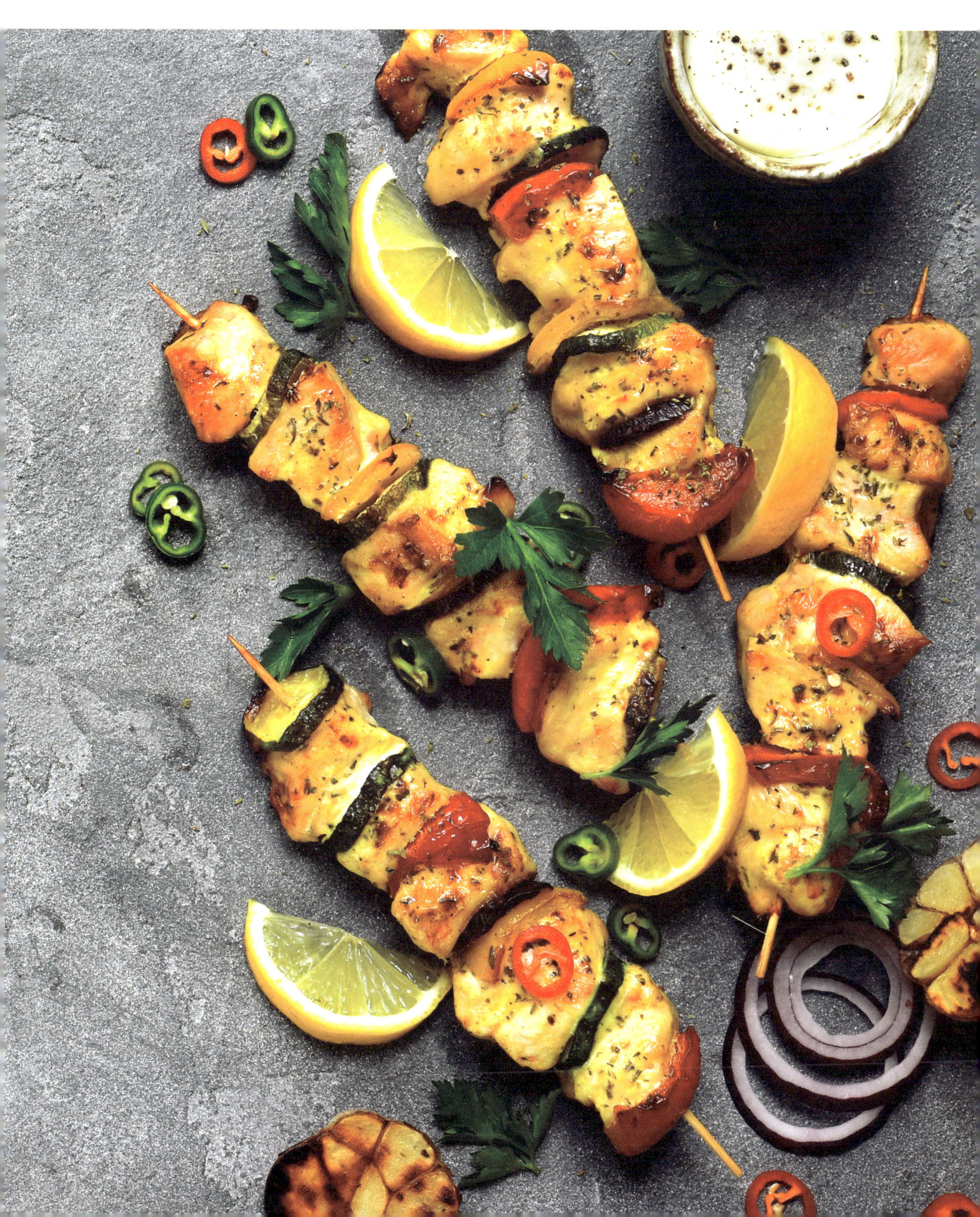

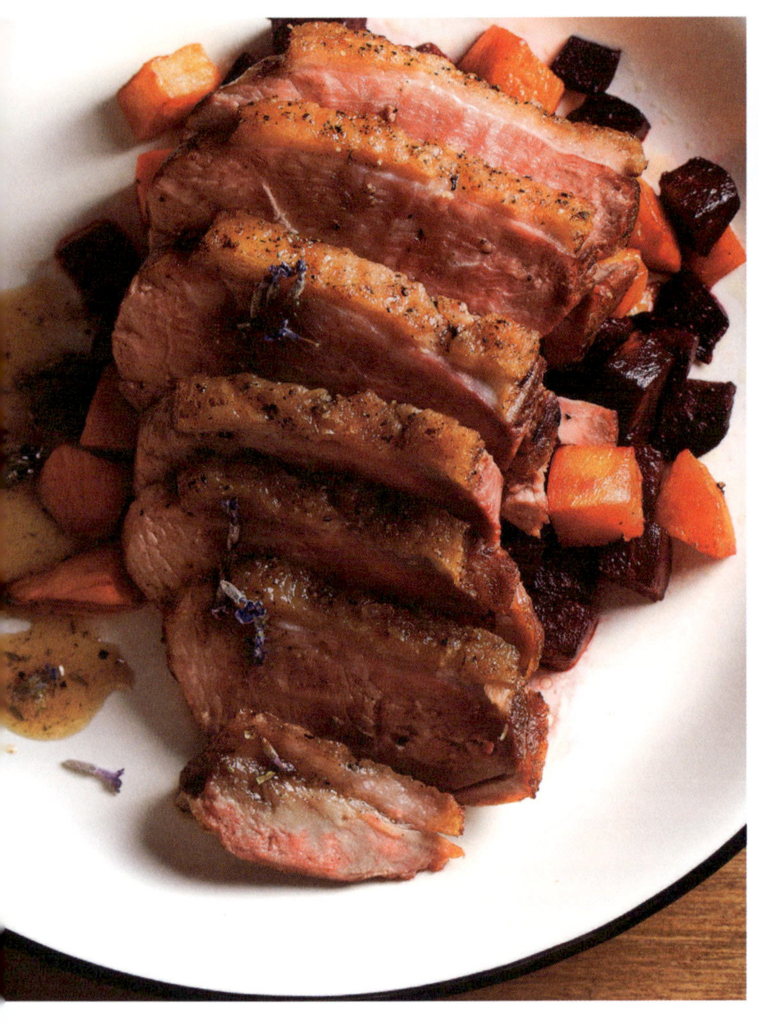

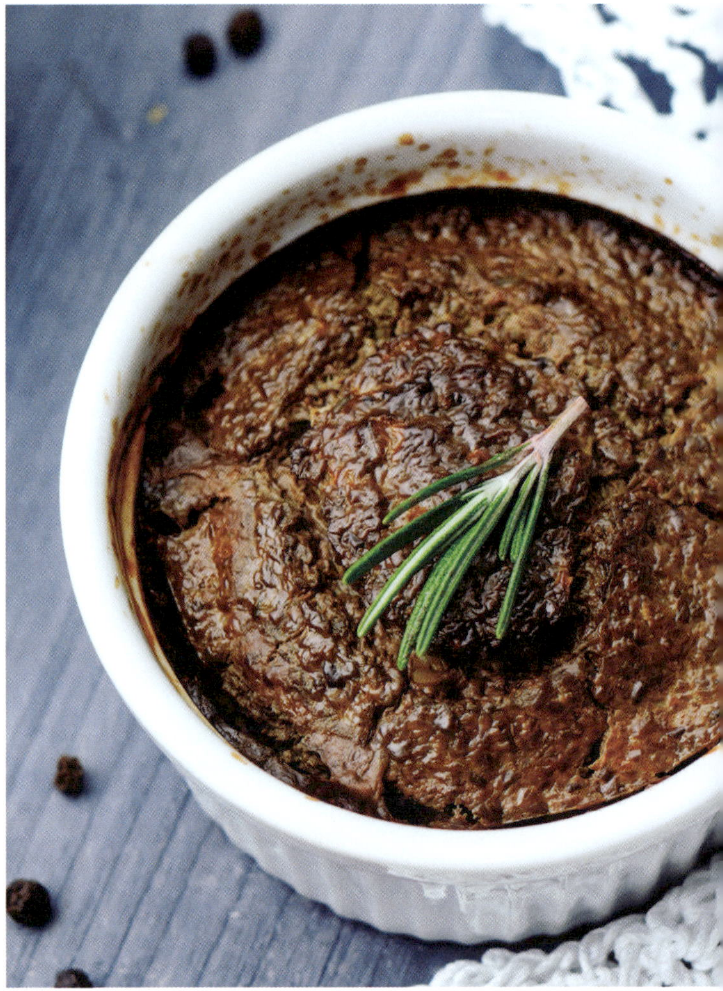

Maple Duck Breast

SERVES 2

PREP + COOK TIME: 1 HOUR

GLUTEN FREE • DAIRY FREE

Chicken Liver & Mushroom Souffle

SERVES 4

PREP + COOK TIME: 45 MINS + 1 HOUR CHILLING

GLUTEN FREE

MAPLE DUCK BREAST

2 medium beetroots, peeled and chopped

1 medium sweet potato, peeled and chopped

1 tbsp olive oil

Salt and pepper to taste

2 duck breasts, skin on

2 tbsps maple syrup

¼ tsp cayenne pepper

2 tsps brown sugar

Preheat the air fryer to 200°C.

Place beetroot and sweet potato in a bowl with olive oil, salt and pepper. Toss to coat.

Place beetroot in air fryer basket. Cook for 30 minutes, shaking every 10 minutes. After 5 minutes add in sweet potatoes. When tender set aside and keep warm.

Score duck fat several times and rub with salt and pepper.

Combine the maple syrup, cayenne pepper, and sugar in a small pan. Place over medium-low heat and stir until the sugar dissolves.

Place duck in basket skin-side up. Spray with cooking spray. Cook for 10 minutes at 200°C. Flip over and spray once more, and cook for 6-8 minutes.

Flip over once more, brush with the maple glaze and cook for a further 2 minutes. Transfer duck breast to a cutting board and allow to rest for a few minutes.

Slice duck and pour over any remaining sauce. Serve with roast vegetables.

CHICKEN LIVER AND MUSHROOM SOUFFLE

3 tbsps olive oil

300g mushrooms, finely diced

600g chicken livers, cleaned

¾ cup (200ml) kefir

1 egg

1 onion, diced

1 tbsp fresh rosemary

2 tbsps almond meal

½ tsp garlic powder

Salt and pepper to taste

25g butter

4 ramekins

Heat oil in a large frying pan over medium heat. Add mushrooms and fry for 4-6 minutes until all the liquid evaporates from the pan. Set aside to cool.

Place chicken livers in a large bowl with the kefir, egg, diced onion and rosemary. Use a stick blender to blend until smooth.

Stir in almond meal, garlic powder and salt and pepper. Cover and refrigerate for 1 hour.

Add the cooled mushrooms to the bowl and stir to combine.

Grease four ramekins with the butter.

Pour mixture into ramekins and place in air fryer basket.

Cook at 160°C for about 30 minutes or until completely set.

CHICKEN SCHNITZEL

3 tbsps vegetable oil
1⅔ cups (200g) breadcrumbs
½ tsp salt
1 egg
400g thin chicken schnitzels
1 tbsp butter
8 large sage leaves
Lemon slices, to serve

Preheat air fryer to 180°C.

Combine the oil, breadcrumbs and salt together until a crumbly mixture forms. Place on a plate or in a shallow bowl.

Beat the egg in another shallow bowl.

Dip each schnitzel into the egg, shaking off any excess. Then dip into the crumb mix, pressing to ensure they are evenly and fully covered.

Place the schnitzel in the air fryer basket. (Be careful not to overcrowd the basket. Cook in batches or use a double-layer accessory if needed.)

Cook for 8 minutes until golden, removing and shaking the basket halfway.

A few minutes before serving, heat the butter in a small pan until it begins to sizzle. Add sage leaves and cook for 30 seconds until just crispy. Serve on top of the schnitzel with lemon wedges.

FRENCH FRIES

1kg frozen French fries
Salt to taste

Preheat the air fryer to 200°C.

Place the frozen fries in the air fryer basket and spread evenly over the base.

Cook for 15 minutes, removing and shaking the basket a couple of times during cooking.

Continue to cook for a few extra minutes if needed to crisp up the fries.

Season with salt before serving.

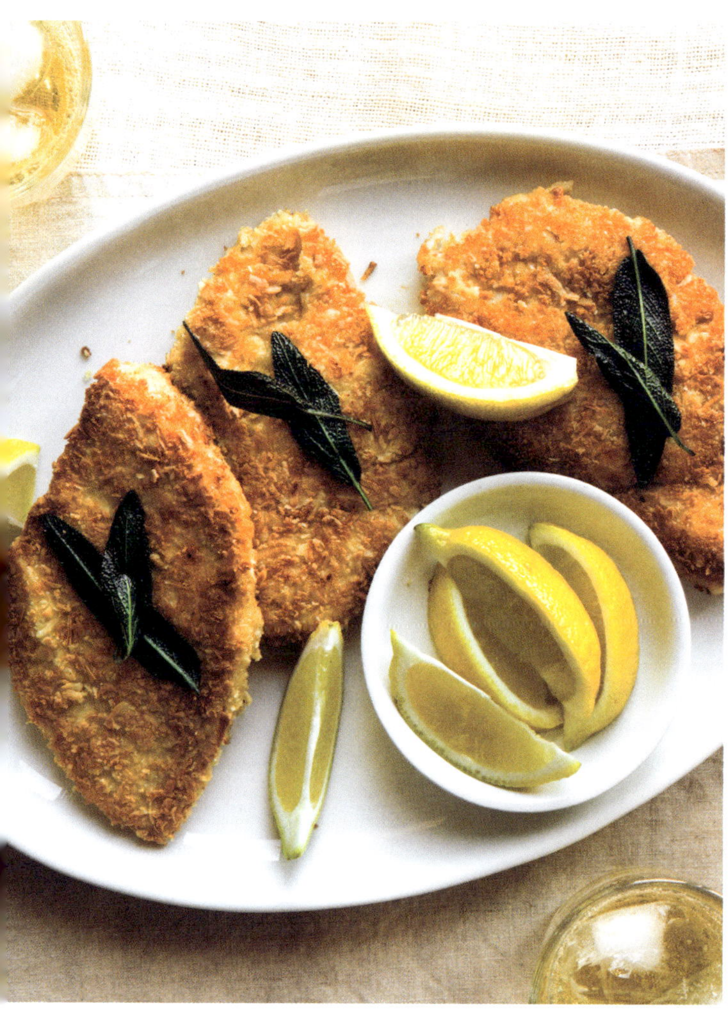

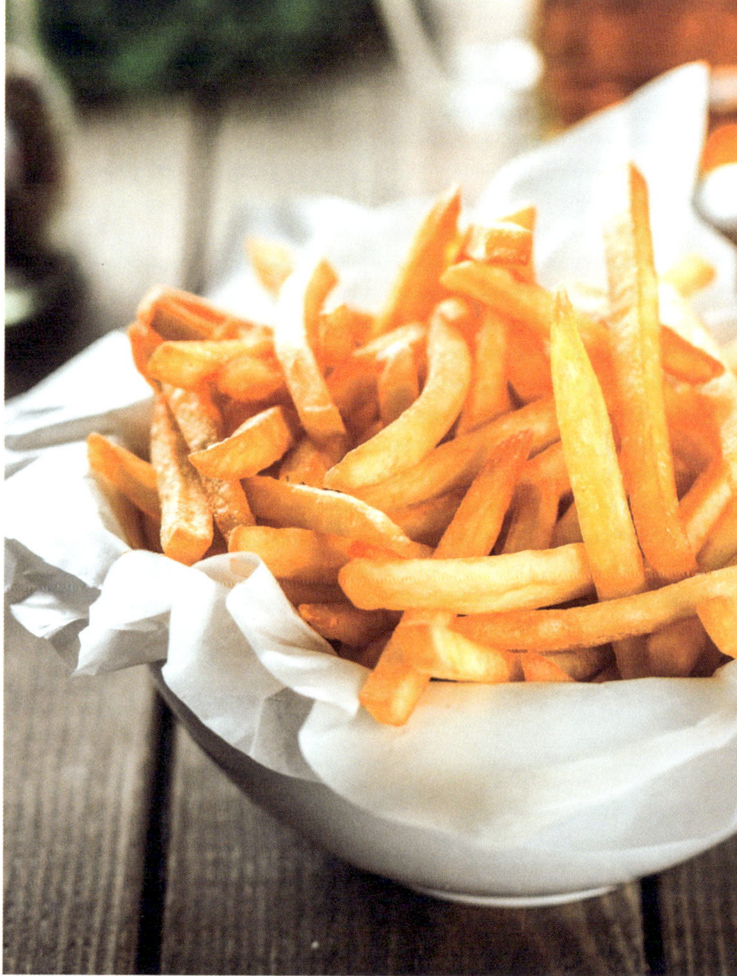

Chicken Schnitzel

SERVES 4

PREP + COOK TIME: 15 MINS

DAIRY FREE

French Fries

SERVES 4

PREP + COOK TIME: 20 MINS

VEG • GLUTEN FREE • DAIRY FREE

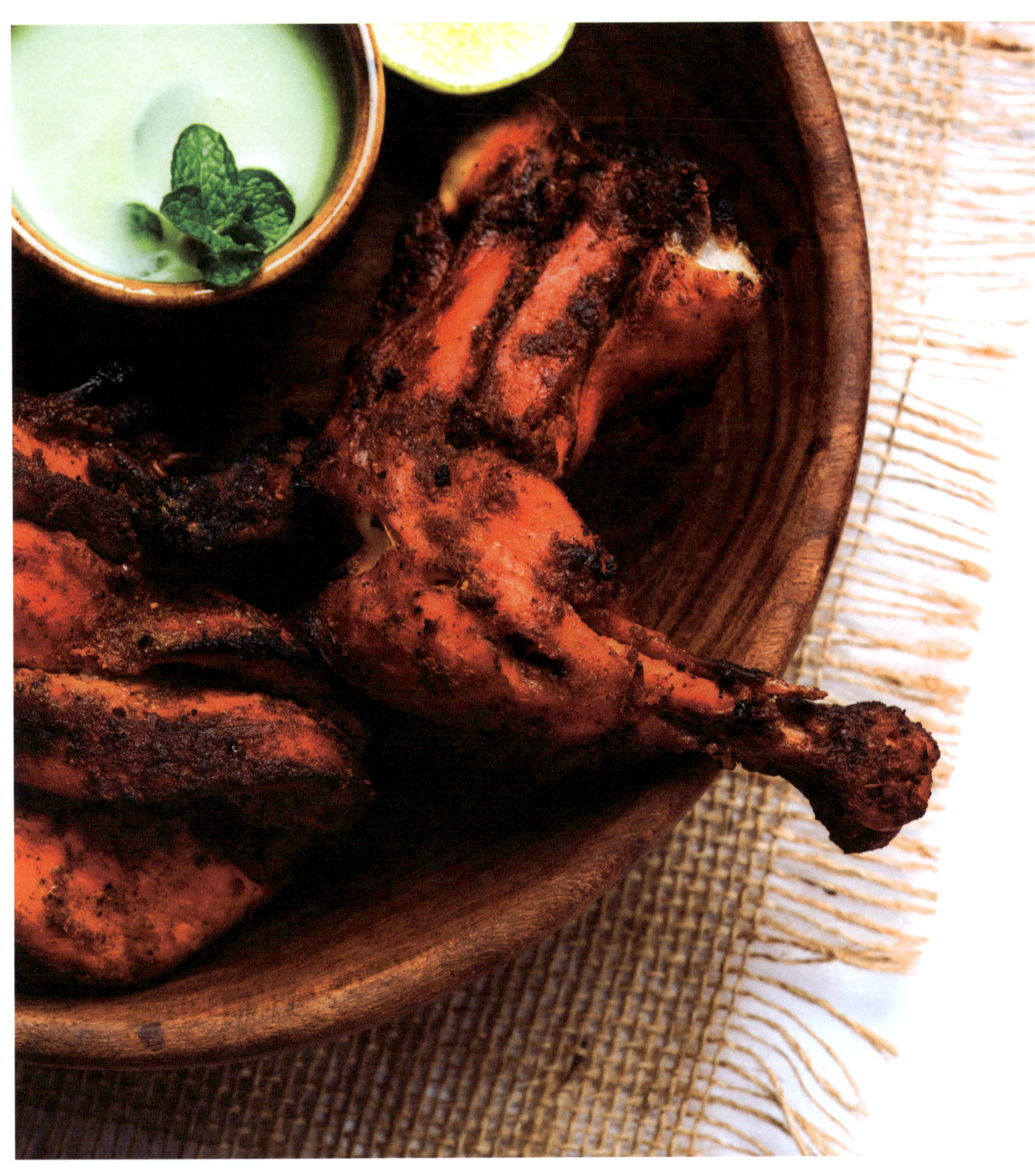

Tandoori Roasted Chicken Legs

SERVES 2

PREP + COOK TIME: 50 MINS + MARINATING

GLUTEN FREE

TANDOORI ROASTED CHICKEN LEGS

2 chicken Marylands

MARINADE

1 cup (250ml) Greek yoghurt

1 tbsp peanut oil

1 tbsp lemon juice

Small piece ginger, grated

3 cloves garlic, minced

2 tsps garam masala

1 tbsp smoked paprika

½ tsp ground turmeric

2 tsps ground cumin

2 tsps ground coriander

½ tsp chilli powder

½ tsp salt

MINT YOGHURT

⅔ cup (160ml) Greek yoghurt

⅓ cup (5g) mint leaves

Salt and pepper to taste

1 tsp olive oil

Place all the marinade ingredients in a large bowl. Mix well then add the chicken. Coat the chicken in the marinade, then cover and refrigerate for 12-24 hours.

Preheat air fryer to 200°C.

Remove chicken from marinade (retaining marinade for later). Place chicken in air fryer basket, in a single layer, skin-side down. Cook for 10 minutes.

Baste with marinade and cook for a further 15 minutes.

Flip over and baste once more. Cook for a further 10-12 minutes or until cooked through.

Allow the chicken to rest for 5 minutes before serving.

To make the mint yoghurt, place all of the ingredients into a food processor and blitz until smooth. Serve with the chicken.

GARLIC PRAWN KEBABS

500g raw prawns, peeled and deveined
¼ tsp garlic powder
½ chilli, finely chopped
1 tbsp avocado or olive oil
2 tbsps chopped fresh coriander
Salt and pepper to taste
Juice of 1 lime
Skewer rack

Place the prawns in a large bowl with garlic, chilli, oil and coriander. Season with salt and pepper and toss to coat.

Thread the prawns onto skewers and arrange in air fryer basket.

Cook for 10-14 minutes at 200°C until just pink.

Squeeze over lime juice to serve.

CHICKEN LIVERS WITH ONIONS

400g chicken livers, washed
1 onion, sliced
25g butter or 2 tbsps olive oil
Salt and pepper to taste
1 tbsp chopped parsley, to serve
Baking pan

Place chicken livers, onion and butter or olive oil in baking pan.

Cook for 15-20 minutes at 190°C, stirring after 2 minutes then again after 10 minutes.

Season well with salt and pepper, then spoon onto plates and sprinkle with chopped parsley to serve.

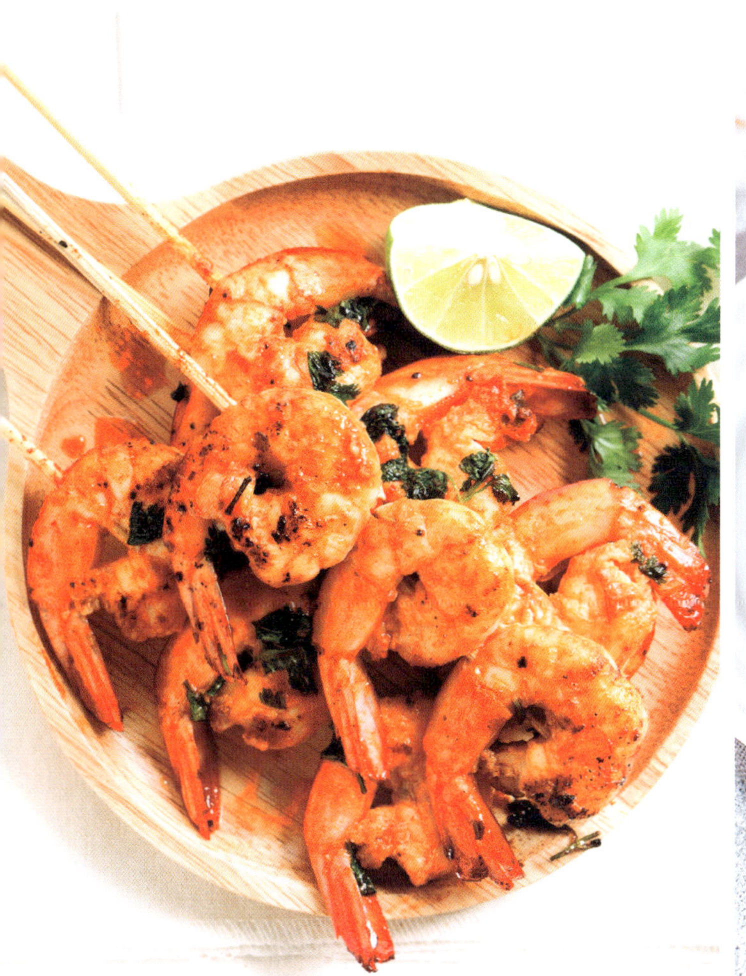

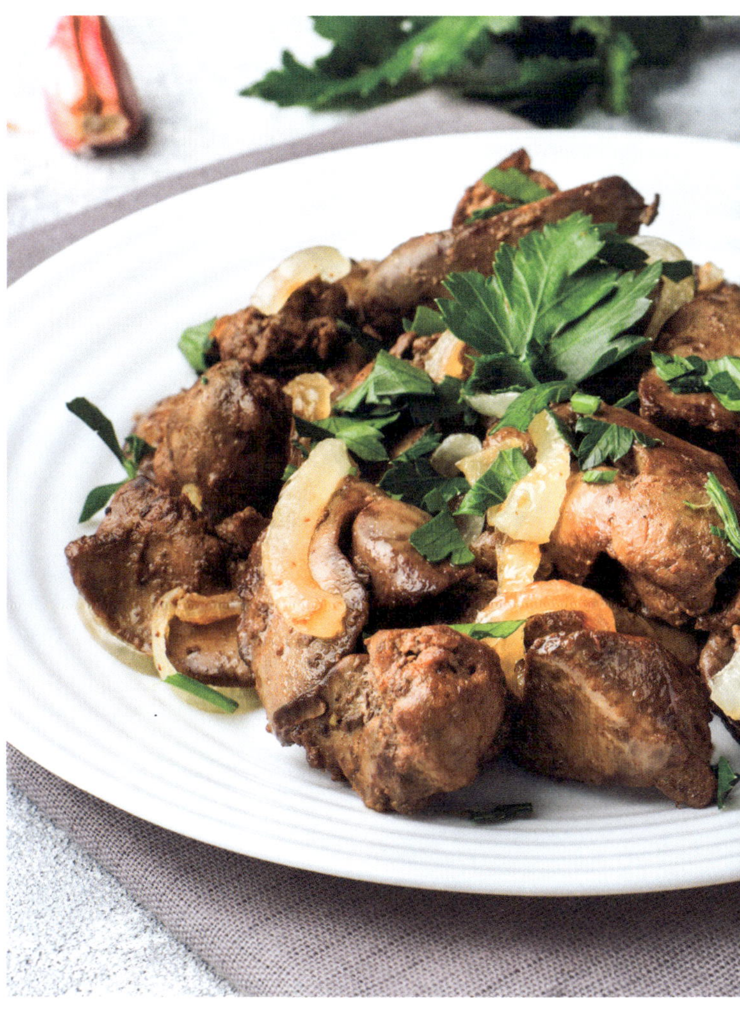

Garlic Prawn Kebabs

SERVES 2

PREP + COOK TIME: 20 MINS

GLUTEN FREE • DAIRY FREE

Chicken Livers with Onions

SERVES 2

PREP + COOK TIME: 25 MINS

GLUTEN FREE

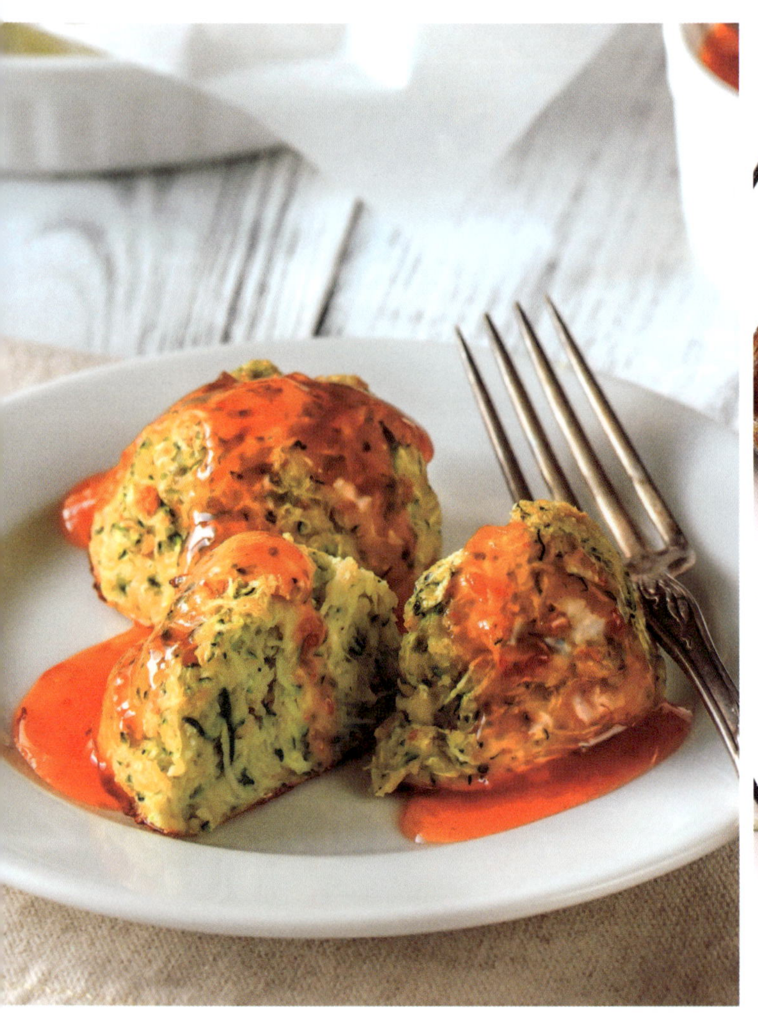

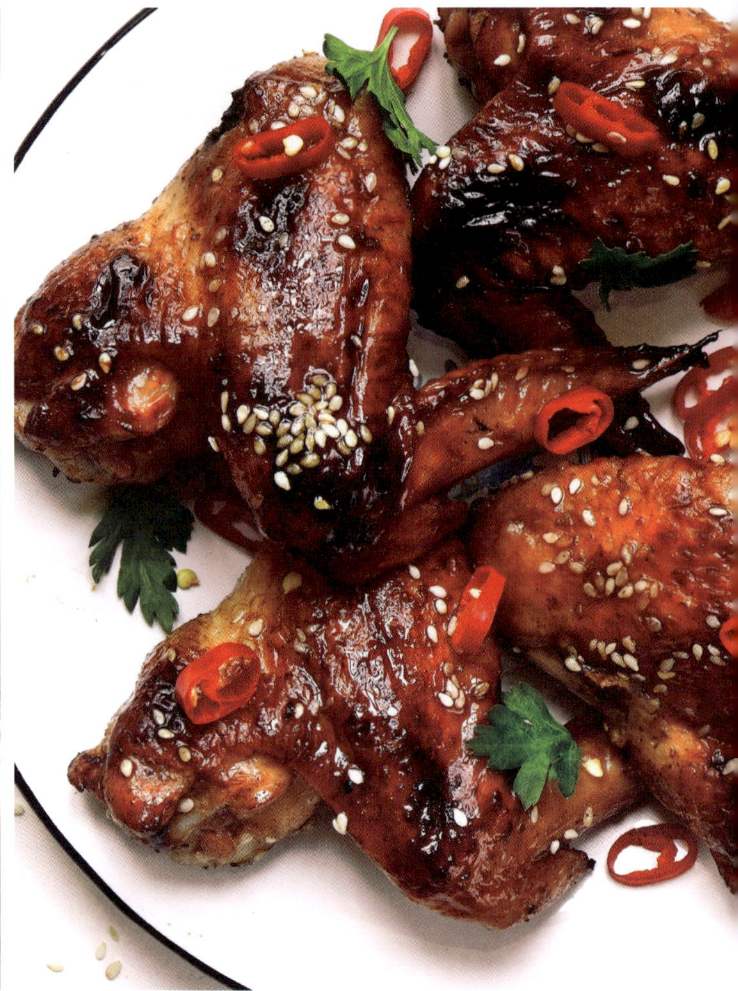

Vegetable Tots

SERVES 2

PREP + COOK TIME: 20 MINS + 1 HOUR CHILLING

VEG

Honey Chicken Wings

SERVES 2

PREP + COOK TIME: 25 MINS + 2 HOURS MARINATING

DAIRY FREE

VEGETABLE TOTS

½ cup (60g) plain flour

¼ tsp salt

1 tsp garlic powder

2 tsp dried basil

2 medium zucchinis

1 small onion, peeled

2 eggs + 1 egg white

½ cup (50g) Parmesan cheese, finely grated

Sweet chilli sauce, to serve

Preheat the air fryer to 200°C.

Grate the zucchinis and onion. Squeeze the liquid out by placing the grated vegetables in a tea towel, rolling up the towel and twisting it.

In a medium bowl, combine all the ingredients.

The mixture should be thick but quite soft. For best results, cover the bowl and place the mixture in the refrigerator to chill for 1 hour.

Form balls using wet hands, and place in the air fryer in a single layer. (Be careful not to overcrowd the basket. Cook in batches or use a double layer accessory if needed.)

Cook for 10 minutes.

Serve with sweet chilli sauce.

HONEY CHICKEN WINGS

6 chicken wings

3 tsps honey

1 tsp sesame oil

2 tsps soy sauce

1 tsp dark soy sauce

Pinch of pepper

1 tbsp sesame seeds

Whisk all the ingredients except the chicken wings in a large bowl. Add the chicken wings and stir to fully coat them.

Cover and transfer to the refrigerator to marinate for 2 hours.

Place the wings in the air fryer basket and cook for 20 minutes at 180°C, turning halfway.

Sprinkle with sesame seeds to serve.

Lemon Cauliflower Chicken

SERVES 2

PREP + COOK TIME: 30 MINS

GLUTEN FREE • DAIRY FREE

2 chicken breasts, each cut into 4 equal pieces

1½ cups (150g) cauliflower florets

4 tbsps olive oil

1 tbsp fresh rosemary, minced

1 tbsp fresh thyme, minced

1 tsp grated lemon zest

2 tbsps lemon juice

½ tsp salt

¼ tsp pepper

¼ tsp dried chilli flakes

Garden salad, to serve

Preheat air fryer to 175°C.

Place chicken and cauliflower in a large bowl with olive oil, rosemary, thyme, lemon zest, lemon juice, salt, pepper and chilli flakes. Toss to coat.

Remove chicken from the bowl and place in air fryer basket. Cook for 10-12 minutes until cooked through, flipping halfway. Remove chicken from air fryer and cover with foil to keep warm.

Add cauliflower to air fryer. Cook for 8-10 minutes, stirring halfway through, until florets are tender and edges are browned.

Serve chicken and cauliflower together with a garden salad.

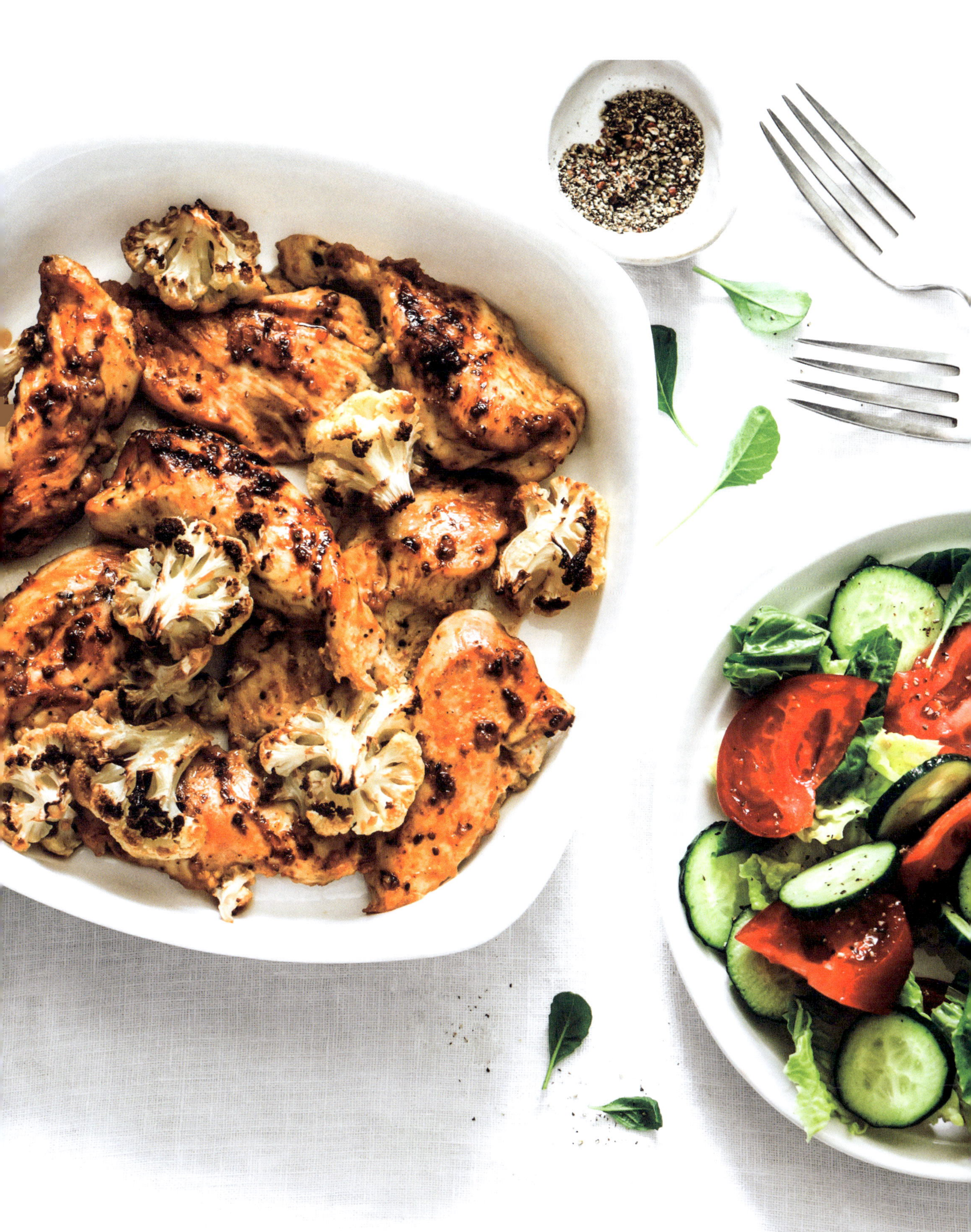

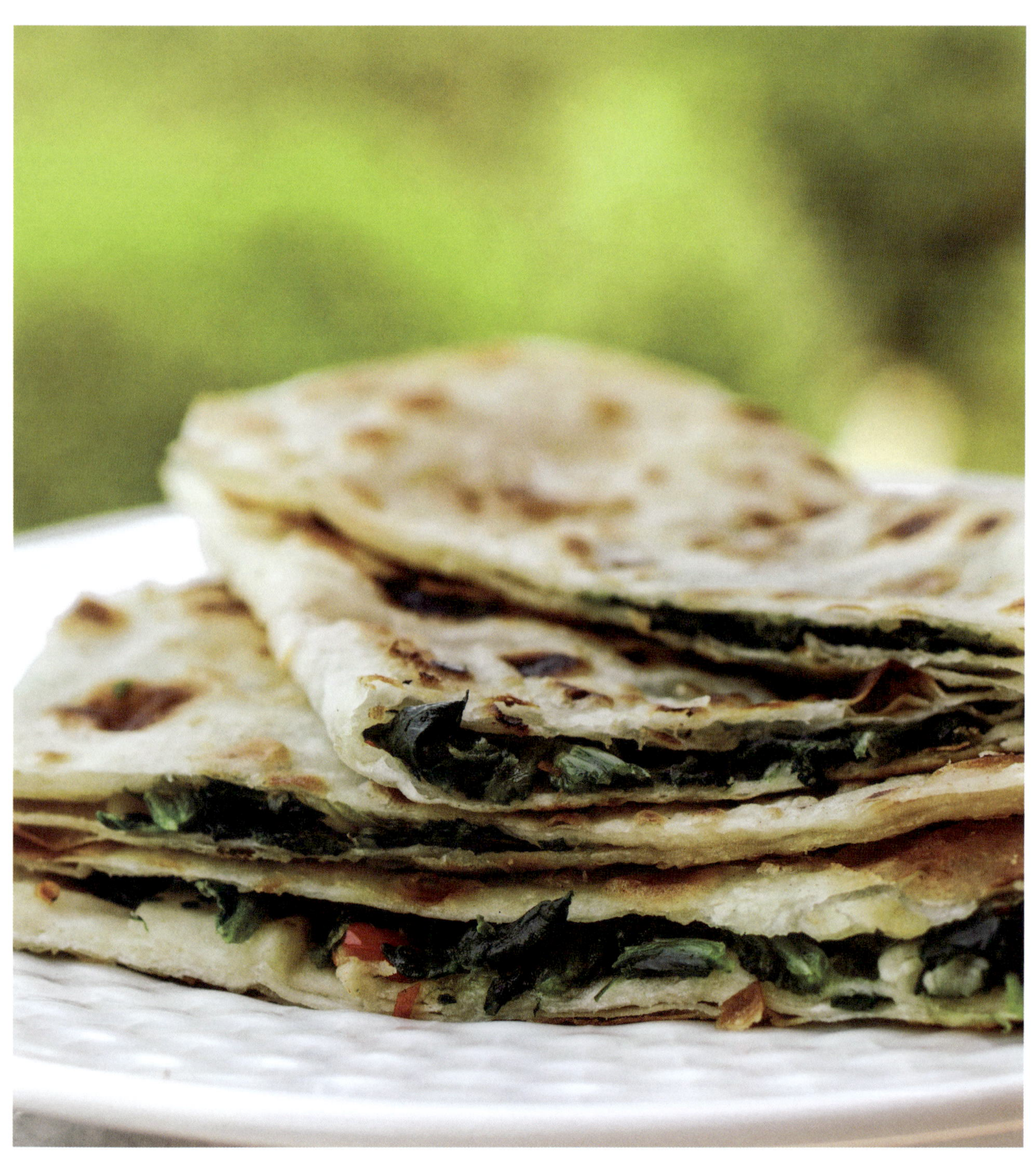

Spinach Gozleme

SERVES 6

PREP + COOK TIME: 1 HOUR + RESTING

VEG

SPINACH GOZLEME

2 cups (270g) plain flour
3 tbsps Greek yoghurt
½ tsp baking powder
½ tsp dry yeast
½ tsp salt flakes
½ cup (150ml) warm water
2 tbsps olive oil
2 cups (60g) baby spinach leaves, chopped
1 cup (245g) crumbled feta
1 red chilli, chopped (optional)
Lemon wedges, to serve

Combine flour, yoghurt, baking powder, yeast, salt and water in a large bowl. Stir to combine, then turn onto a floured work surface and knead until smooth.

Return to the bowl and set in a warm place for 30 minutes.

Knead in the olive oil to get a smooth dough ball. Cover and set aside for another 30 minutes.

Divide dough into six balls. Roll each ball into a large rectangle. as thin as you can without tearing the pastry. Scatter spinach, feta and chilli (if using) in the centre of the pastry. Fold the ends over like an envelope, brushing with water to seal. Spray with cooking spray.

Cook one at a time in the air fryer for 5 minutes each side at 210°C until golden brown. Serve with lemon wedges.

BAKED TROUT WITH LEMON & HERBS

1 whole trout, deboned
Salt and pepper to taste
1 lemon, sliced
3-4 sprigs fresh dill
3-4 sprigs fresh parsley
1 tbsp olive oil

Season the inside of the trout with salt and pepper.

Arrange half the lemon slices in a single layer inside the fish and top with the herbs. Drizzle the outside of the fish with olive oil. Rub all over the skin.

Place trout in air fryer basket. Lay the remaining lemon slices on top of the skin.

Cook for 15 minutes at 170°C or until the flesh flakes easily with a fork.

GLUTEN-FREE MEATBALLS

500g beef mince
1 cup (100g) grated Parmesan cheese
¼ cup (60ml) milk
2 cloves garlic, minced
2 tsps Italian seasoning
Salt and pepper to taste
Homemade or store-bought pasta sauce, to serve

Combine mince, cheese, milk, garlic and herbs in a bowl. Season with salt and pepper and mix well. Roll into golf-ball-sized meatballs.

Place meatballs into air fryer basket in a single layer, making sure they are spaced apart.

Air fry the meatballs at 190°C for 15 minutes.

Serve meatballs with warmed pasta sauce.

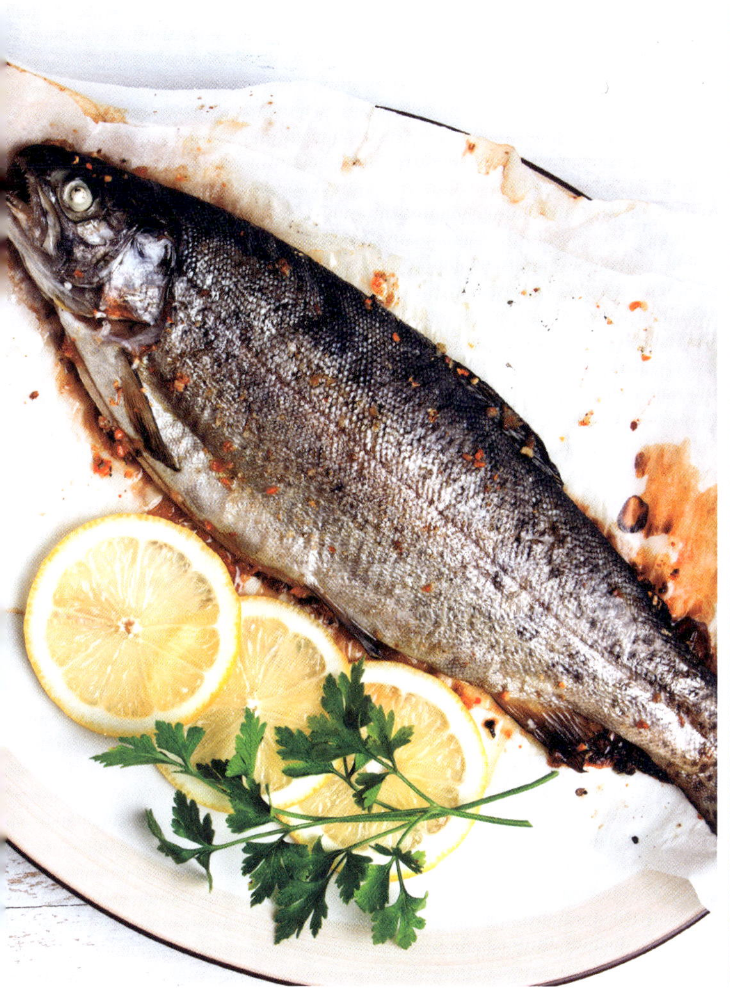

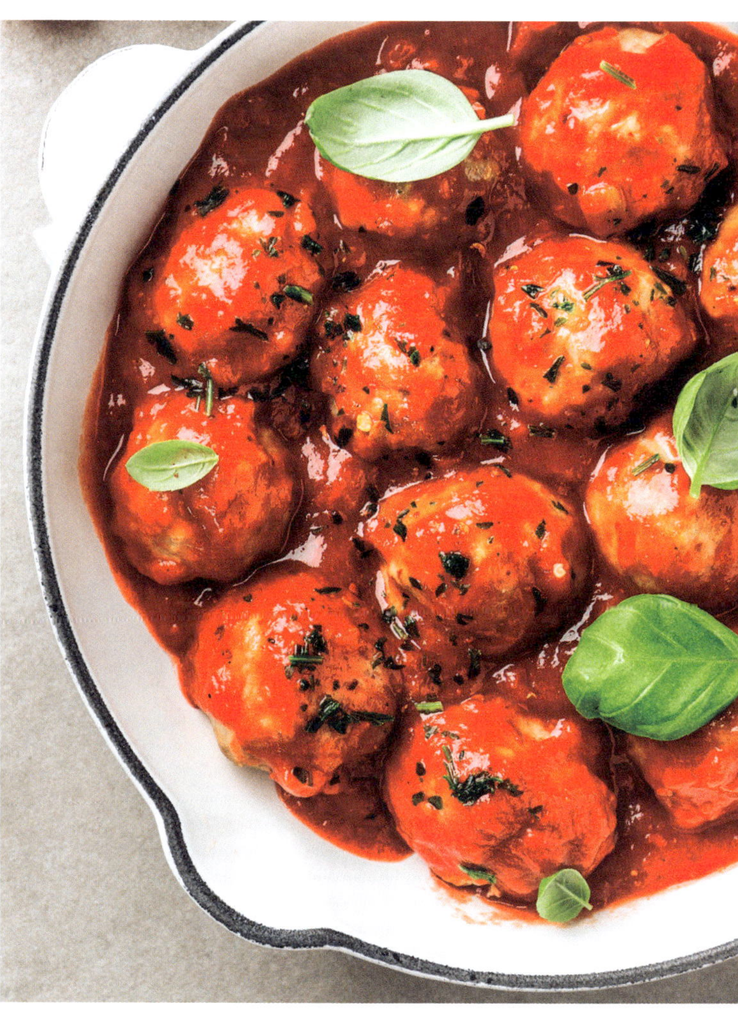

Baked Trout with Lemon & Herbs

SERVES 2

PREP + COOK TIME: 20 MINS

GLUTEN FREE • DAIRY FREE

Gluten-Free Meatballs

SERVES 4

PREP + COOK TIME: 25 MINS

GLUTEN FREE

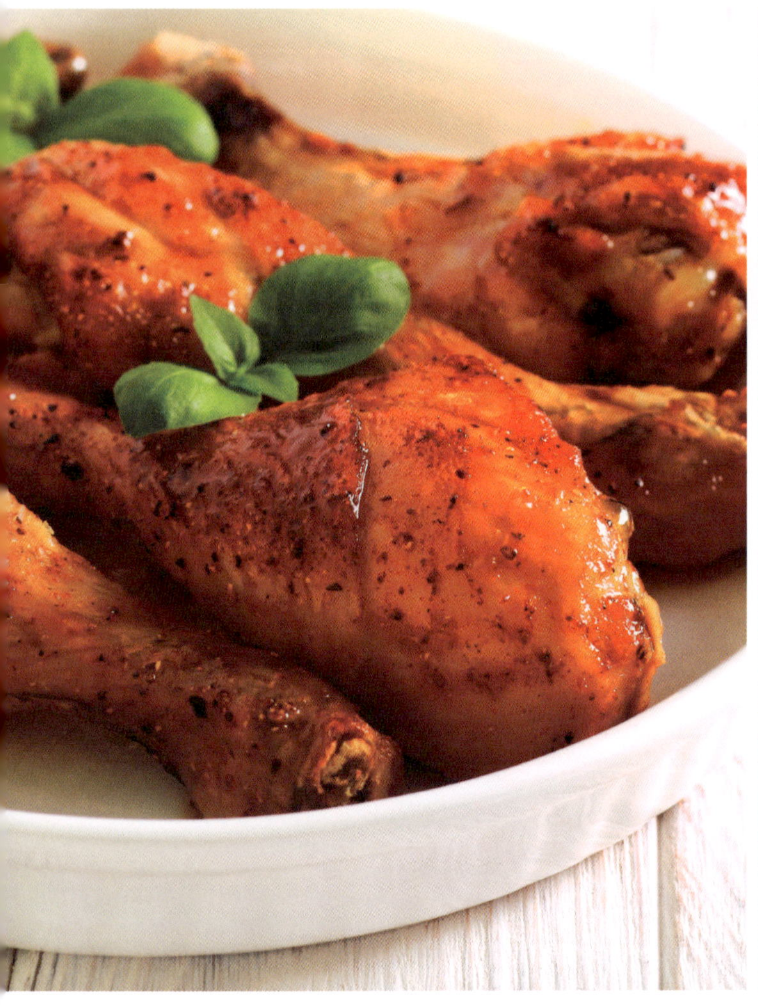

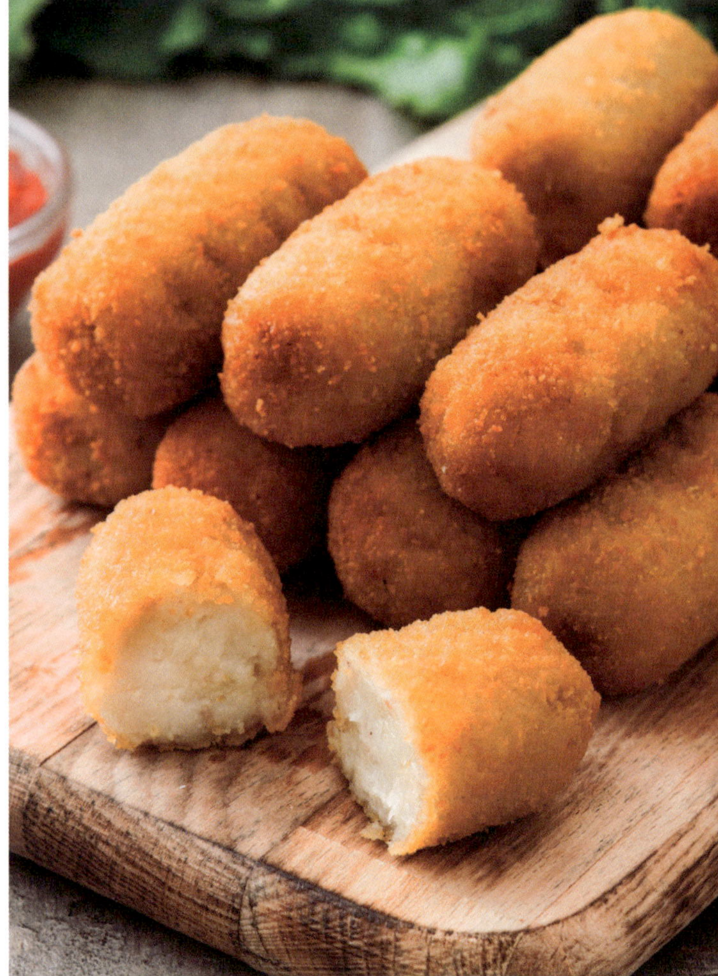

Chicken Tikka Drumsticks

SERVES 4

PREP + COOK TIME: 35 MINS + 1 HOUR MARINATING

GLUTEN FREE • DAIRY FREE

Cheese & Ham Croquettes

SERVES 4

PREP + COOK TIME: 15 MINS

VEG

CHICKEN TIKKA DRUMSTICKS

8 chicken drumsticks
1 x 280g jar tikka masala curry paste (such as Patak's)

Place the chicken drumsticks in a large bowl. Add the curry paste and stir to coat thoroughly and evenly. Cover with plastic wrap and transfer to the fridge to marinate for 1 hour.

Preheat the air fryer to 180°C.

Remove the drumsticks from the fridge and shake off any excess marinade.

Transfer to the air fryer basket.

Cook for 30 minutes.

CHEESE & HAM CROQUETTES

300g (8-pack) frozen cheese and ham potato croquettes

Preheat the air fryer to 180°C.

Place all the frozen potato croquettes in the air fryer basket.

Cook for 13 minutes, turning halfway.

Salmon & Green Beans

SERVES 4
PREP + COOK TIME: 20 MINS
GLUTEN FREE

SALMON

4 x 175g salmon fillets

Salt and pepper to taste

1 tbsp olive oil

Lemon wedges to serve

GREEN BEANS

500g green beans

2 tsps olive oil

Salt and pepper to taste

Preheat air fryer to 190°C.

Season salmon all over with salt and pepper and rub with olive oil.

Place skin-side down in the air fryer basket and cook for 6-8 minutes until salmon is opaque and flakes easily with a fork. Cover the salmon with foil and set aside to rest while you cook the green beans.

Drizzle the green beans with olive oil and season with salt and pepper. Transfer to the air fryer and cook at 190°C for 7-8 minutes, shaking the basket halfway through cooking.

Serve the salmon with green beans and lemon wedges.

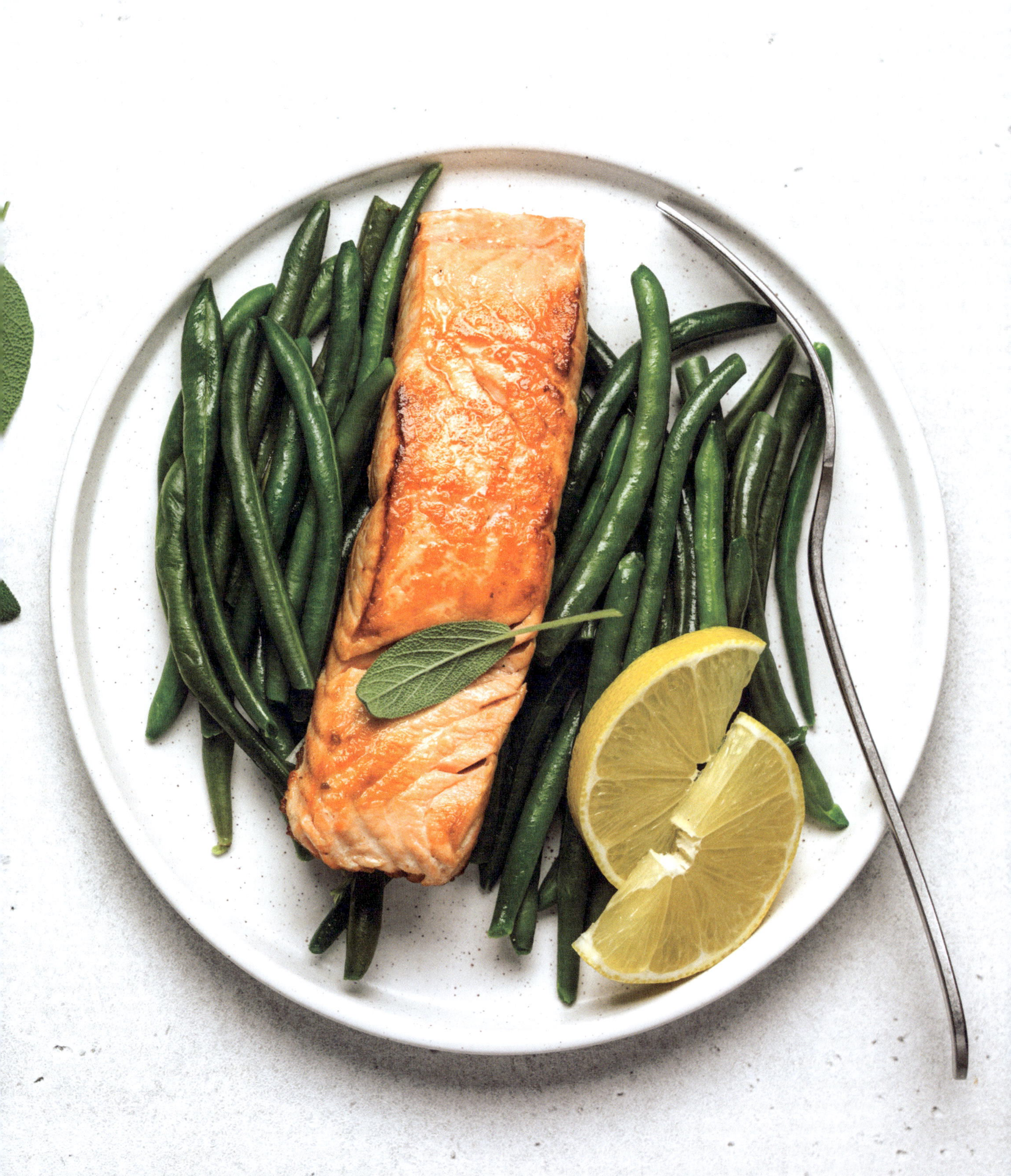

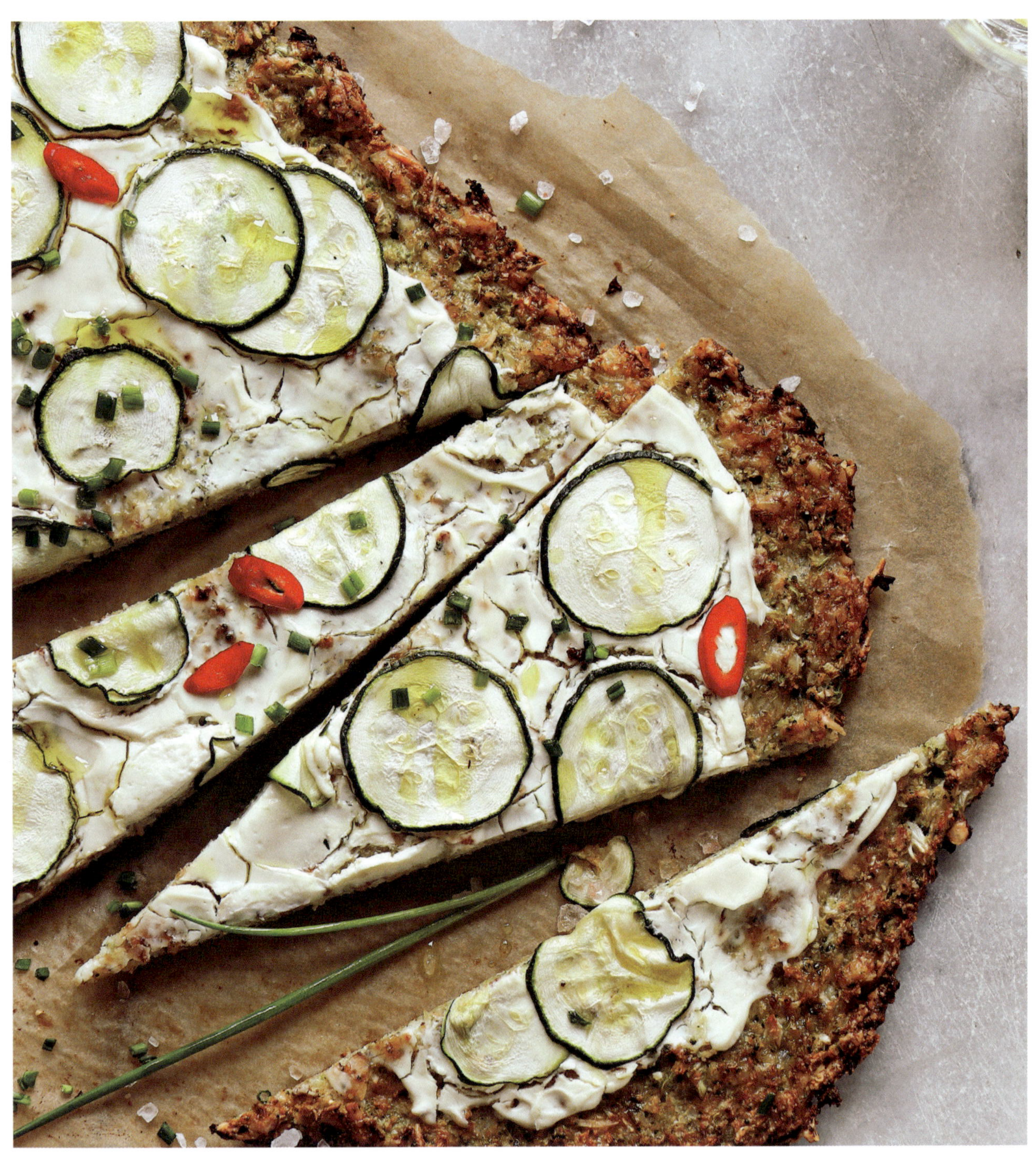

Cauliflower Crust Pizza

SERVES 2

PREP + COOK TIME: 50 MINS

VEG • GLUTEN FREE

CAULIFLOWER CRUST PIZZA

1 head of cauliflower, broken into florets

½ cup (60g) shredded mozzarella cheese

¼ cup (25g) grated Parmesan cheese

½ tsp dried oregano

¼ tsp salt

¼ tsp garlic powder

2 eggs, lightly beaten

100g cream cheese

1 zucchini, thinly sliced

1 tbsp olive oil

1 tbsp chives, chopped

½ red chilli, sliced

Place cauliflower in a food processor and pulse until it resembles rice.

Steam cauliflower in a steamer basket for 5 minutes until tender or microwave for 5 minutes in a covered bowl. Drain well. Pat dry with a clean tea towel or paper towels.

In a large bowl, combine mozzarella, Parmesan, oregano, salt, garlic powder and eggs. Add the cauliflower and use a rubber spatula to mix.

Transfer mixture to a piece of greaseproof paper and shape into a pizza crust that will fit into your air fryer. If you have a regular-sized air fryer you will need to make two crusts and cook one at a time.

Use the greaseproof paper to lift the pizza crust into the air fryer.

Cook for 14 minutes at 175°C.

Using the greaseproof paper, gently lift the crust out of the air fryer. Place an upturned plate on top of the crust. With one hand under the greaseproof paper and one hand on the plate, flip the crust over onto the plate, then carefully slide back onto the greaseproof paper, so now the bottom side is up.

Spread the crust with cream cheese. Arrange zucchini slices on the cream cheese and drizzle with oil.

Return crust to air fryer and cook for 3-4 minutes at 175°C.

Remove from air fryer and scatter with chives and chillies to serve.

Fish Tacos with Salsa & Slaw

SERVES 2 (MAKES 4)
PREP + COOK TIME: 30 MINS
DAIRY FREE

2 white fish fillets (such as snapper)
1 tsp chilli powder
1 tsp ground cumin
1 tsp smoked paprika
½ tsp garlic powder
½ tsp onion powder
½ tsp salt
4 tortillas
1 avocado, chopped
Lime wedges, to serve
2 tbsps chopped fresh coriander, to serve

SALSA

2 medium ripe tomatoes, finely diced
½ green capsicum, finely diced
1 tbsp finely diced red onion
2 tbsps chopped fresh coriander
1 tbsp lime juice
Pinch of salt

SLAW

½ cup (50g) red cabbage, sliced
½ cup (50g) green cabbage, sliced
1 tbsp mayonnaise
2 tsps lime juice
½ clove garlic, minced
Pinch of salt

Prepare the fish by cleaning and cutting into four small fillets.

Place the chilli powder, cumin, paprika, garlic powder, onion powder and salt in a large ziplock bag and then add the fish. Seal the bag and gently rub the seasoning mix into the flesh of the fish.

Place tomatoes, capsicum, red onion, coriander, lime juice and a pinch of salt in a bowl and mix well to combine. Set aside.

In another bowl combine red and green cabbage, mayonnaise, lime juice, garlic and salt. Toss to coat.

Preheat the air fryer to 180°C.

Remove fish from the bag and place in air fryer basket. Cook for 10 minutes.

To serve place each fish piece inside a tortilla, then top with salsa, slaw and avocado slices. Squeeze over lime wedges and scatter with fresh coriander to serve.

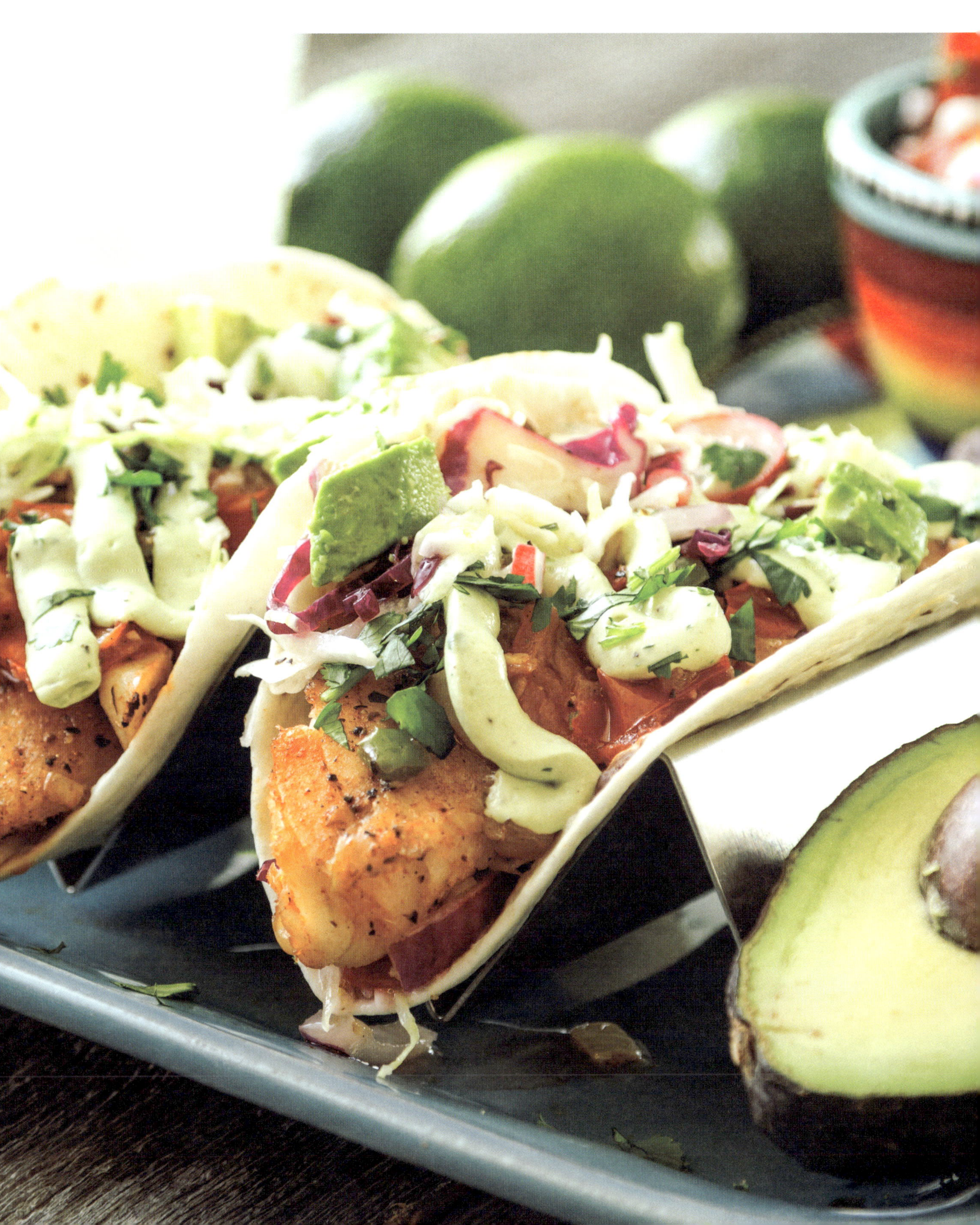

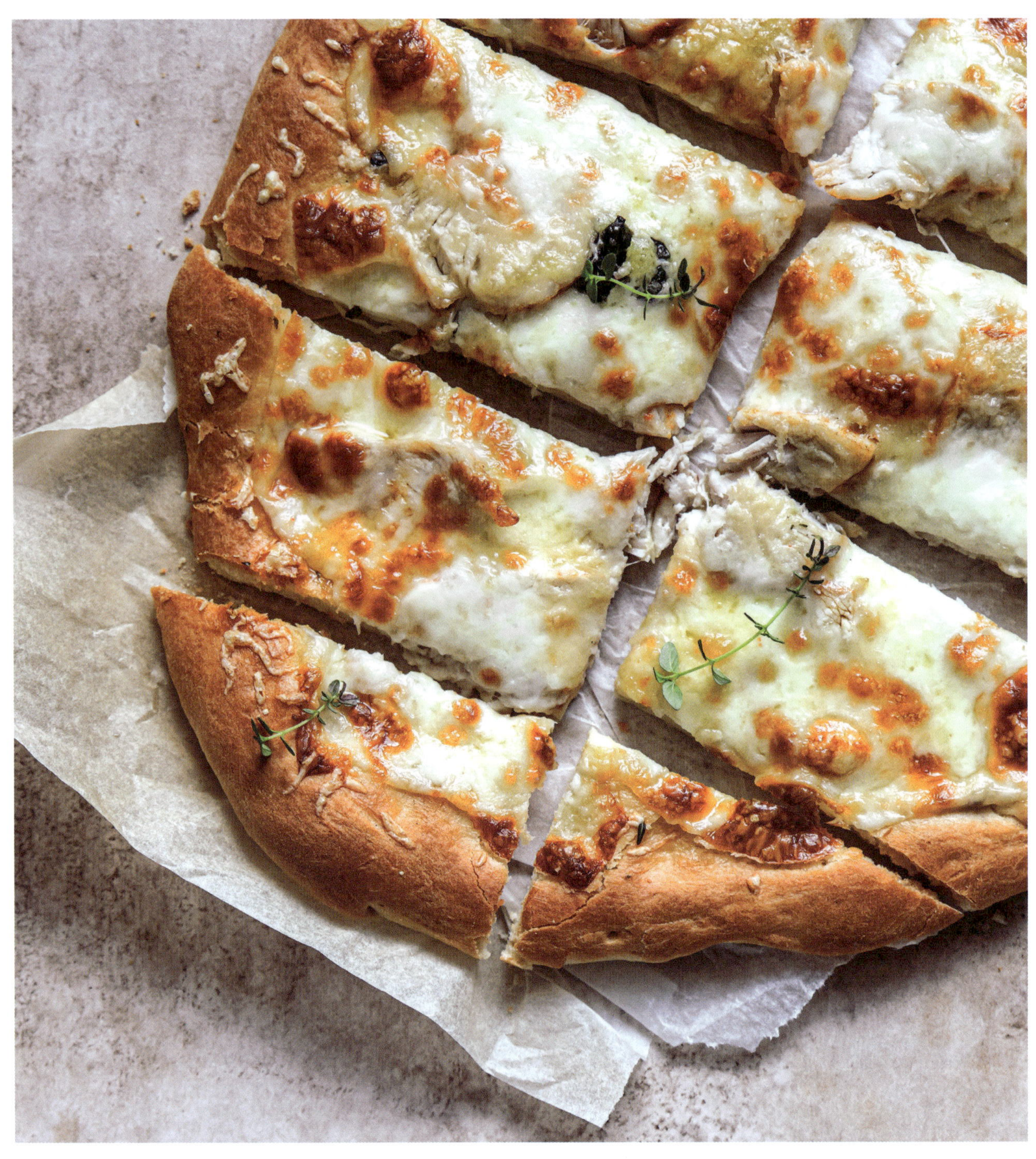

Garlic Chicken Pizza

SERVES 1-2

PREP + COOK TIME: 25 MINS

GARLIC CHICKEN PIZZA

2 chicken thigh fillets
2 tsps olive oil
2 cloves garlic, minced
2 tsps fresh thyme leaves
Salt and pepper to taste
1 x 16-20cm pizza base
100g mozzarella cheese, grated or sliced

Place the chicken thighs in a bowl along with olive oil, garlic and thyme. Season with salt and pepper and toss to coat.

Place chicken thighs into the air fryer basket cook for 10 minutes at 180°C.

Transfer the chicken to a cutting board and shred with two forks.

Scatter the chicken on top of the pizza base, then top with mozzarella cheese.

Place the pizza in the air fryer and cook at 190°C for 7-8 minutes until the crust is brown and crispy and the cheese is melted.

Rack of Lamb with Macadamia & Rosemary Crust

SERVES 4

PREP + COOK TIME: 30 MINS

DAIRY FREE

2 tbsps olive oil

2 cloves garlic, minced

750g rack of lamb

½ tsp salt

Pinch of pepper

¾ cup (90g) macadamia nuts

½ cup (60g) breadcrumbs

1 tbsp rosemary, finely chopped (or use dried)

1 egg

Combine the olive oil and garlic in a small bowl. Using a pastry brush, coat the lamb rack with garlic oil and season with salt and pepper.

Grind the nuts in a spice grinder or blender into a coarse crumble. Transfer to a shallow bowl and add the breadcrumbs and rosemary.

Beat the egg in another bowl.

Preheat the air fryer to 180°C.

Dip the meat into the egg mixture, shaking off any excess. Then roll the lamb through the macadamia crumb, ensuring the top side is well coated.

Place the lamb rack in the air fryer basket.

Cook for 10 minutes. Increase the temperature to 200°C and cook for a further 5 minutes.

Remove the meat and cover with foil. Rest for 5-10 minutes before serving.

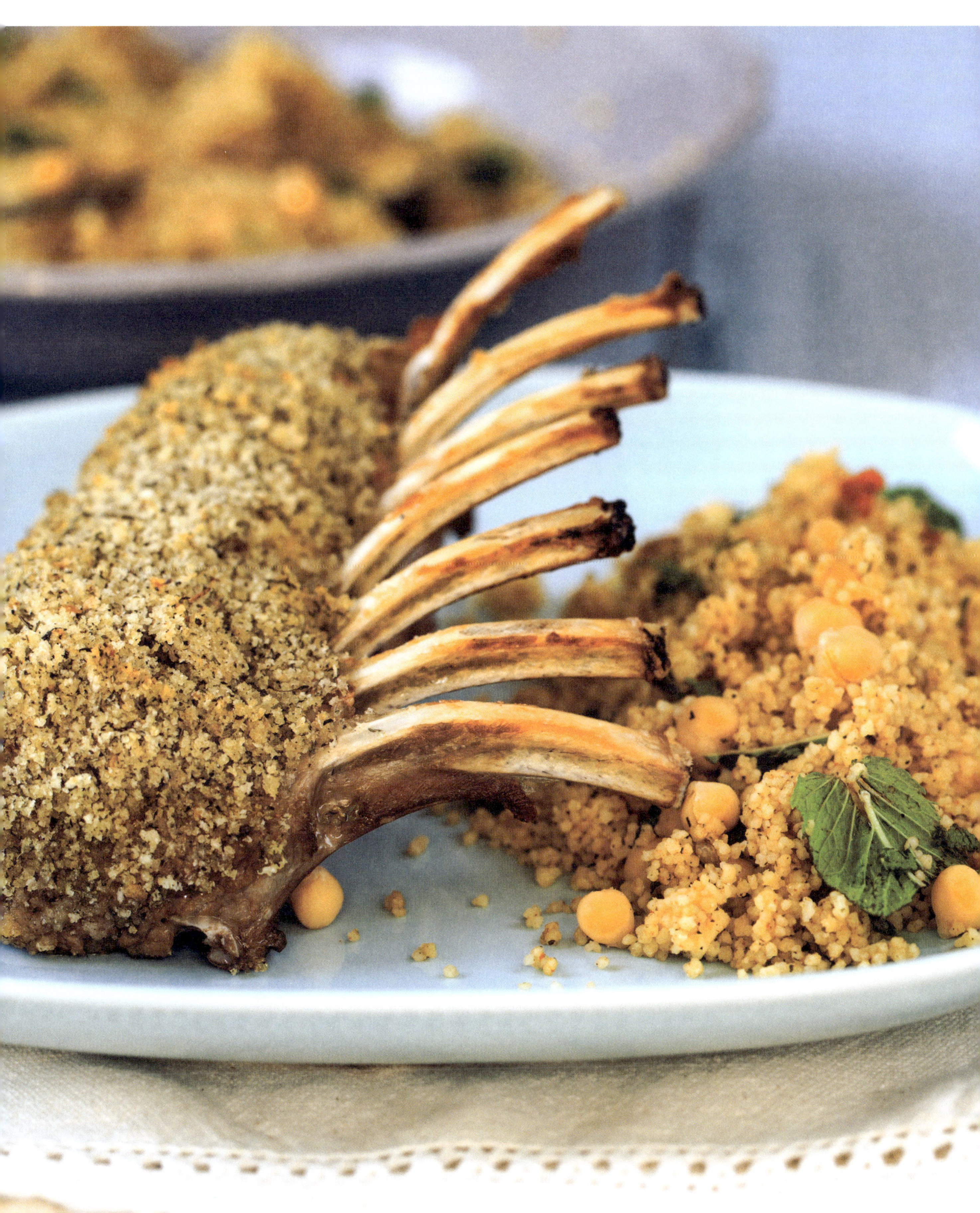

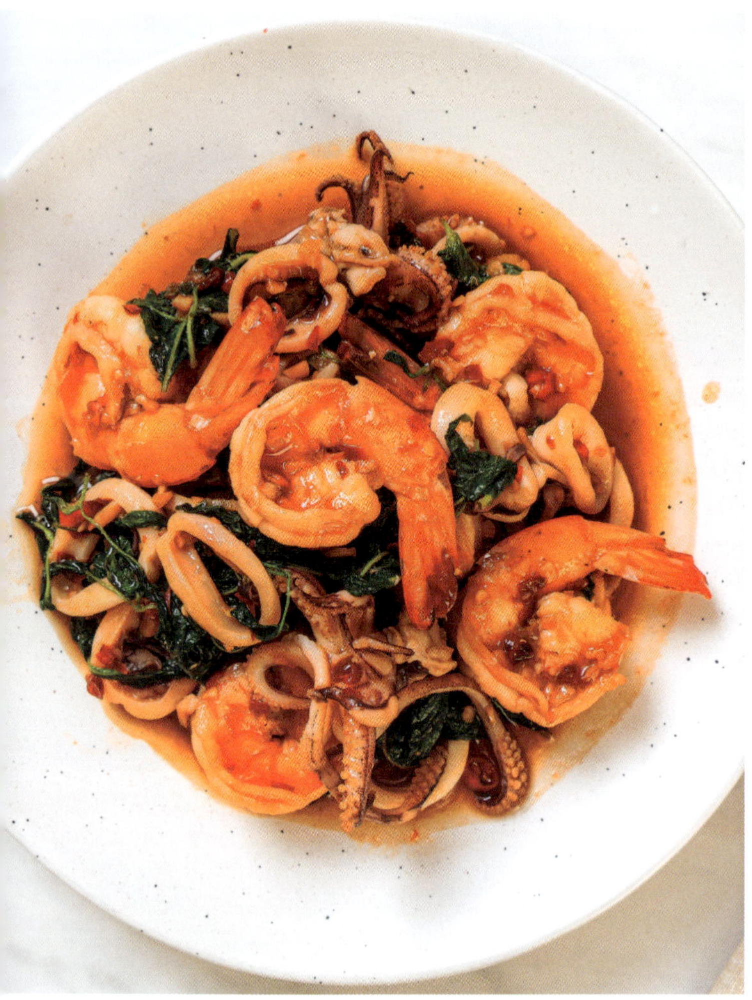

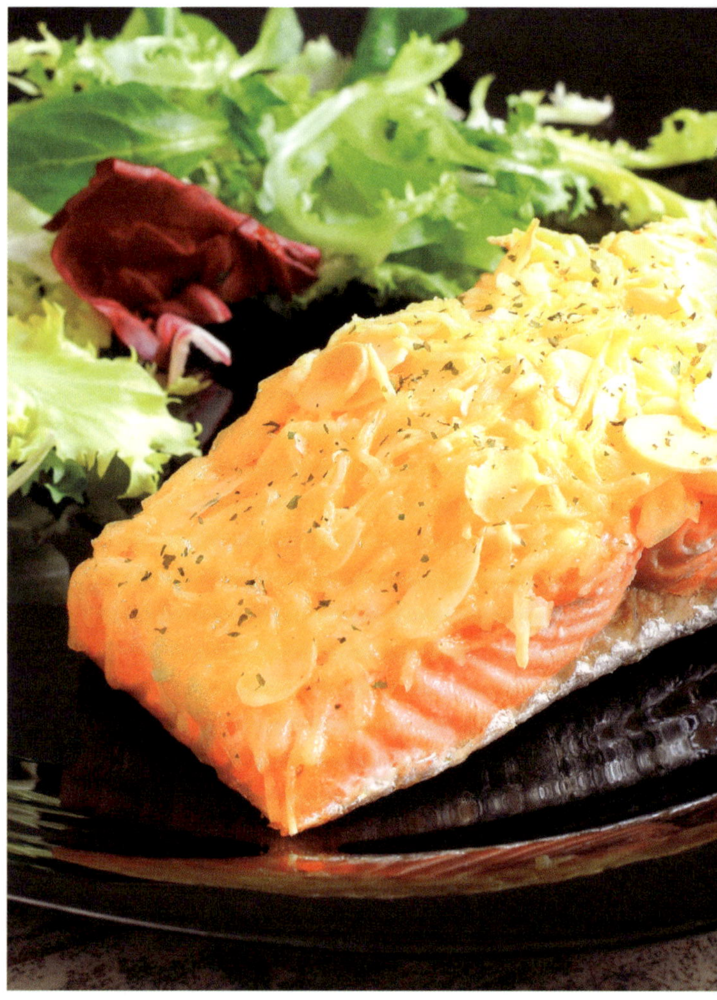

Thai Seafood Stir-Fry

SERVES 4

PREP + COOK TIME: 15 MINS

DAIRY FREE

Baked Salmon with Almond & Cheese Crust

SERVES 2

PREP + COOK TIME: 25 MINS

GLUTEN FREE

THAI SEAFOOD STIR-FRY

3 tbsps Thai chilli paste (nam prik pao)

1½ tbsps soy sauce

1½ tbsps fish sauce

1 tsp brown sugar

1 tbsp water

2 tbsps peanut or avocado oil

500g prawns, shelled and deveined

500g squid, cleaned and cut into tentacles and rings

4 cloves garlic, minced

Small piece ginger, chopped

1 small chilli, chopped

1 cup (15g) Thai basil

Baking pan

In a small bowl, mix together Thai chilli paste, soy sauce, fish sauce, brown sugar and water. Set aside.

Place oil and prawns in pan. Toss to coat then place pan in air fryer basket. Cook for 5 minutes at 175°C.

Add squid, garlic, ginger and chilli. Stir to combine, then cook for 3 minutes until squid is almost cooked.

Add reserved sauce and Thai basil. Stir to combine and cook for 1-2 more minutes until squid is just cooked and sauce is heated through. Take care not to overcook squid.

Spoon onto plates to serve.

BAKED SALMON WITH ALMOND & CHEESE CRUST

2 skin-on salmon fillets

Salt and pepper to taste

25g butter, softened

4 tbsps slivered or flaked almonds

¾ cup (100g) grated Gruyere or Emmental cheese

1 tsp dried parsley

150g mixed salad leaves, to serve

Preheat air fryer to 160°C.

Season salmon fillets with salt and pepper. Place skin-side down, then smear with softened butter.

Combine almonds, cheese and parsley in a large bowl. Mix gently.

Press cheese mixture onto salmon fillets.

Spray air fryer basket with cooking spray.

Place salmon fillets skin-side down in air fryer basket.

Cook for 12-15 minutes, until the topping is crisp and golden and the salmon cooked.

Allow to rest for 5 minutes before serving with mixed leaf salad.

Pork Belly with Stir-Fried Greens

SERVES 4

PREP + COOK TIME: 1 HOUR 20 MINS + 6 HOURS DRYING

GLUTEN FREE • DAIRY FREE

750g pork belly

1½ tsps salt

¼ tsp five-spice powder

2 tsps olive oil

500g Chinese greens, such as gai lan, bok choy or choi sum

1 tbsp peanut oil

2 cloves garlic, finely chopped

Small piece ginger, grated

1 long red chilli, deseeded, finely chopped

3 tbsps tamari

¼ cup (60ml) chicken stock

Place pork belly in a pan of boiling water and simmer for 15 minutes. Pat dry with a paper towel and place uncovered in fridge for 6-8 hours to dry out.

When ready to cook, remove from fridge and pat dry once again. Score the top of the rind. Mix together ½ teaspoon of the salt and the five-spice powder and rub the base of the pork belly with the spice mix.

Rub the top rind with remaining salt and olive oil, massaging into the creases.

Preheat air fryer to 200°C.

Place pork belly in air fryer basket for 30 minutes.

Reduce temperature to 185°C and bake for another 30 minutes. Allow to rest for 10 minutes.

Meanwhile cut greens into 5cm lengths. Heat a wok over high heat. Add peanut oil and swirl to coat. Add garlic, ginger and chilli. Stir-fry for 1 minute or until fragrant.

Add stems of the greens. Stir-fry for 2-3 minutes or until bright green and just tender. Add leaves, tamari and chicken stock. Stir-fry for 1-2 minutes or until leaves wilt.

Slice pork belly and serve with cooked greens.

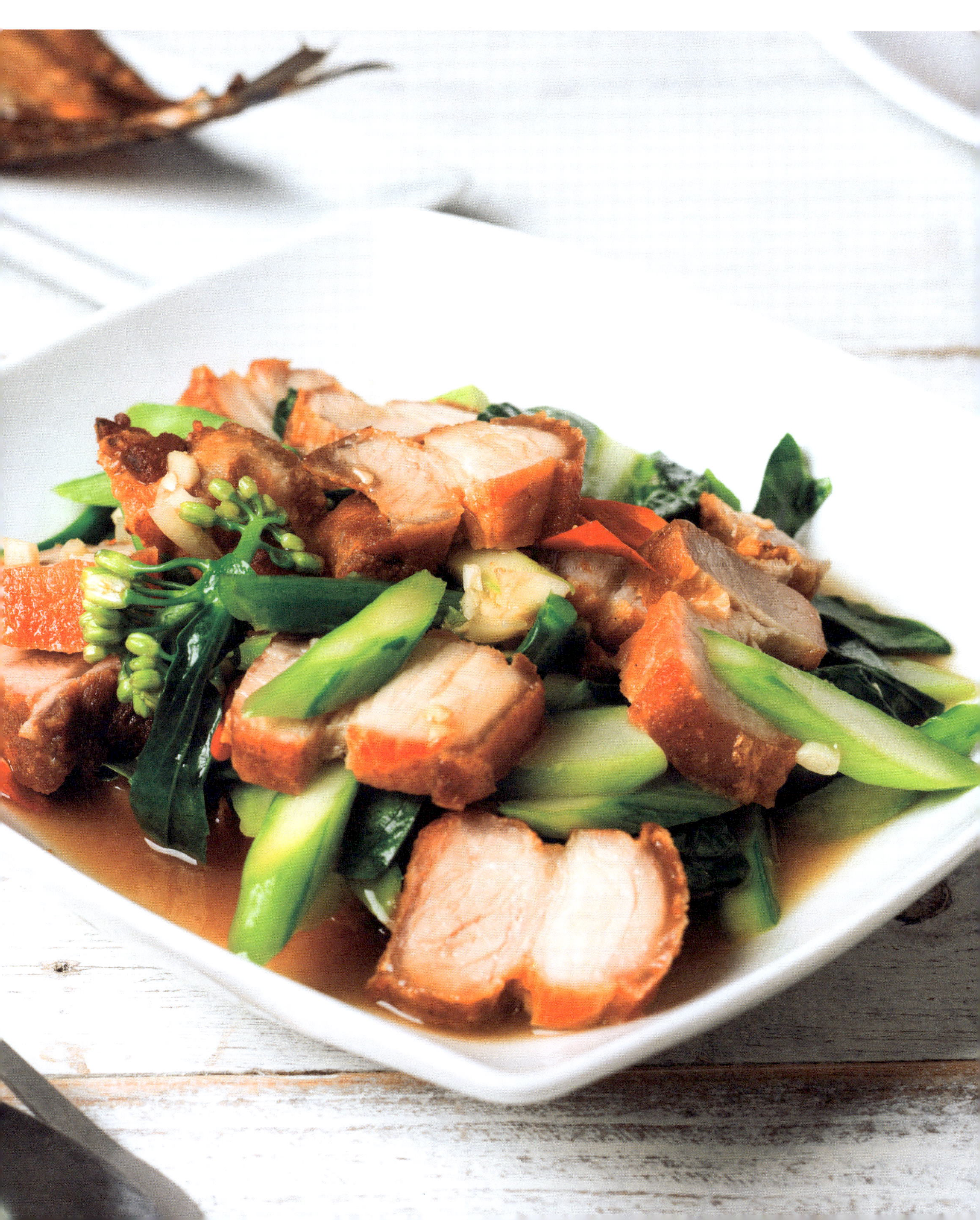

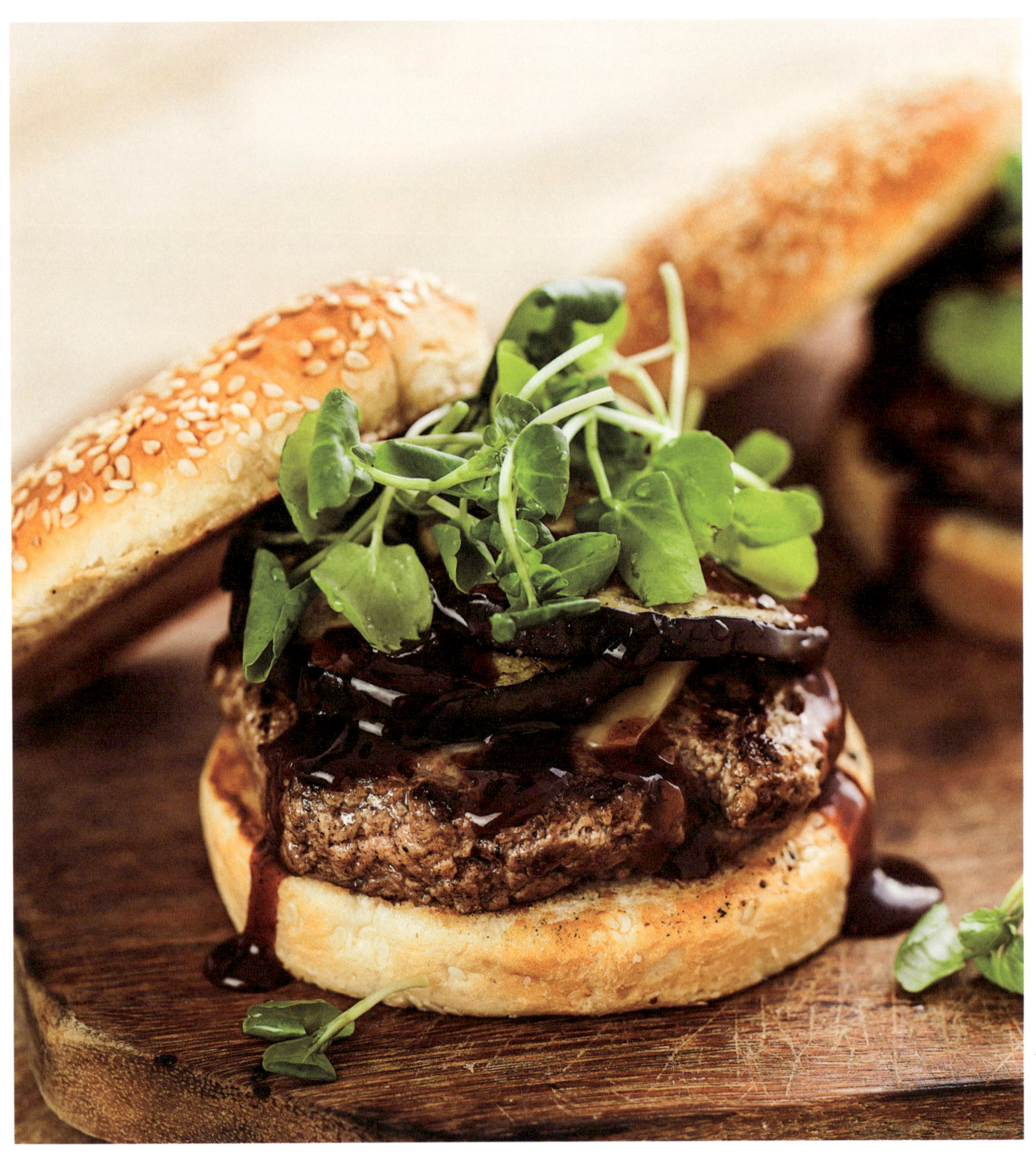

Lamb Burgers

SERVES 6

PREP + COOK TIME: 40 MINS

LAMB BURGERS

1 eggplant
2 tbsps olive oil
1 tsp garlic powder
1 tsp sweet paprika
½ tsp dried oregano
Salt and pepper to taste
6 square slices cheese
6 burger buns
⅓ cup (75g) barbecue sauce
1½ cups (50g) watercress

BURGER PATTIES

1kg lamb mince
1 onion, finely chopped
2 cloves garlic, finely chopped
2 tsps ground cumin
1 tsp ground coriander
¼ tsp ground cinnamon
½ tsp ground allspice
½ tsp dried chilli flakes
2 tbsps chopped parsley
1 egg

Preheat the air fryer to 190°C.

Cut the eggplant in to 1cm-thick slices. Place in a bowl with olive oil, garlic powder, paprika and oregano. Season with salt and pepper. Toss to coat.

Put the eggplant in the air fryer basket.

Air fry for 20 minutes, until tender, shaking the basket halfway through cooking. Set aside and keep warm.

Place all the burger patty ingredients together in a large bowl and mix well to combine.

Shape the mixture into six burger patties with your hands.

Spritz the patties on both sides with cooking spray and place into the air fryer basket.

Cook for 10 minutes at 180°C.

Place a slice of cheese on top of each burger and cook for a further minute.

Fill the burger buns with cheese-topped patties, eggplant slices, barbecue sauce and watercress. Serve immediately.

SPINACH & RICOTTA LASAGNE

4 sheets lasagne noodles

1 cup (225g) passata

¾ cup (200g) ricotta

1 cup (30g) baby spinach leaves, chopped

½ zucchini, grated

½ cup (10g) basil, chopped

Loaf tin

Cook the lasagne sheets according to the directions on the packet. Drain and set aside to cool slightly.

Line the bottom of the loaf tin with 2 tablespoons of passata and place a lasagne sheet over the top. Next add a similar amount each of the ricotta, spinach and zucchini. Place another lasagne sheet on top. Continue like this until all ingredients have been used up, finishing with a layer of the passata.

Cover the loaf tin with foil and transfer to the air fryer.

Cook for 10 minutes on 200°C, then remove the foil and return to the air fryer to cook for a further 3 minutes.

Transfer to a plate to serve.

Note:

A large air fryer can accommodate two loaf tins.

BACON-WRAPPED CHICKEN BREAST

2 skinless chicken breasts

Salt and pepper to taste

½ tsp garlic powder

½ tsp paprika

4-6 rashers streaky bacon

Fresh green vegetables to serve (optional)

Pound chicken breasts into an even 2cm thickness.

Rub chicken breasts with salt, pepper, garlic powder and paprika.

Wrap bacon strips around chicken, tucking the ends on the underside of the chicken breasts.

Spray air fryer basket with cooking spray then carefully transfer chicken to basket. Make sure bacon is still tucked under firmly.

Cook at 200°C for 20-25 minutes or until chicken is cooked through and internal temperature reaches 74°C.

Serve with fresh green vegetables.

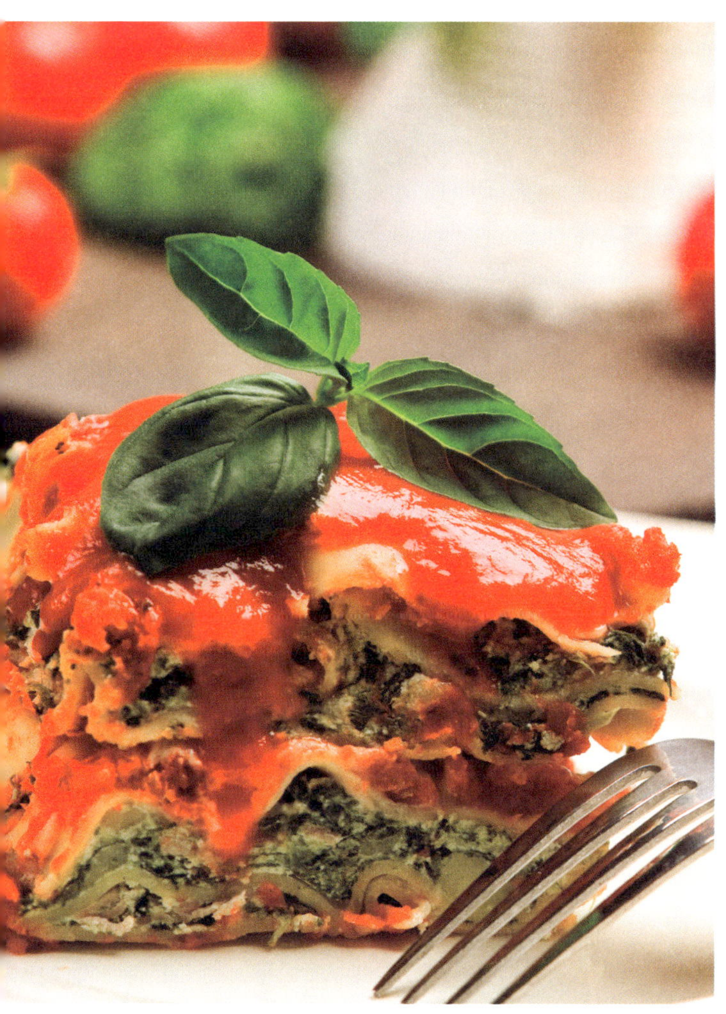

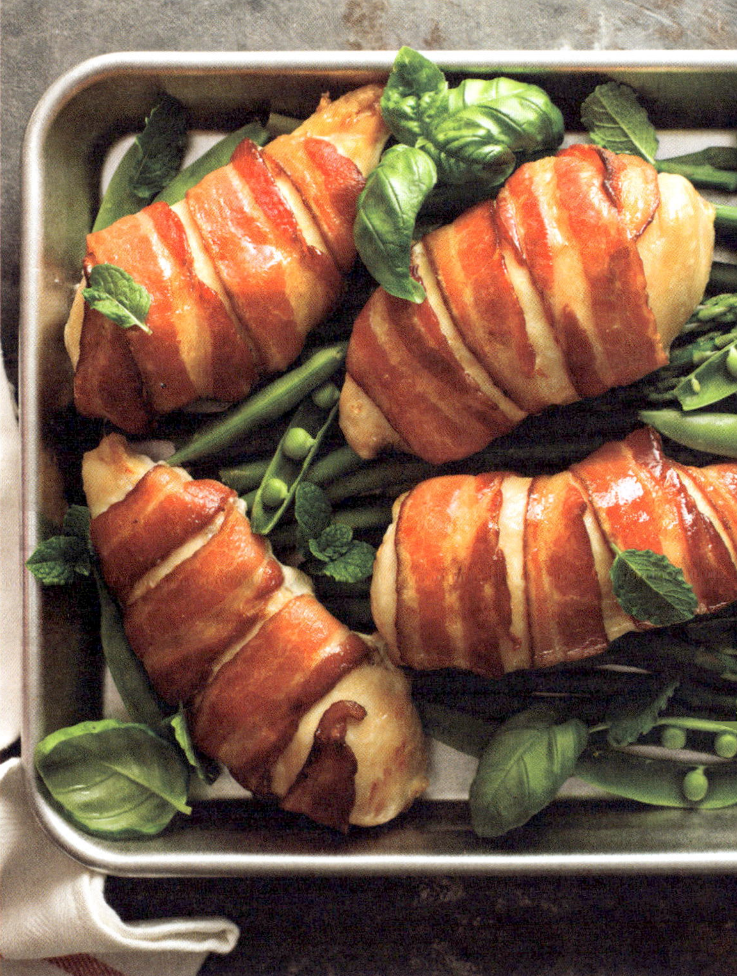

Spinach & Ricotta Lasagne

SERVES 2

PREP + COOK TIME: 30 MINS

VEG

Bacon-Wrapped Chicken Breast

SERVES 2

PREP + COOK TIME: 35 MINS

GLUTEN FREE • DAIRY FREE

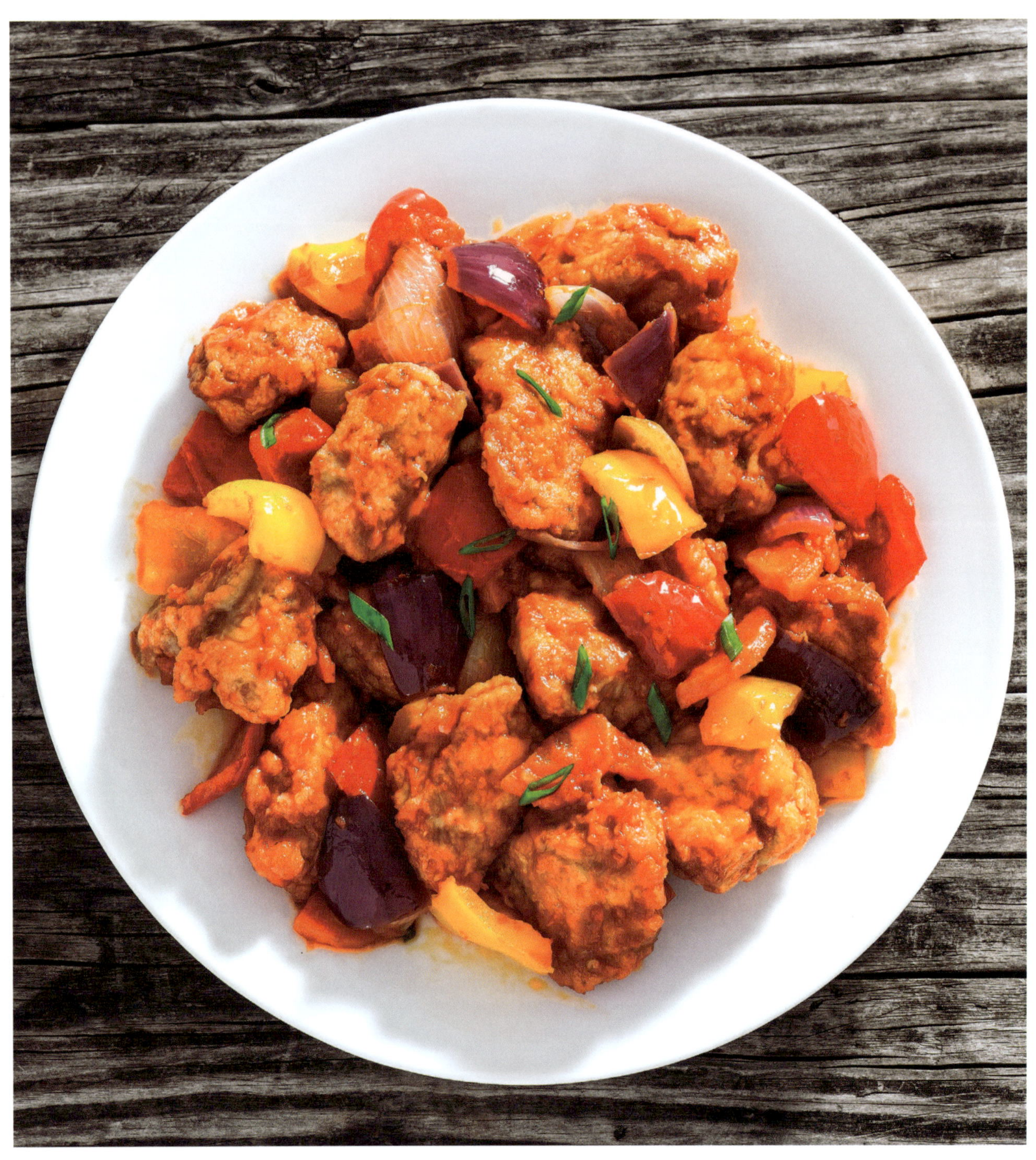

Sweet & Sour Pork

SERVES 4

PREP + COOK TIME: 30 MINS + 45 MINS MARINATING

DAIRY FREE

SWEET & SOUR PORK

500g pork belly

1 tbsp potato starch

3 tbsps soy sauce, divided

1 tsp five-spice powder

1 tsp pepper

2 tbsps oil

⅔ cup (100g) red onion, chopped

1 red capsicum + 1 yellow capsicum, seeded and diced

⅓ cup (75g) tomato puree

1 tbsp apple cider vinegar

⅓ cup (80ml) water

2 tbsps sugar

4 tomatoes, diced

Ovenproof bowl

Remove the skin from the pork belly, cut into chunks and place into a large bowl. Add potato starch, 1 tablespoon soy sauce, five-spice powder and pepper, and stir until well coated. Cover and transfer to the fridge; marinate for 45 minutes.

Preheat the air fryer to 200°C and spritz the air fryer basket with cooking spray.

Transfer the pork to the air fryer basket and cook for 5 minutes. Take out and set aside.

Place the oil, onion and capsicums in the ovenproof bowl and cook in the air fryer for 5 minutes.

In a small bowl, prepare the sauce. Mix together the tomato puree, vinegar, water, sugar and remaining soy sauce.

Pour the sauce into the ovenproof bowl with the onion and capsicum. Add tomatoes, stir well and return to the air fryer to cook for 8 minutes. Add the pork cubes and cook for a final 2 minutes.

Chilli Sesame Salmon

SERVES 2
PREP + COOK TIME: 25 MINS
DAIRY FREE

2 tbsps Sriracha
2 tbsps soy sauce
1 tbsp sesame oil
1 tbsp rice wine
1 clove garlic, minced
Small piece ginger, grated
2 salmon fillets
1 tbsp sesame seeds
1 spring onion, chopped
Boiled rice to serve
1 avocado, sliced, to serve
Wilted greens to serve

In a shallow dish, mix together Sriracha, soy sauce, sesame oil, rice wine, garlic and ginger. Lay the pieces of salmon in the marinade, skin-side up, and set aside for 15 minutes.

Preheat air fryer to 200°C.

Spray air fryer basket with cooking spray.

Place salmon fillets in air fryer, skin-side down. Cook for 6-8 minutes until flesh flakes away easily with a fork.

Sprinkle salmon with sesame seeds and chopped spring onion.

Serve with boiled rice, avocado and wilted greens.

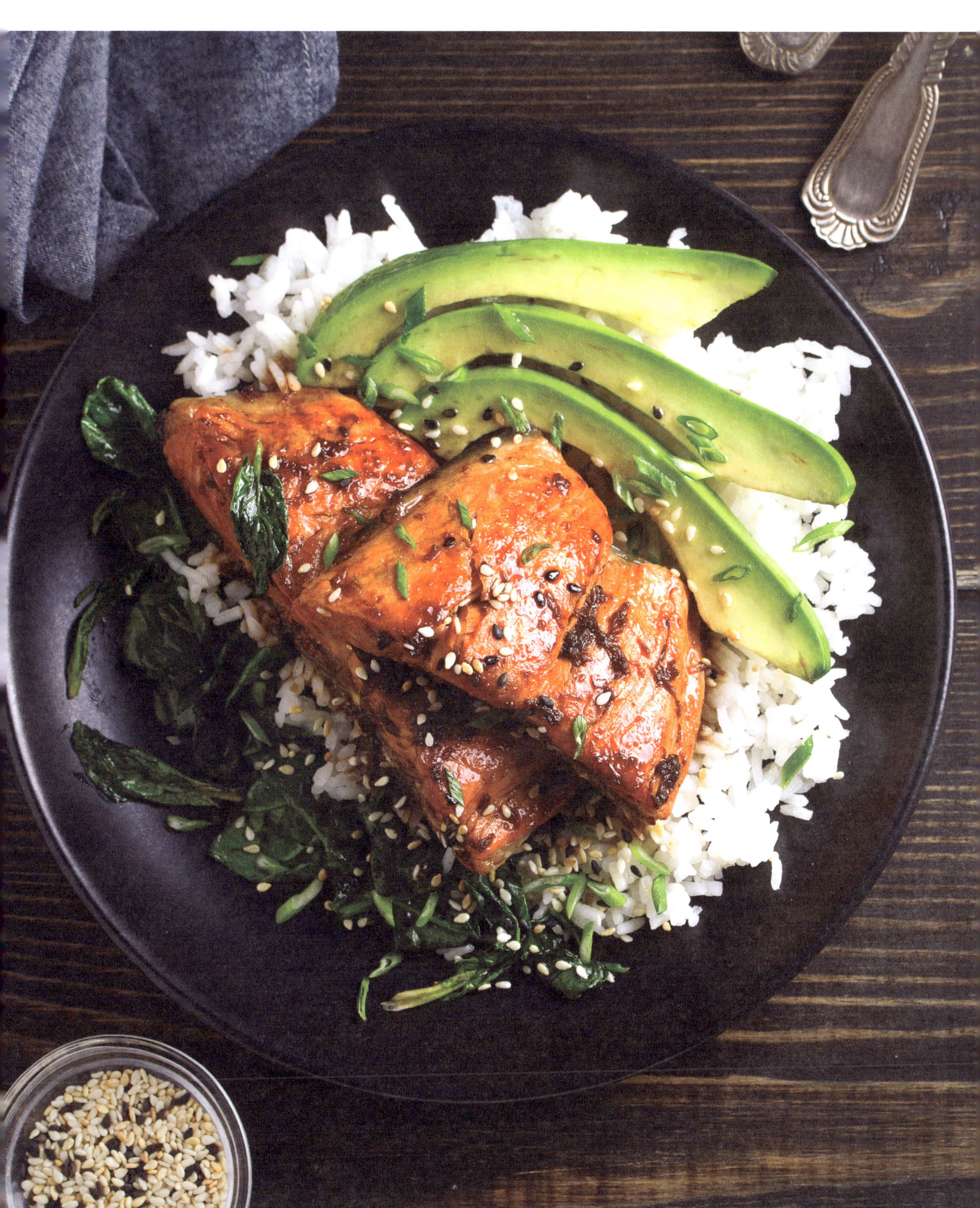

Chapter Four

Sweets and Desserts

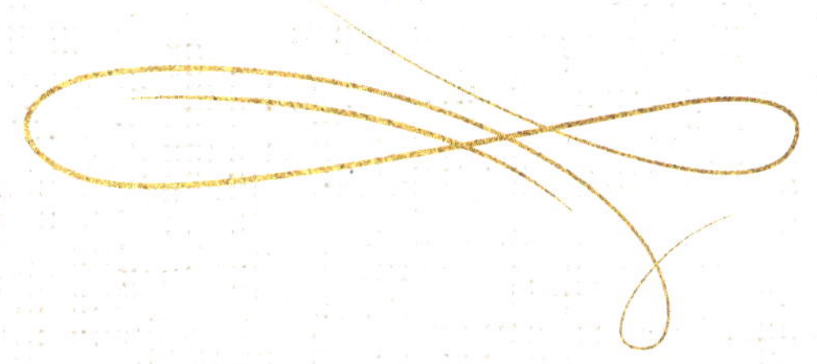

CHOCOLATE MUG CAKE

¼ cup (30g) self-raising flour

2 tbsps caster sugar

1 tbsp cocoa powder

3 tbsps milk

2 tsps mild-tasting oil (such as canola)

Ovenproof mug, greased

Combine all the ingredients together in a bowl until well mixed.

Transfer to the prepared mug.

Place the mug in the air fryer and cook for 10 minutes at 200°C.

BAKED CAMEMBERT

1 x 250g Camembert

2 tsps honey

Pinch of salt

3 thyme sprigs

¼ cup (30g) toasted walnuts

Remove any packaging then return the Camembert to its wooden box, or place on greaseproof paper in a small ovenproof dish. Score a deep cross or a crosshatch pattern on the top rind of the cheese. Drizzle with 1 teaspoon honey and sprinkle with salt and the leaves of one sprig of thyme.

Place in the air fryer and cook at 160°C for 8-10 minutes until soft and gooey.

Remove from the air fryer. Scatter with nuts and drizzle over remaining honey. Top with thyme sprigs to serve.

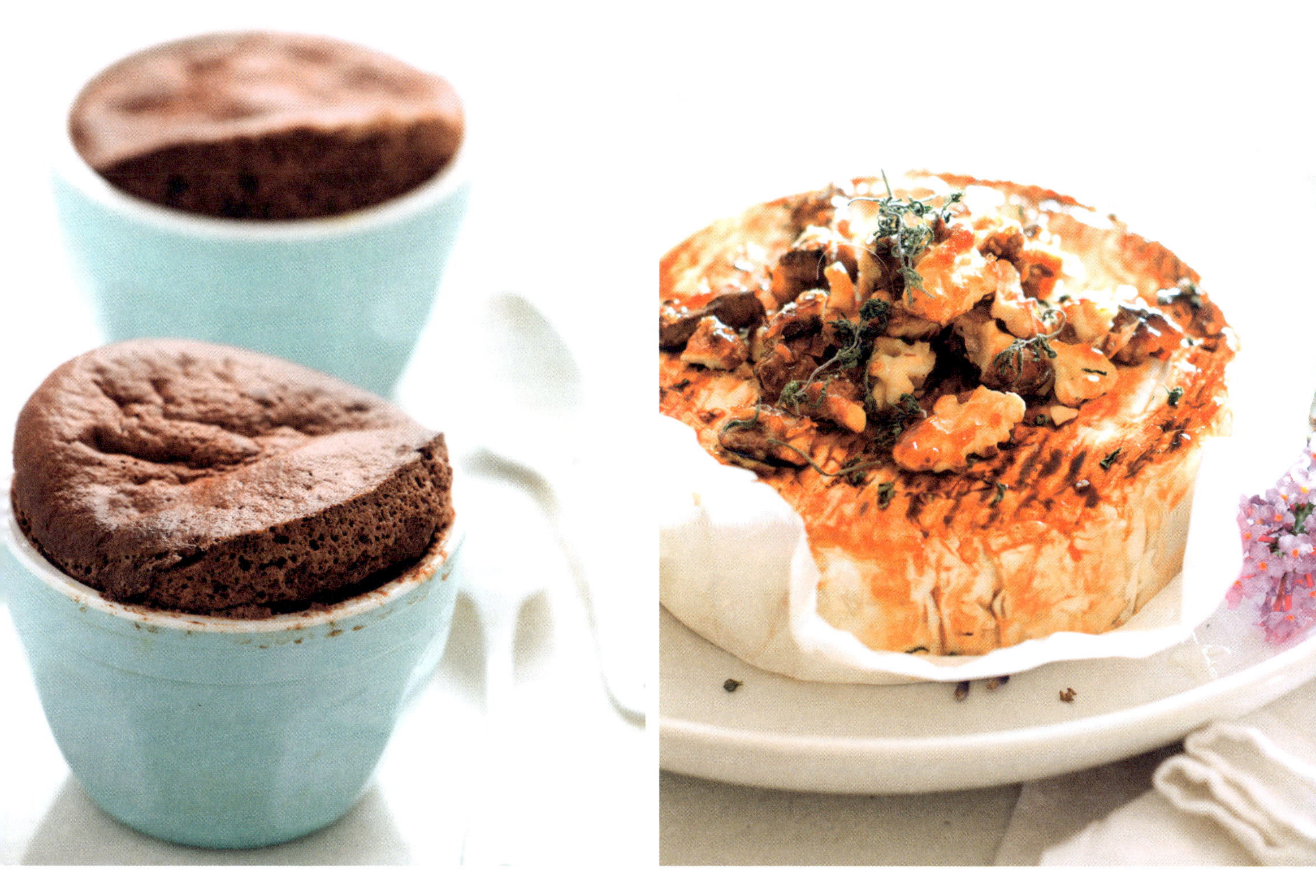

Chocolate Mug Cake

SERVES 1

PREP + COOK TIME: 15 MINS

VEG

Baked Camembert

SERVES 4

PREP + COOK TIME: 15 MINS

VEG • GLUTEN FREE

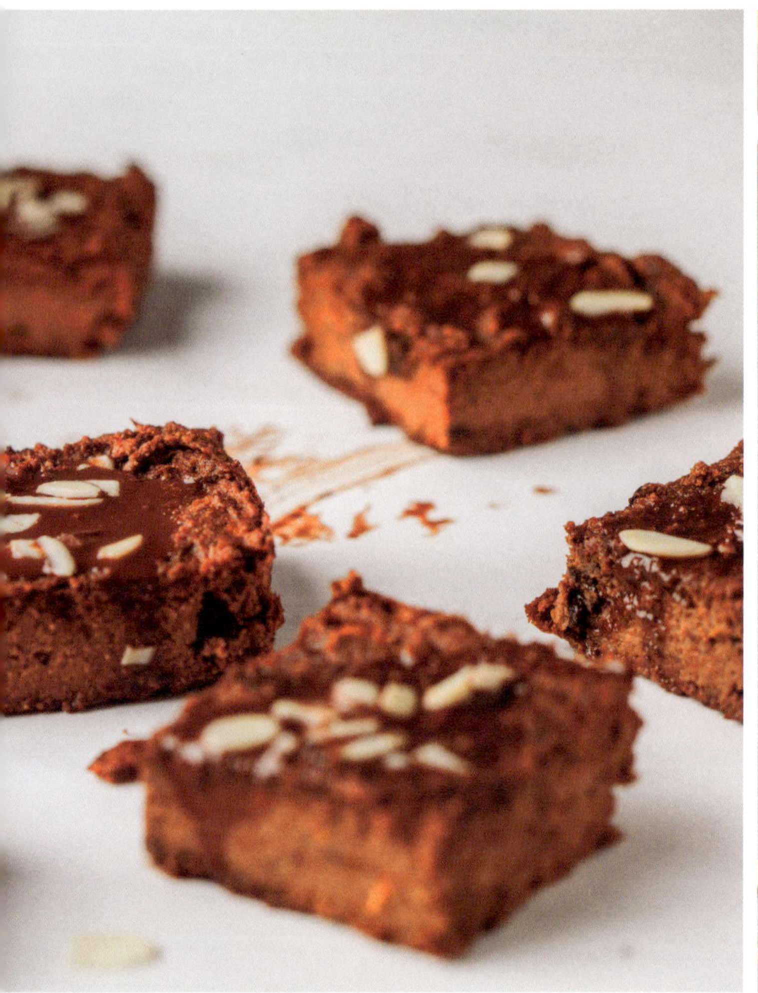

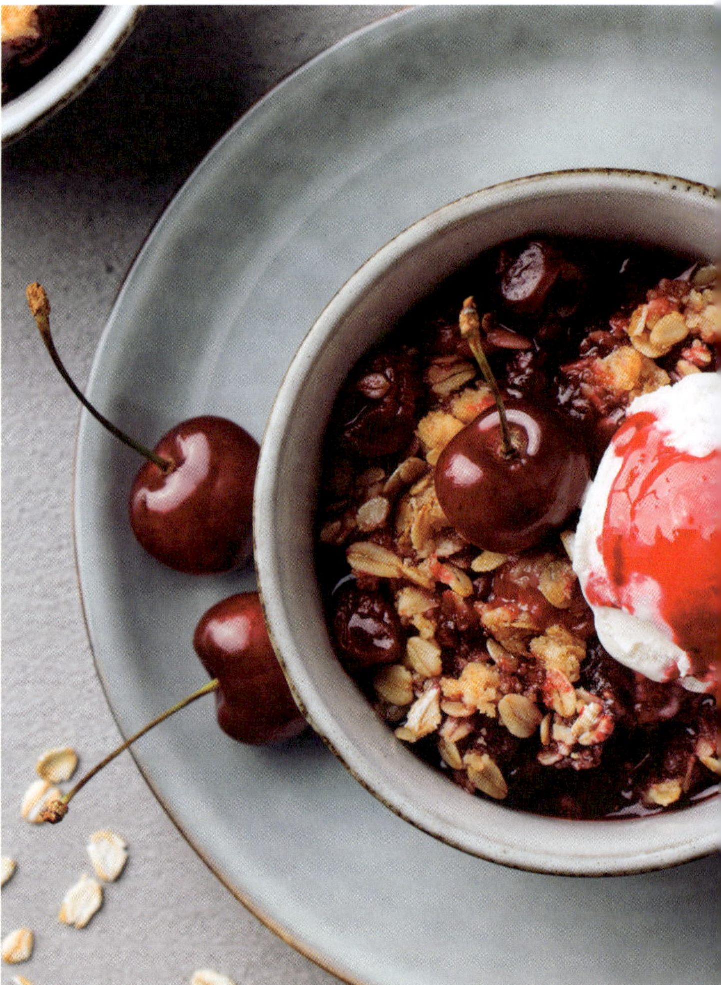

Sweet Potato Brownies

MAKES 10

PREP + COOK TIME: 40 MINS

VEG • GLUTEN FREE • DAIRY FREE

Baked Cherry Crunch

SERVES 2

PREP + COOK TIME: 25 MINS

VEG

SWEET POTATO BROWNIES

1 medium sweet potato, grated
½ cup (125ml) coconut oil, melted
⅓ cup (115g) honey
2 tsps vanilla extract
½ cup (60g) cocoa powder or raw cacao powder
1 tsp baking powder
1 tsp bicarbonate of soda
3 tbsps coconut flour
1 cup (150g) chocolate chips, to serve
Flaked almonds, to serve
Cake tin

Grease and line cake tin. Preheat air fryer to 160°C.

In a large bowl place grated sweet potato, coconut oil, honey and vanilla extract. Mix well.

Add cocoa, baking powder, bicarb and coconut flour. Stir to combine.

Pour into prepared tin and place in air fryer.

Cook for 20-30 minutes until firm on the outside and soft in the centre.

Melt chocolate chips in a microwave or small saucepan over a low heat. Pour over cooked brownie. Scatter with flaked almonds.

Cool slightly before cutting into squares to serve.

BAKED CHERRY CRUNCH

3 cups (450g) cherries, halved and pitted
2 tbsps maple syrup
1 tbsp butter, melted
½ tsp almond extract (optional)
4 tbsps granola or toasted muesli
Vanilla ice cream, to serve
2 ramekins

Preheat air fryer to 180°C.

Mix together cherries, maple syrup, butter and almond extract (if using) and divide between ramekins.

Place ramekins into the air fryer and cook for 15 minutes, until cherries are soft, stirring once halfway through cooking.

Sprinkle granola over the cooked cherries.

Cook for a further 2-3 minutes.

Serve warm with ice cream.

Vegan Buckwheat Bars

MAKES 14

PREP + COOK TIME: 30 MINS + COOLING AND CHILLING

VEG • GLUTEN FREE • DAIRY FREE

⅔ cup (100g) dried cranberries
1 cup (110g) pepitas (pumpkin seeds)
1 cup (90g) desiccated coconut
1 cup (170g) raw activated buckwheat
½ cup (60g) tapioca flour
½ cup (155g) rice malt syrup
⅔ cup (160ml) coconut oil
2 tsps ground flaxseed
1 tsp vanilla powder
1 tbsp cinnamon
150g vegan dark chocolate, chopped
Cake tin

Line cake tin with greaseproof paper.

Place cranberries and pepitas in a food processor and pulse to finely chop.

Add remaining ingredients, except for the chocolate, to the food processor and pulse to combine.

Pour mixture into tin and press down evenly.

Place tin in air fryer and cook for 18-20 minutes at 160°C until golden brown and fragrant.

Allow to cool then cut into bars.

Melt chocolate in a small bowl in a microwave or over a pan of simmering water on a low heat.

Dip each bar into the melted chocolate and turn to coat both sides.

Arrange on a baking tray lined with greaseproof paper and transfer to the fridge to set.

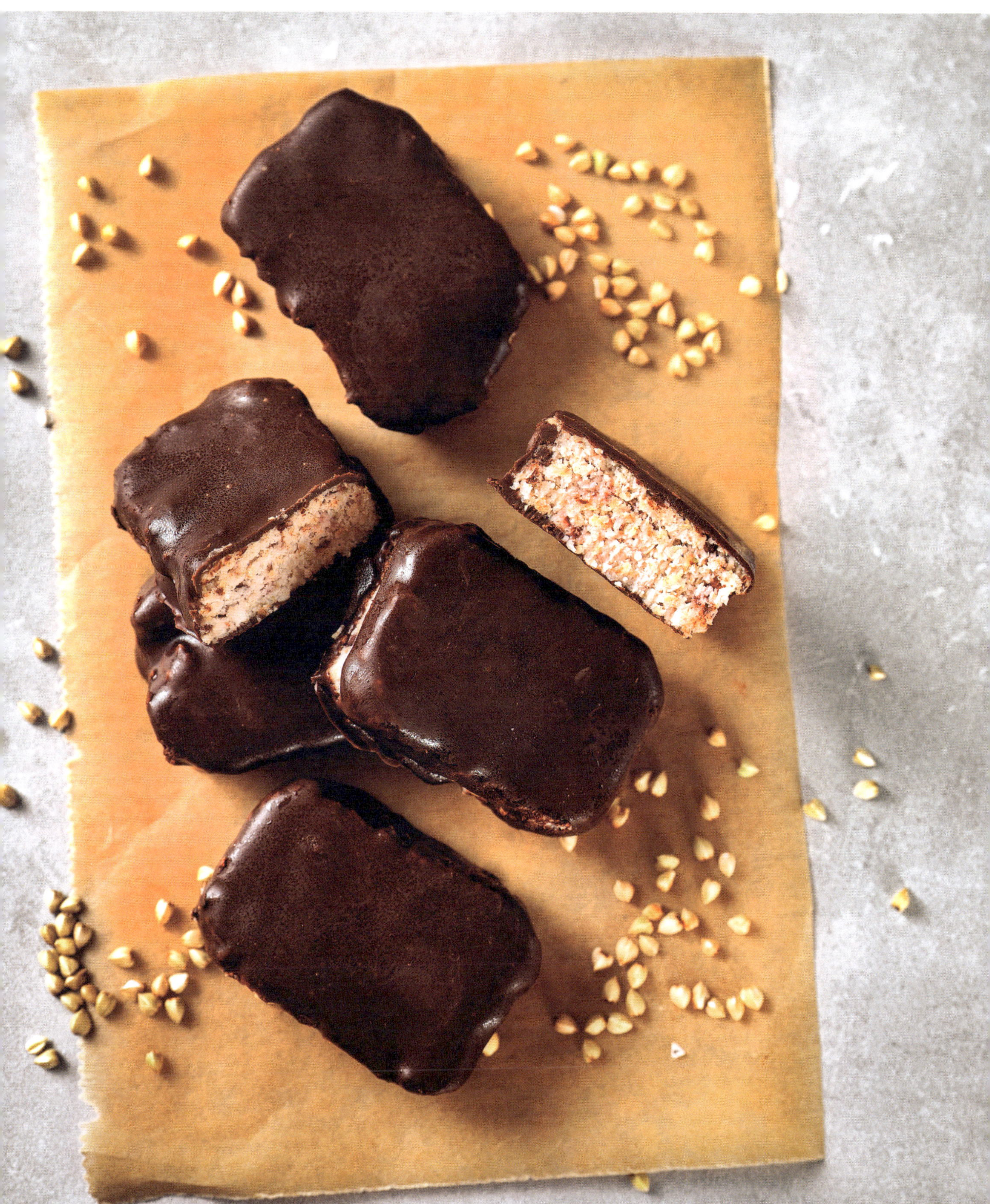

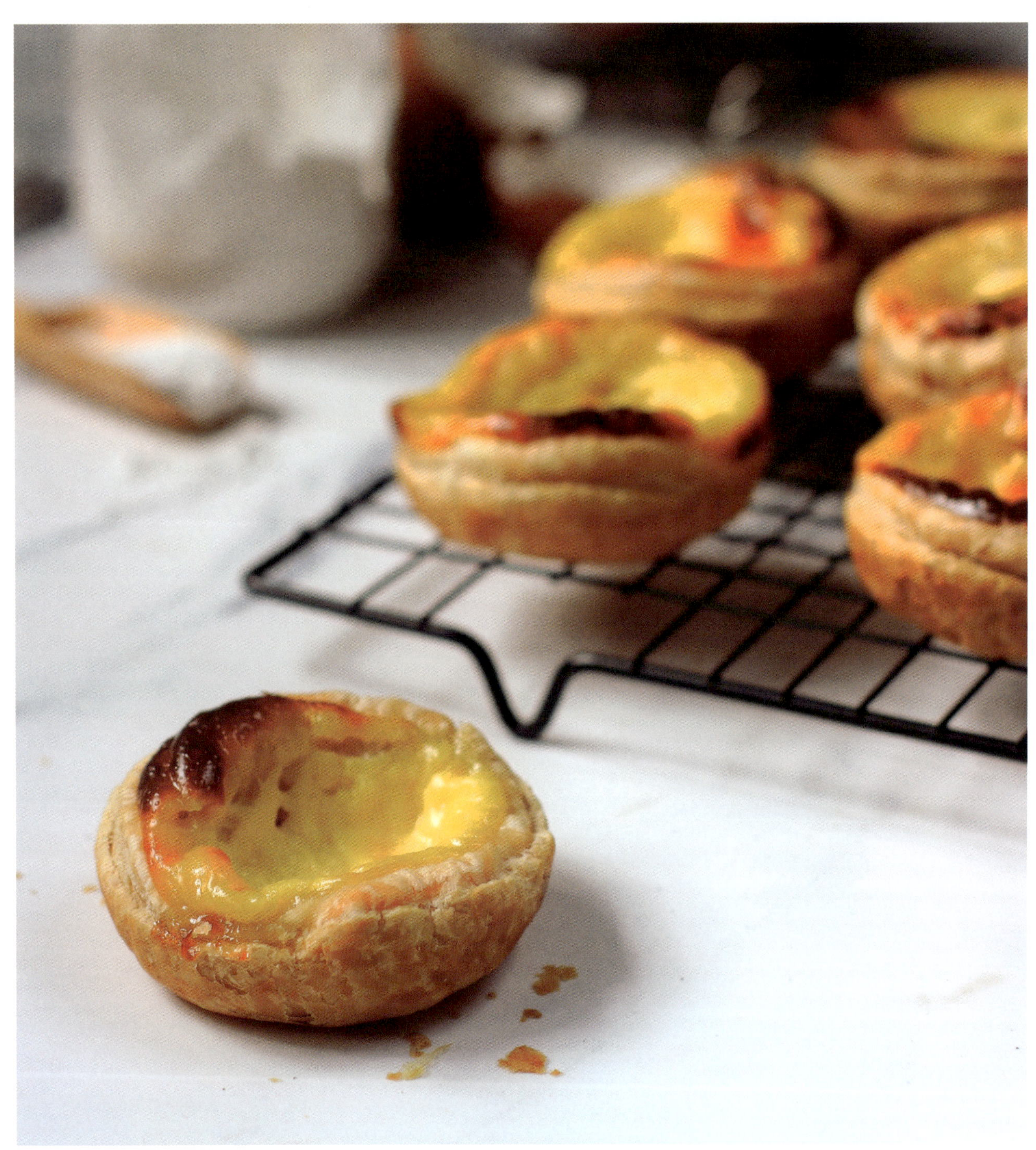

Portuguese Tarts

MAKES 12

PREP + COOK TIME: 30 MINS

VEG

PORTUGUESE TARTS

2 sheets puff pastry
2 tbsps honey
½ cup (135ml) milk
3 eggs
1 tsp cinnamon
Muffin tray or silicone moulds

Use a large round cookie cutter or cut around a coffee mug to create 12 even circles of pastry. Press into silicone cupcake moulds or a greased muffin tray. You will need to cook in batches or use a double layer accessory.

Combine honey and milk in a small pan over medium heat. Bring to a boil, stirring regularly. Set aside to cool.

Whisk the eggs and cinnamon in a medium bowl.

When milk is cool, whisk into eggs.

Pour filling into pastry cases, ensuring you don't fill more than three-quarters full.

Cook in air fryer at 150°C for 15 minutes. Reduce temperature to 130°C and cook for a further 3 minutes.

Repeat with remaining mixture.

STRAWBERRY TARTS

2 sheets frozen puff pastry, thawed

1½ cups (300g) strawberries, sliced

1 tbsp sugar

Icing sugar to serve

Cut the pastry into six 12½ x 9cm rectangles, rerolling the scraps as needed.

Score a border around each rectangle, 1cm from the edge, using a sharp knife.

Arrange the sliced strawberries within the border and sprinkle with sugar.

Place as many pastries into your air fryer as will fit in one layer.

Cook at 180°C for 10-12 minutes until golden.

Repeat with the remaining pastries. Dust with icing sugar to serve.

JAM & BERRY TARTS

1 sheet shortcrust pastry

½ cup (160g) raspberry jam

1 cup (125g) mixed berries

¼ cup (30g) fresh raspberries

Tart tins

Lay the pastry on a flat work surface and cut out rounds with a pastry cutter or glass.

Press pastry rounds into greased tart tins.

Spoon equal amounts of jam into each pastry case, then top with a spoonful of mixed berries.

Transfer to the air fryer and cook for 10 minutes at 180°C.

Allow to cool slightly then top with fresh raspberries to serve.

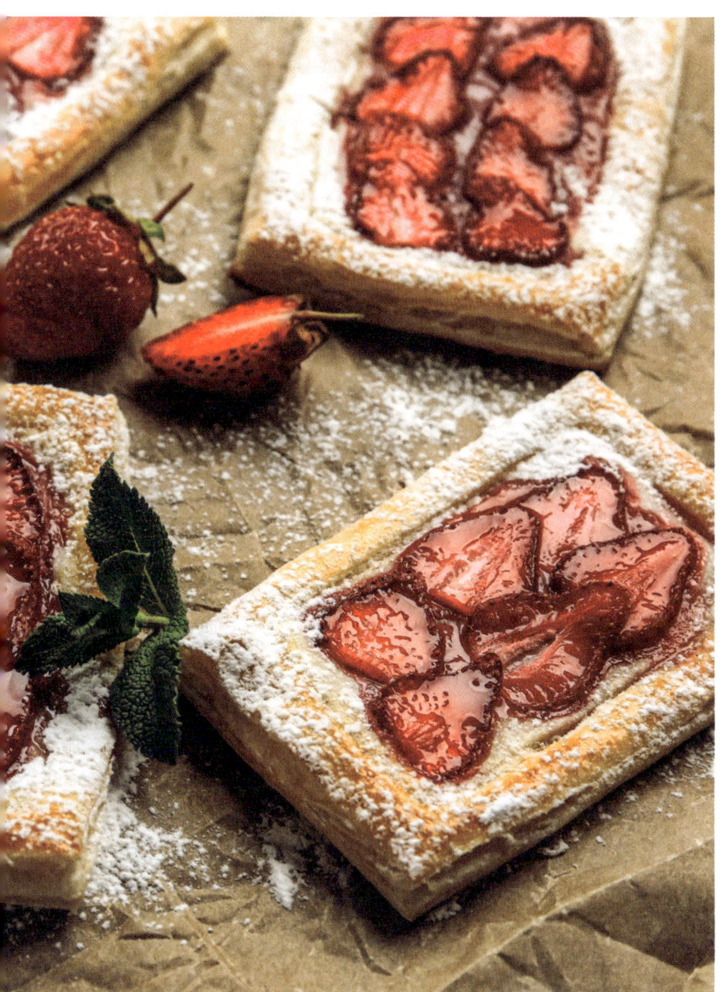

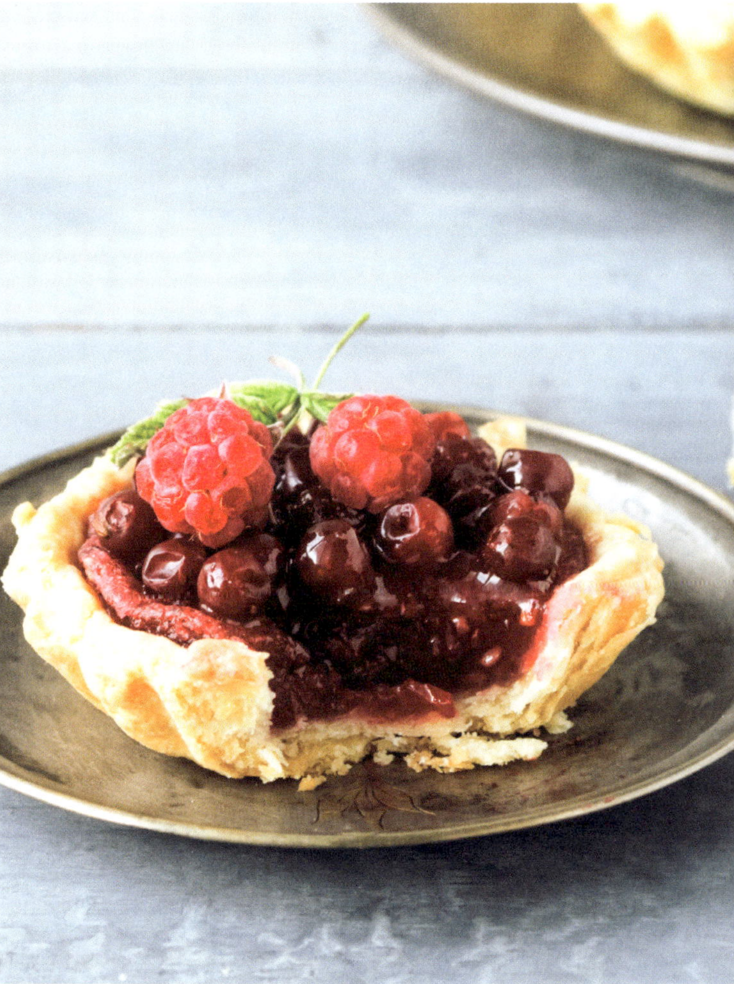

Strawberry Tarts

SERVES 6

PREP + COOK TIME: 15 MINS

VEG

Jam & Berry Tarts

MAKES 12

PREP + COOK TIME: 15 MINS

VEG

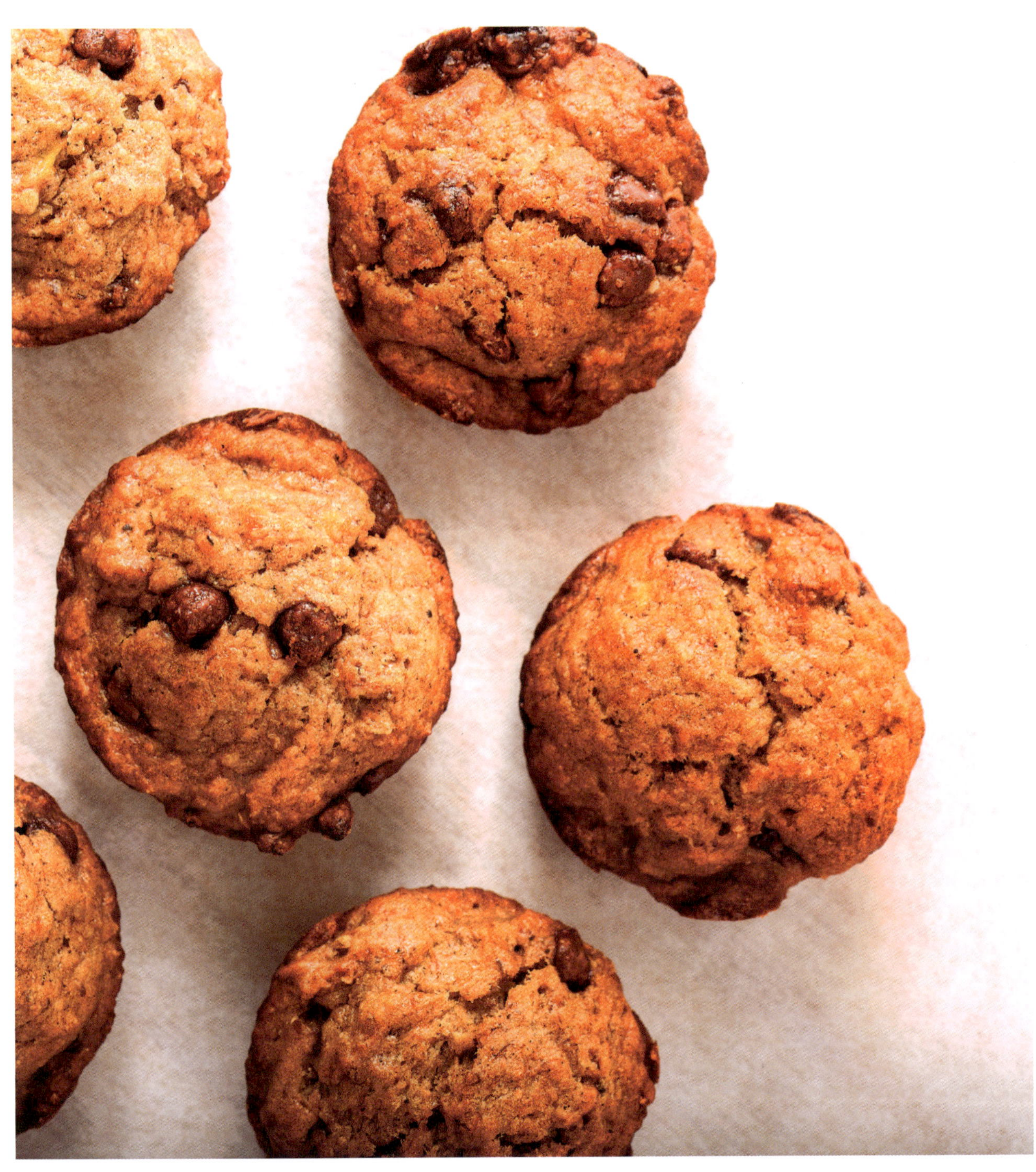

Banana Choc Chip Muffins

MAKES 12

PREP + COOK TIME: 30 MINS

VEG

BANANA CHOC CHIP MUFFINS

1¾ cups (225g) self-raising flour
1 cup (225g) caster sugar
100g butter, cold, cut into cubes
2 eggs
5 tbsps milk
1 tsp vanilla essence
3 very ripe bananas, mashed
⅔ cup (100g) milk chocolate chips
Muffin tray or silicone moulds

Combine the flour and sugar in a large mixing bowl.

Add butter. Rub mixture together with fingertips until it forms a crumble.

Whisk the eggs and milk together in a small bowl.

Pour egg mixture into the crumble mixture and add the vanilla essence. Stir well. Add bananas and chocolate chips and stir to combine thoroughly.

Preheat the air fryer to 180°C.

Line a muffin tray with paper liners. Spoon the batter into the tray and place in the basket of the air fryer. (You may need to cook in batches.)

Cook for 10 minutes. Reduce heat to 160°C and cook for a further 5 minutes.

Remove and test with a wooden skewer, which should come out clean when the muffins are cooked. When cooked, cool for 5 minutes in the tray then remove and cool on a wire rack.

Apple Rose Pastries

MAKES 6
PREP + COOK TIME: 50 MINS
VEG

2 tbsps lemon juice
2 red apples
1 sheet frozen puff pastry, thawed
1 tsp ground cinnamon
Icing sugar, to serve
Muffin tray or silicone moulds

Prepare a bowl half-filled with water and the lemon juice. Cut the apples in half, remove the core and cut the apples in paper-thin slices leaving the peel intact. Place sliced apples in the bowl of lemon water.

Microwave the apples in the bowl for 3 minutes, to soften slightly.

Lay the pastry on a lightly floured work surface. Using a rolling pin stretch the pastry into a 30 x 22cm rectangle. Cut the pastry into six strips, each about 5 x 22cm.

Arrange the apple slices on the strips, overlapping one another. Make sure the top (skin side) of the slices sticks a little out of the strip. Sprinkle with cinnamon. Fold up the bottom part of the dough.

Starting from one end, carefully roll the dough, keeping the apple slices in place. Seal the edge at the end, pressing with your finger, and place in a silicone muffin cup or a greased muffin tray.

Transfer to air fryer and cook for 30-35 minutes at 175°C until golden brown. Dust with icing sugar to serve.

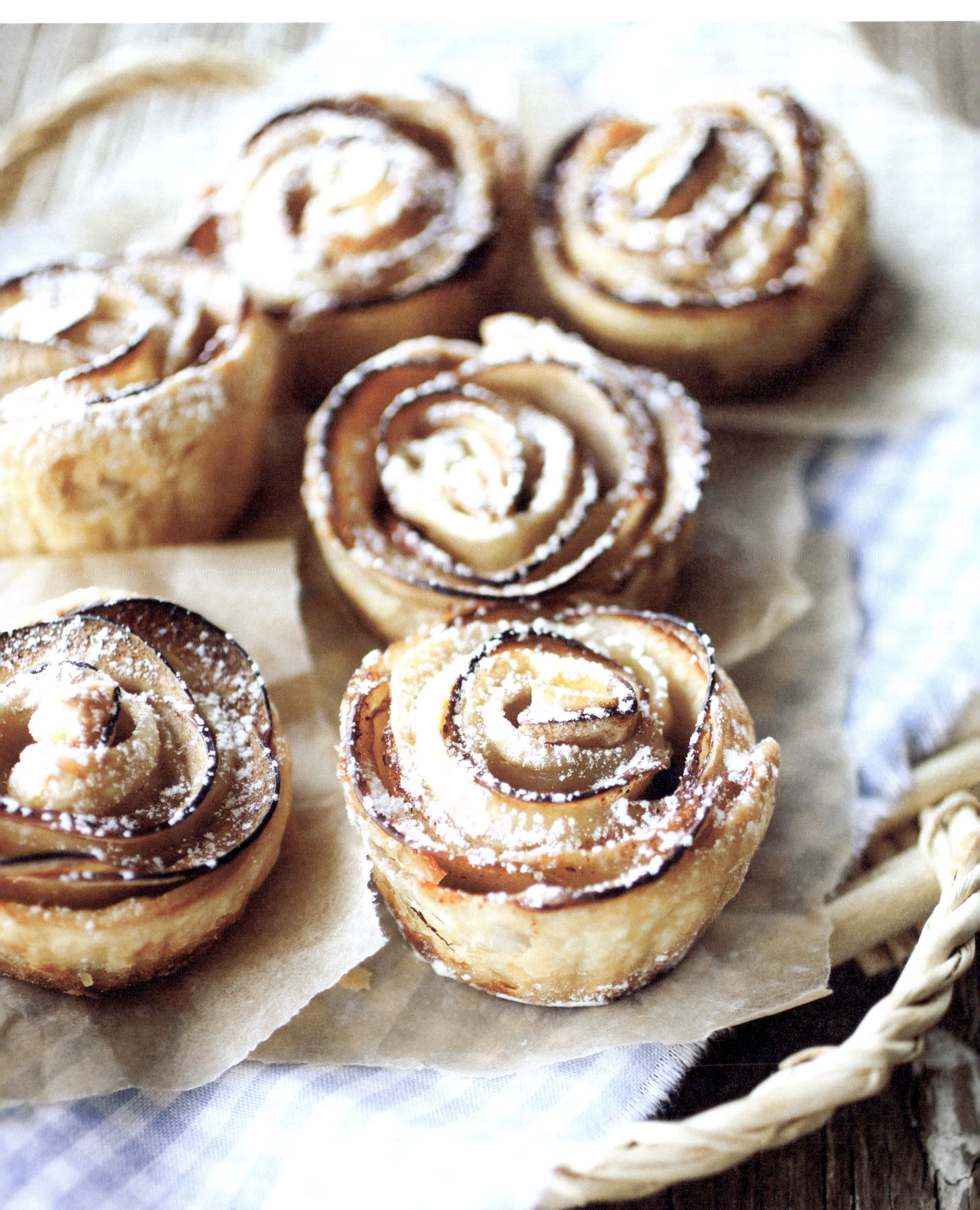

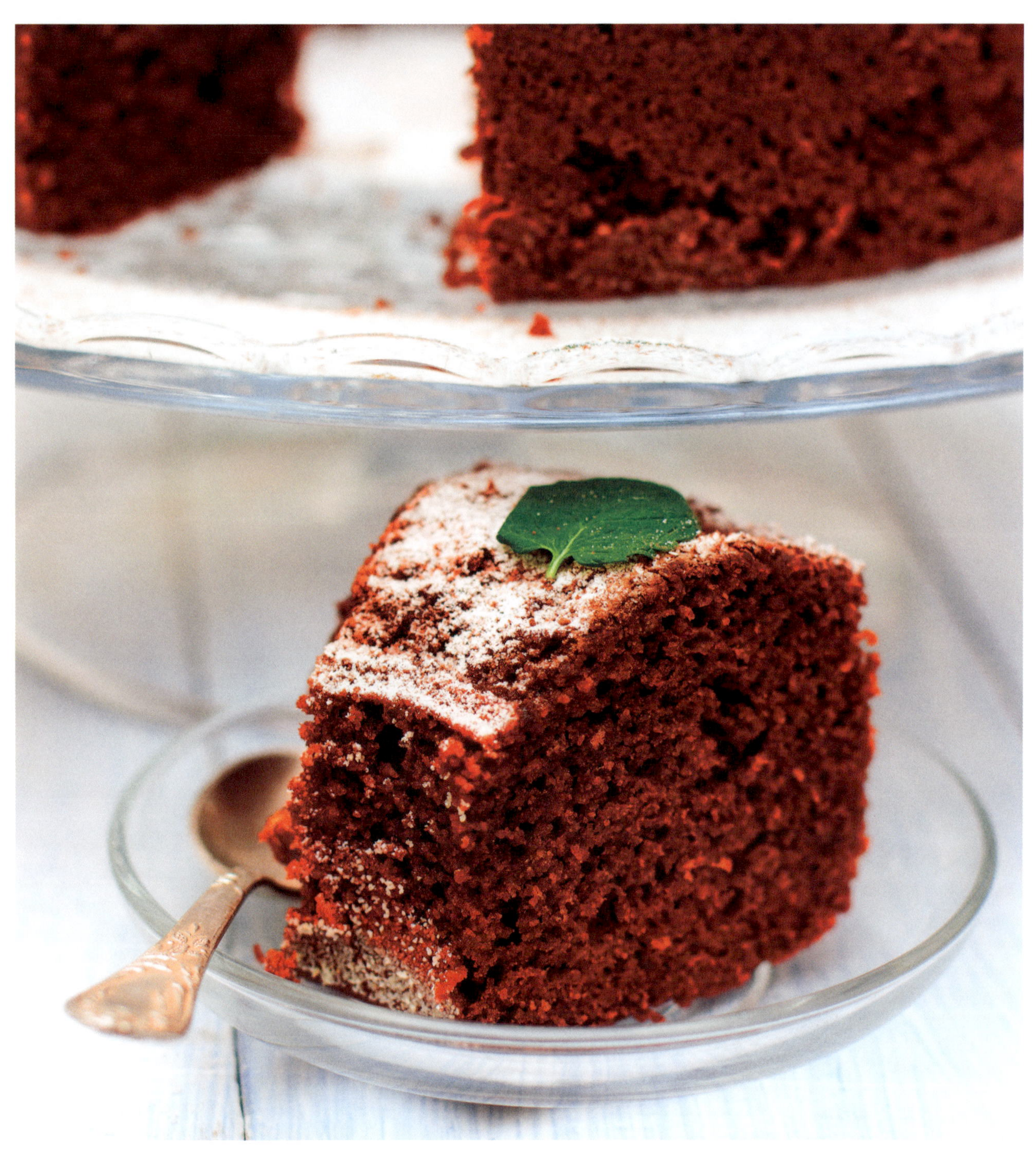

Beetroot Chocolate Cake

SERVES 6

PREP + COOK TIME: 40 MINS

VEG

BEETROOT CHOCOLATE CAKE

125g raw beetroot

2 tbsps milk

1 tsp lemon juice

¾ tsp white wine vinegar

1 tsp vanilla extract

65g unsalted butter, softened

1 large egg

¾ cup (90g) self-raising flour

⅓ cup (50g) rapadura or coconut sugar

2 tbsps cocoa powder

1½ tsps baking powder

Cake tin

Grease and line cake tin with greaseproof paper.

Peel and finely chop the beetroot, place into a food processor with milk and lemon juice, vinegar and vanilla extract. Blend to a fine, smooth puree.

Add butter and egg and pulse to combine. Transfer to a large mixing bowl.

Sift flour, sugar, cocoa powder and baking powder into the beetroot mixture and stir to combine.

Preheat the air fryer to 160°C.

Transfer the batter to the cake tin and use a spatula to smooth the surface.

Put the cake tin in the air fryer basket and slide the basket into the air fryer. Cook for 20 25 minutes until cake is nicely browned and an inserted skewer comes out clean.

Allow the cake cool in the tin for 5 minutes, then turn out onto a wire rack to cool.

Chocolate Hazelnut Twists

SERVES 4
PREP + COOK TIME: 25 MINS
VEG

1 egg

1 tsp water

1 sheet frozen puff pastry, thawed

¼ cup (75g) chocolate hazelnut spread

Spray air fryer basket with cooking spray.

In a small mixing bowl, beat together the egg and water.

Lay out puff pastry on a flat work surface and then brush with egg wash. Spread with chocolate hazelnut spread.

Fold the puff pastry in half. Using a pizza cutter, cut the filled puff pastry into long strips.

Holding each strip at both ends twist the dough two or three times.

Place the twists into the air fryer basket.

Cook at 175°C for 10-12 minutes, until golden brown, flipping halfway through cooking.

Allow to cool slightly before serving.

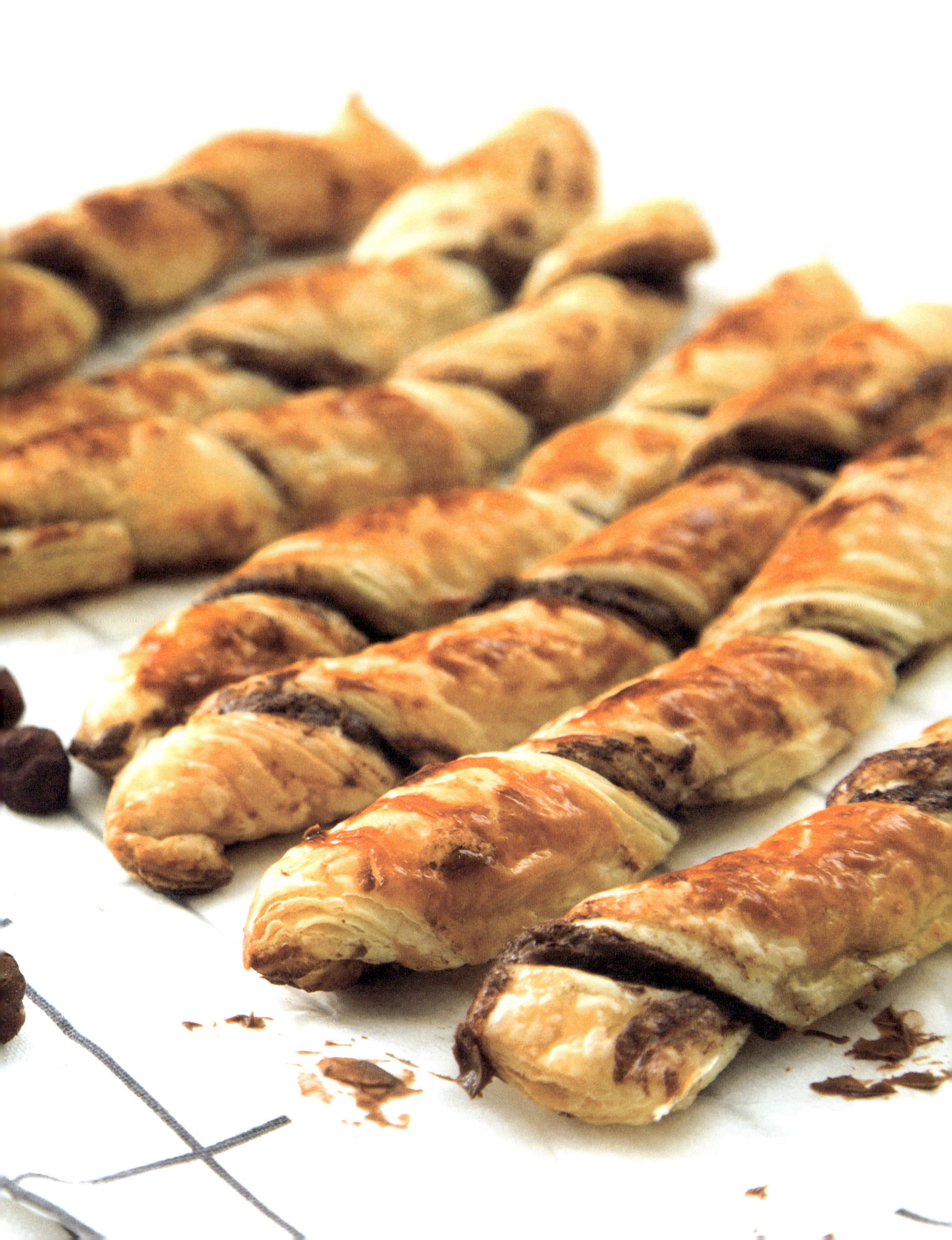

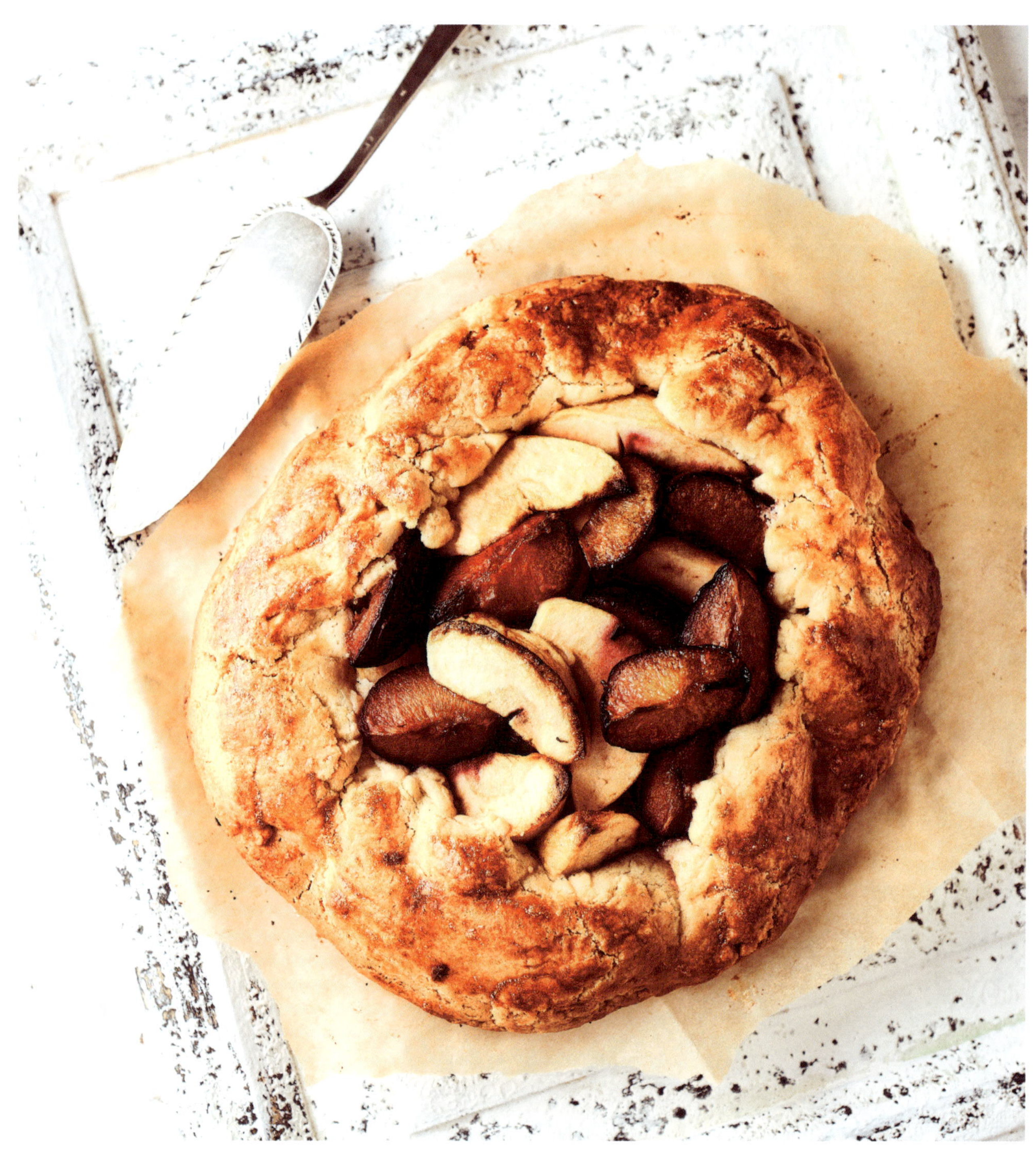

Plum & Apple Galette

SERVES 3

PREP + COOK TIME: 30 MINS + 30 MINS CHILLING

VEG • GLUTEN FREE

PLUM & APPLE GALETTE

¾ cup (90g) almond meal
¼ cup (30g) tapioca flour
2 tsps coconut sugar
⅛ tsp salt
75g cold butter, diced
2 eggs
2 apples, sliced
4 plums, sliced
Juice and zest from 1 orange
1 tbsp maple syrup
½ tsp vanilla extract
½ tsp cinnamon
2 tsps cornflour

In a food processor, combine almond meal, tapioca flour, coconut sugar, salt and butter and pulse until a breadcrumb consistency is reached.

Add one egg and pulse again until the dough comes together. Form into a flattened disc, wrap in plastic wrap and place in refrigerator for 30 minutes to chill.

Place apple and plum slices in a large bowl with orange juice and zest, maple syrup, vanilla, cinnamon and cornflour. Toss to coat.

Remove dough from fridge. Place dough between two sheets of greaseproof paper. Roll out to roughly 16cm in diameter. Remove top sheet of paper.

Add the fruit to the centre of the dough, leaving about 5cm around the edge. Fold the edges of the dough over the fruit to create the galette.

Beat the other egg and brush it over the dough.

Preheat the air fryer to 160°C. Use the bottom sheet of greaseproof paper to lift the galette into air fryer. Bake for 12-15 minutes until golden brown and cooked through.

Use the greaseproof paper to remove the galette from the air fryer and allow it to cool slightly before serving.

Palmiers

MAKES ABOUT 20
PREP + COOK TIME: 40 MINS
VEG

1 sheet frozen puff pastry, thawed
¼ cup (40g) brown sugar
1 tsp cinnamon

Place pastry on a floured work surface.

Mix brown sugar and cinnamon together in a small bowl.

Sprinkle cinnamon sugar all over the pastry. Then use a rolling pin to gently press the sugar into the pastry.

Take one side of the pastry sheet and roll it toward the middle. Do the same thing on the other side.

Wrap the pastry in plastic wrap and freeze for 15 minutes to firm up the pastry.

Cut into approximately 1cm-thick slices.

Grease the air fryer basket with cooking spray.

Place the cookies in one layer in the air fryer basket. Work in batches if needed.

Air fry at 190°C for 10 minutes total, flipping after 7 minutes.

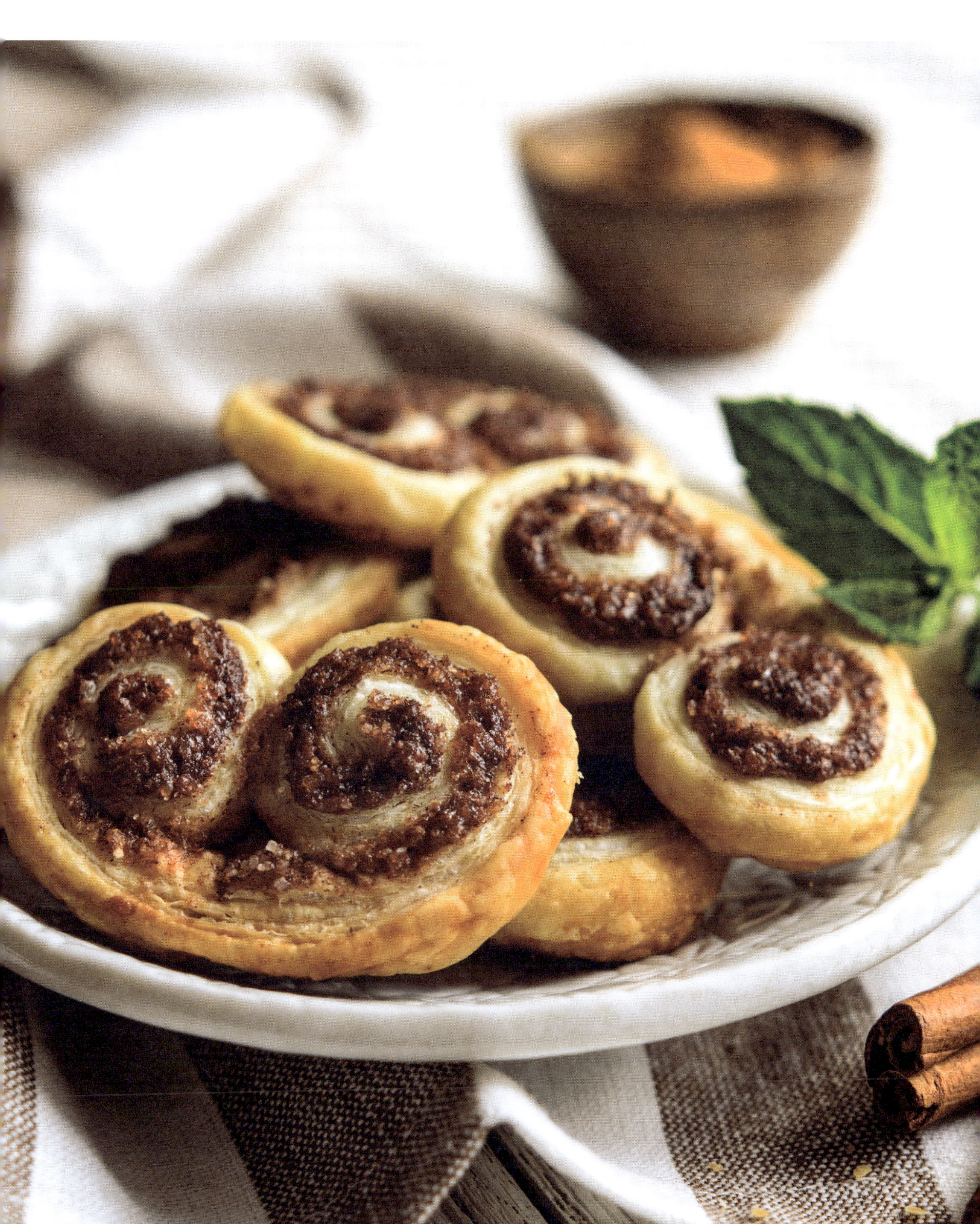

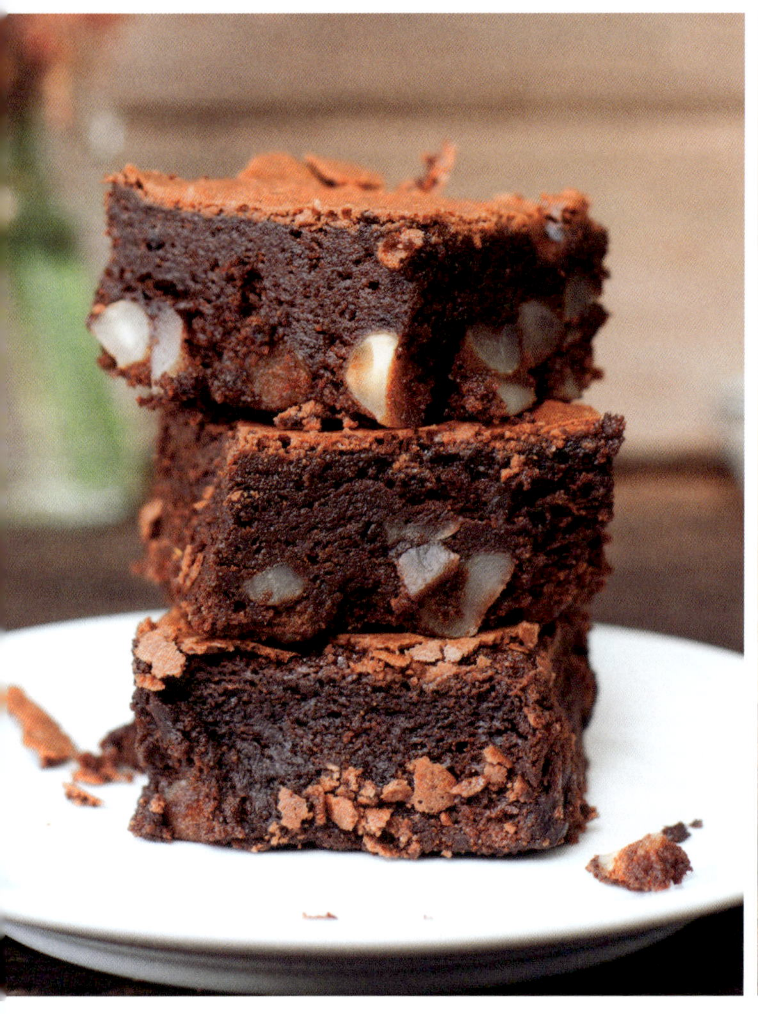

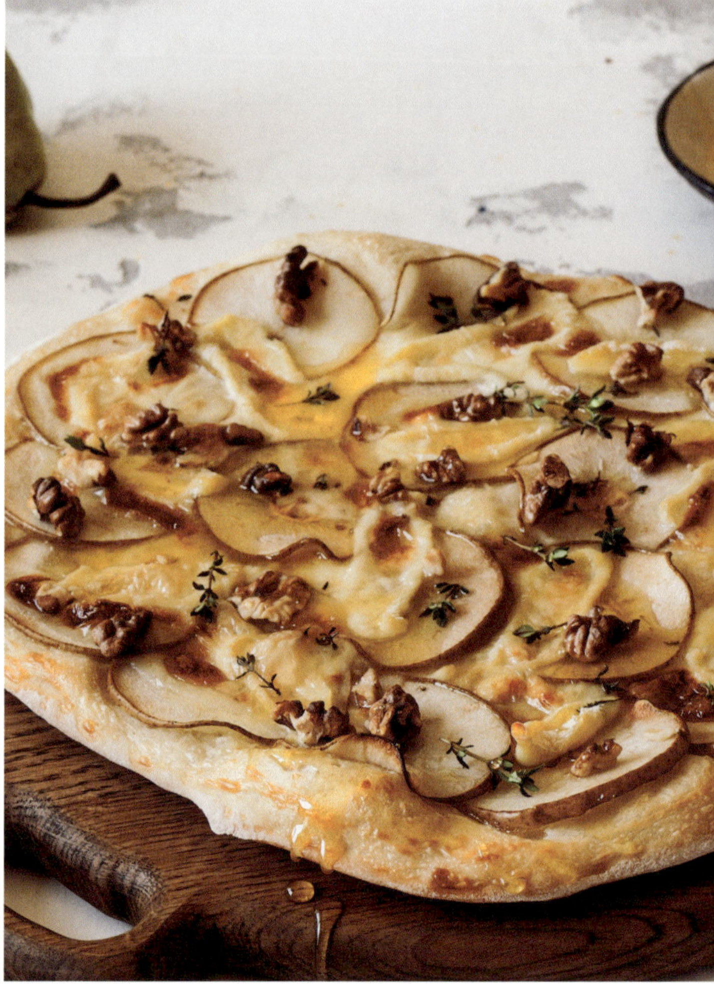

Macadamia Fudge Brownies

SERVES 12

PREP + COOK TIME: 30 MINS

VEG • GLUTEN FREE • DAIRY FREE

Pear Walnut Pizza

SERVES 1-2

PREP + COOK TIME: 15 MINS

VEG

MACADAMIA FUDGE BROWNIES

⅓ cup (80ml) coconut oil, melted
⅓ cup (105g) maple syrup
1 tsp vanilla extract
2 eggs
¼ cup (65g) macadamia butter
⅔ cup (80g) almond meal
⅓ cup (35g) raw cacao powder
1 tsp baking powder
¼ tsp salt
⅓ cup (40g) macadamias, chopped
Cake tin

Grease and line cake tin with greaseproof paper. Preheat the air fryer to 160°C.

Add coconut oil, maple syrup, vanilla extract, eggs and macadamia butter to a large bowl. Mix well, then add remaining ingredients. Stir well to combine.

Pour batter into cake tin and place in air fryer. Cook for 20-25 minutes. Allow to cool before cutting up.

PEAR WALNUT PIZZA

1 medium pizza base
½ cup (60g) shredded mozzarella cheese
1 medium pear, cored and very thinly sliced
⅓ cup (80g) goat's cheese or fresh ricotta
1 tbsp honey
¼ cup (30g) walnut pieces
3 thyme sprigs, broken into pieces

Cover the pizza base with a layer of mozzarella cheese.

Top with a layer of pear slices, dot with goat's cheese or ricotta and drizzle with honey.

Air fry pizza at 190°C for 7 minutes.

Top with walnuts and thyme and cook for a further minute.

Blackcurrant Coconut Slice

SERVES 6
PREP + COOK TIME: 40 MINS
VEG

BASE

¾ cup (100g) plain flour

½ cup (100g) caster sugar

1 cup (85g) desiccated coconut

100g butter

3 large egg yolks

TOPPING

4-5 tbsps blackcurrant jam (with whole blackcurrants)

3 large egg whites

⅓ cup (75g) white caster sugar

½ cup (50g) desiccated coconut

Handful of coconut flakes

Baking pan

Preheat air fryer to 160°C. Grease a baking tin that fits into your air fryer. Line the base with a long strip of greaseproof paper that extends above the rim of the tin.

To make the base, place flour, sugar and coconut into a bowl, stir to combine, then rub in the butter with your fingertips to make coarse crumbs. Stir in the egg yolks with the blade of a knife, then bring the mixture together with your hands to make a dough. Press the dough into the base of the tin, smoothing it with the back of a spoon to make an even layer.

Spread the jam over most of the dough, leaving a 1cm border free around the edges.

Whisk the egg whites with an electric hand whisk until stiff, then gradually add the sugar to make a glossy meringue. Fold in the desiccated coconut, then spoon over the jam layer. Scatter with the coconut flakes and bake for 18-20 minutes until golden.

Leave to cool in the tin, then carefully lift out, using the greaseproof paper to help you, and cut into slices. Will keep in an airtight container for 2 days.

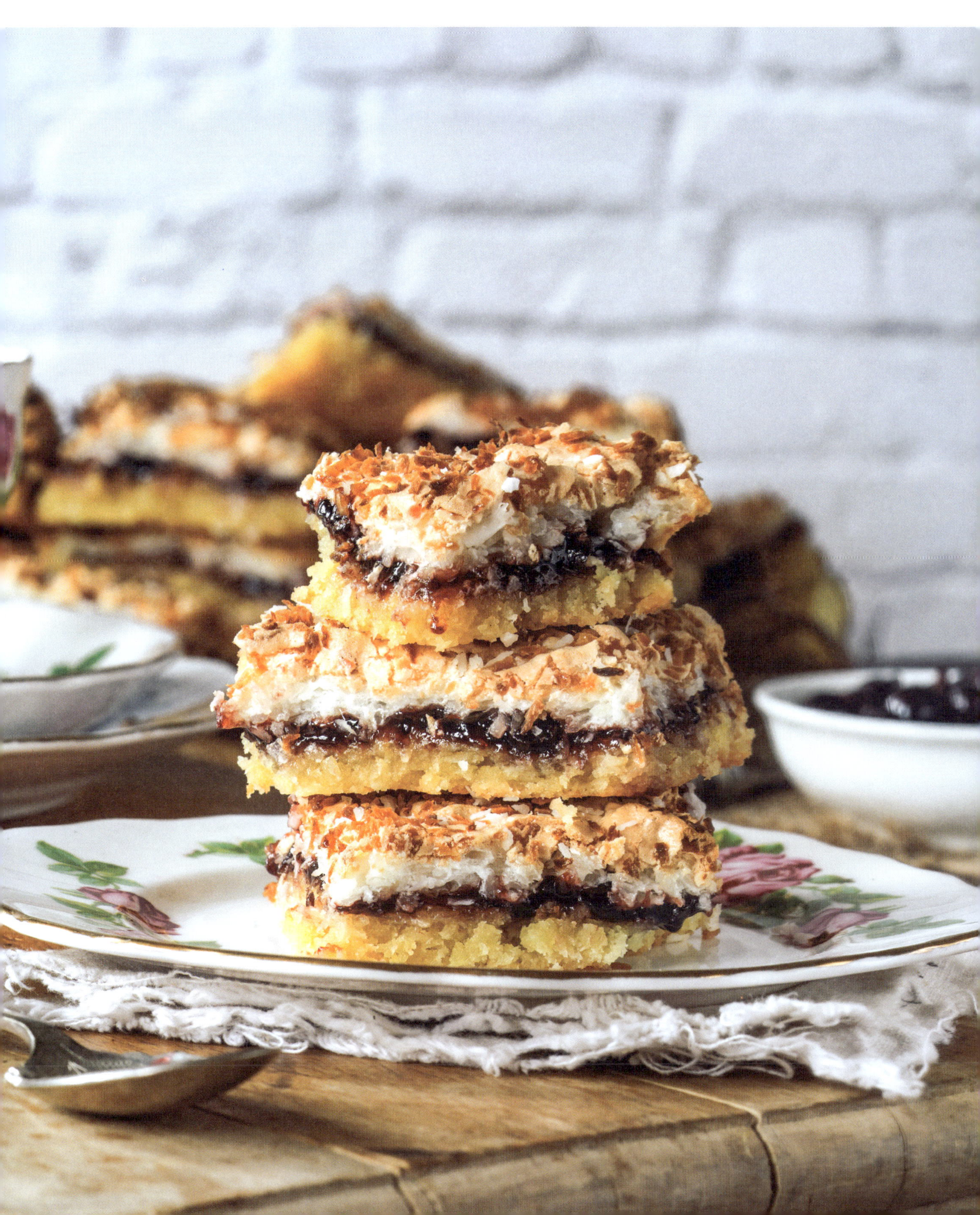

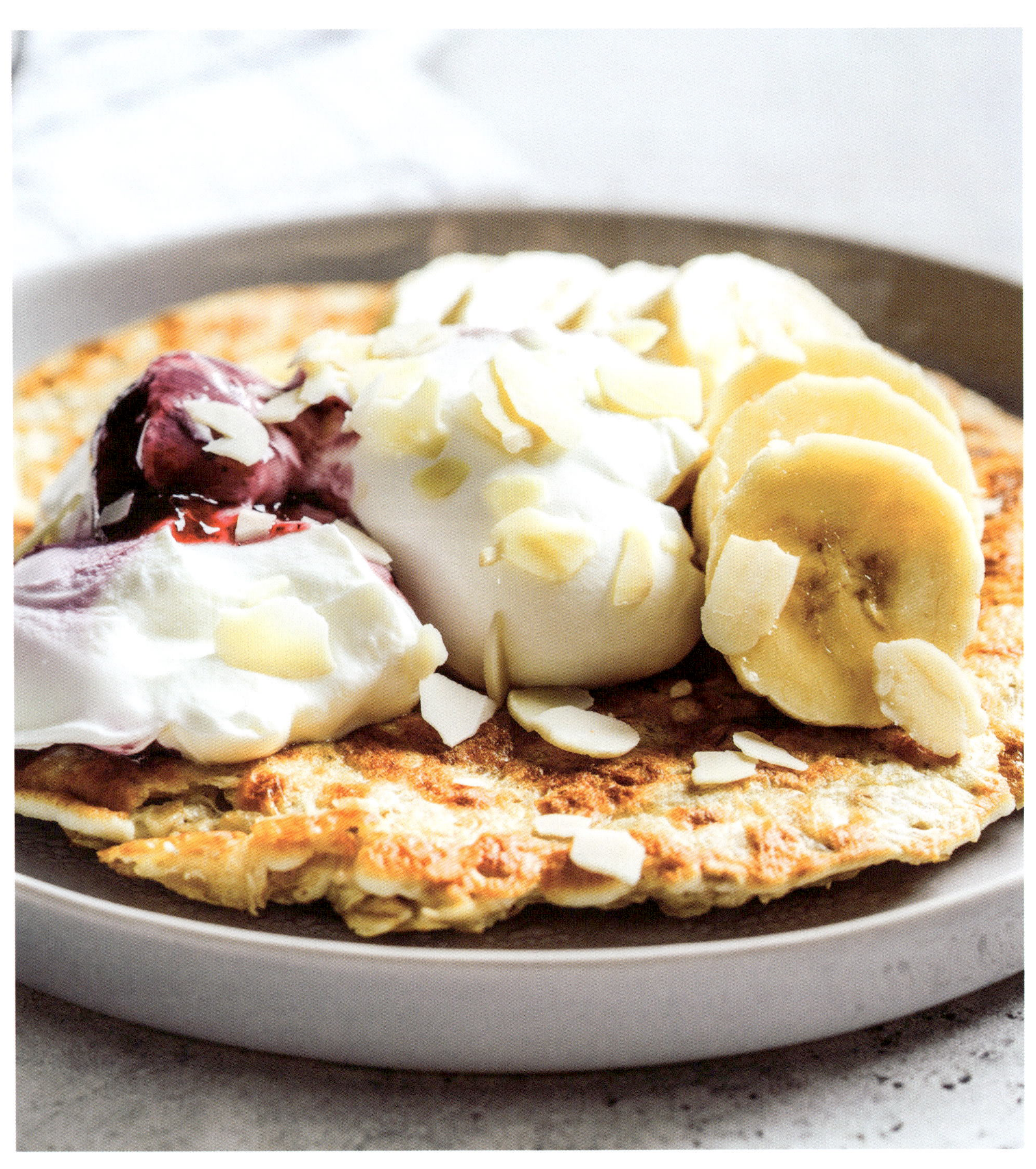

Banana Oat Pancakes

SERVES 4

PREP + COOK TIME: 40 MINS

VEG

BANANA OAT PANCAKES

1 cup (90g) rolled oats

1 cup (250ml) milk

1 tbsp unsalted butter, melted + more for cooking

2 large eggs

1 tbsp sugar

⅔ cup (80g) plain flour

2 tsps baking powder

¼ tsp salt

¼ tsp ground cinnamon

Baking pan

TO SERVE

2 medium bananas, sliced

⅔ cup (160ml) Greek yoghurt

½ cup (50g) frozen blueberries, warmed

2 tbsps flaked almonds

Whisk oats and milk together in a large bowl. Let stand for 10 minutes for the oats to soften.

Add melted butter, eggs and sugar to the oats, and whisk to combine. Add flour, baking powder, salt and cinnamon and whisk until just combined.

Grease the pan with butter. Pour a ladleful of mixture into pan.

Cook for 5-7 minutes at 165°C until golden brown.

Remove from the pan with a spatula and keep warm. Repeat with the remaining mixture.

Serve with sliced banana, yoghurt, blueberries and flaked almonds or other toppings as desired.

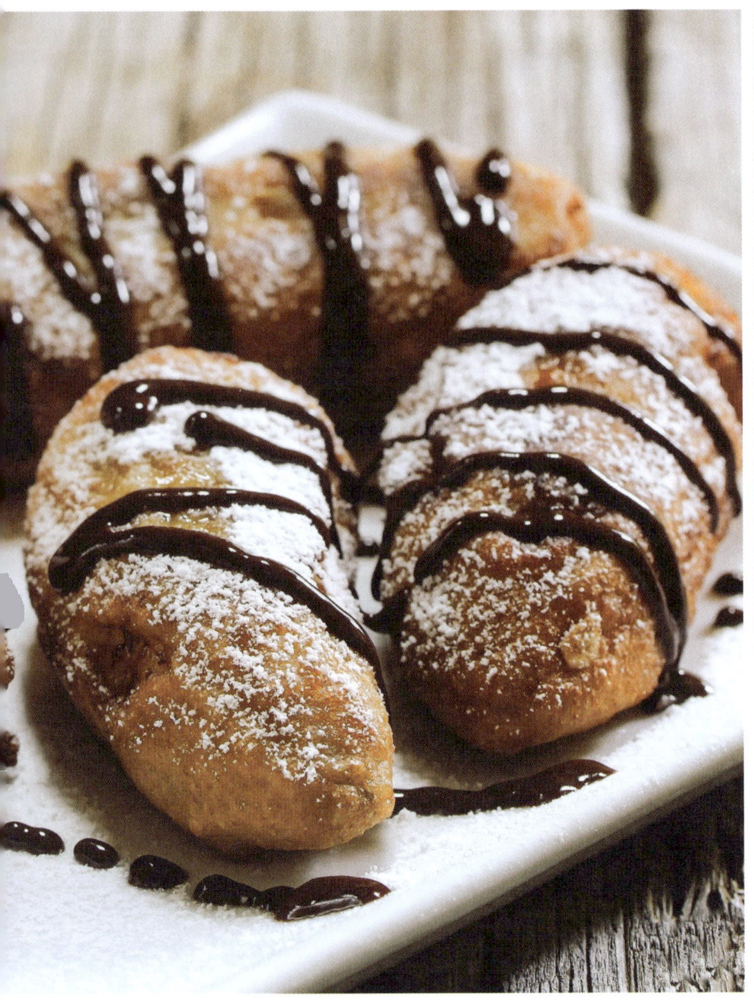

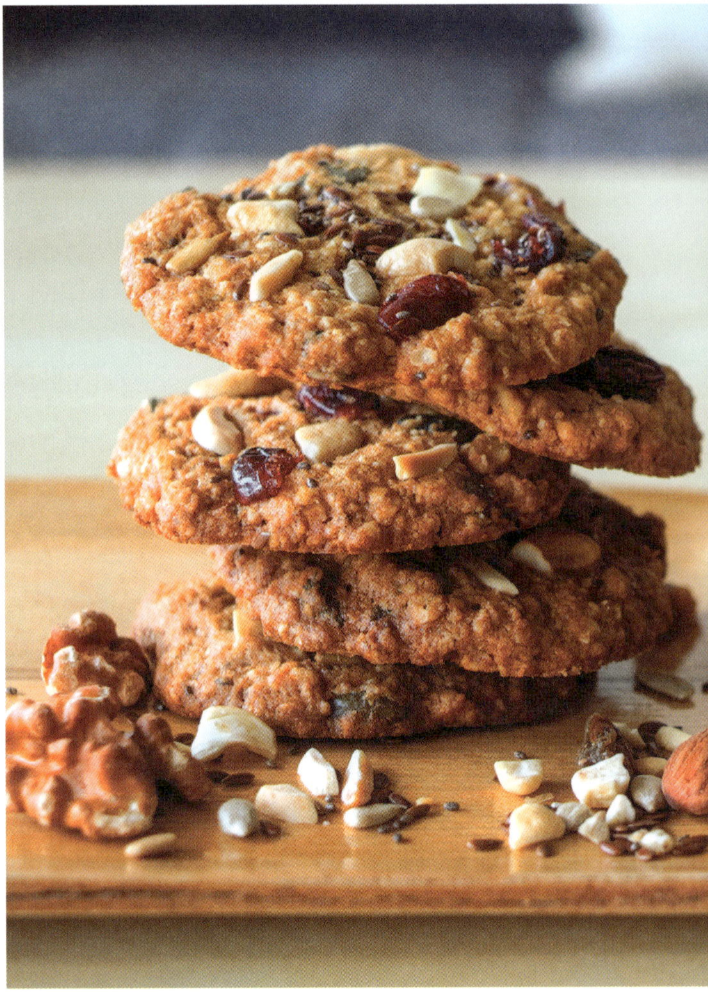

Banana Fritters

SERVES 6-8

PREP + COOK TIME: 25 MINS

VEG • GLUTEN FREE

Cranberry, Nut & Seed Biscuits

MAKES 26

PREP + COOK TIME: 20 MINS

VEG • GLUTEN FREE

BANANA FRITTERS

¾ cup (120g) rice flour

¼ cup (30g) tapioca flour

2 tbsps sugar

1 tsp salt

½ cup (45g) shredded coconut

½ tsp bicarbonate of soda

1 cup (250ml) water

500g lady finger bananas (about 6-8)

100g dark chocolate, broken into squares

Icing sugar, to serve

Cake tin or ovenproof bowl

In a mixing bowl, combine rice flour, tapioca flour, sugar, salt, coconut and bicarb, then add water a little at a time. Mix well to form a thick batter.

Dip the bananas into the batter and shake to remove excess.

Transfer bananas to air fryer and cook at 180°C for 8 minutes until golden brown.

Put chocolate in a cake tin or ovenproof bowl and transfer to air fryer. Cook for 1-2 minutes at 160°C until melted.

Dust bananas fritters with icing sugar and drizzle with melted chocolate to serve.

CRANBERRY, NUT & SEED BISCUITS

2 cups (240g) almond meal

½ tsp salt

1 tsp bicarbonate of soda

⅓ cup (80ml) butter, melted

⅓ cup (105g) maple syrup

1 large egg

1 tsp vanilla extract

½ cup (80g) dried cranberries

½ cup (60g) nuts, roughly chopped (cashews, walnuts and almonds)

1 tsp chia seeds

1 tsp flaxseed

1 tbsp sunflower seeds

Cake tin or baking pan

Preheat air fryer to 155°C. Line cake tin or baking pan with greaseproof paper.

In a medium bowl, combine almond meal, salt and bicarb.

In another bowl, whisk together melted butter, maple syrup, egg and vanilla extract.

Add dry ingredients to the wet mixture and mix to combine. Stir in cranberries, nuts and seeds.

Working in batches, scoop tablespoons of dough into cake tin or baking pan, leaving space between each one. Gently press to flatten slightly.

Place tin into air fryer and cook for 7-10 minutes until edges are slightly golden brown. Set aside to cool.

Repeat with remaining mixture.

CARAMELISED NUT CLUSTERS

1 sheet frozen shortcrust pastry, thawed

1 egg white

¼ cup (80g) maple syrup

¼ tsp cinnamon

¼ cup (30g) macadamia halves

¼ cup (30g) almonds

¼ cup (30g) hazelnuts

¼ cup (30g) cashews

¼ cup (30g) walnut halves

2 tbsps salted butter, melted

Muffin tray or silicone moulds

Use a pastry cutter to cut out fluted circles. Press into silicone moulds or an air fryer muffin tray.

Place in air fryer and cook for 15-18 minutes at 160°C until golden brown. Remove from air fryer and set aside.

Line the air fryer basket with aluminium foil.

Mix egg white, maple syrup and cinnamon together in a bowl. Add nuts and toss to coat.

Pour melted butter into lined air fryer basket. Add the nuts and spread out evenly.

Cook for 5 minutes at 150°C, then shake the basket and cook for a further 5 minutes. Shake basket once again and cook for another 2-4 minutes until golden brown.

Remove nuts from air fryer. Spoon into precooked pastry cases and serve.

BAKED APPLES

4 apples

⅓ cup (50g) raisins

⅓ cup (40g) walnuts, chopped

1 tsp cinnamon

4 tbsps butter, softened

Baking pan

Cut off the tops of the apples, then core using a sharp knife or corer.

Place the raisins, walnuts and cinnamon in a small bowl and stir briefly. Add the butter and mix to combine.

Spoon the filling into the centre of the apples.

Place apples in the baking pan and place in the air fryer.

Cook for 20 minutes at 175°C.

Allow to cool slightly before serving.

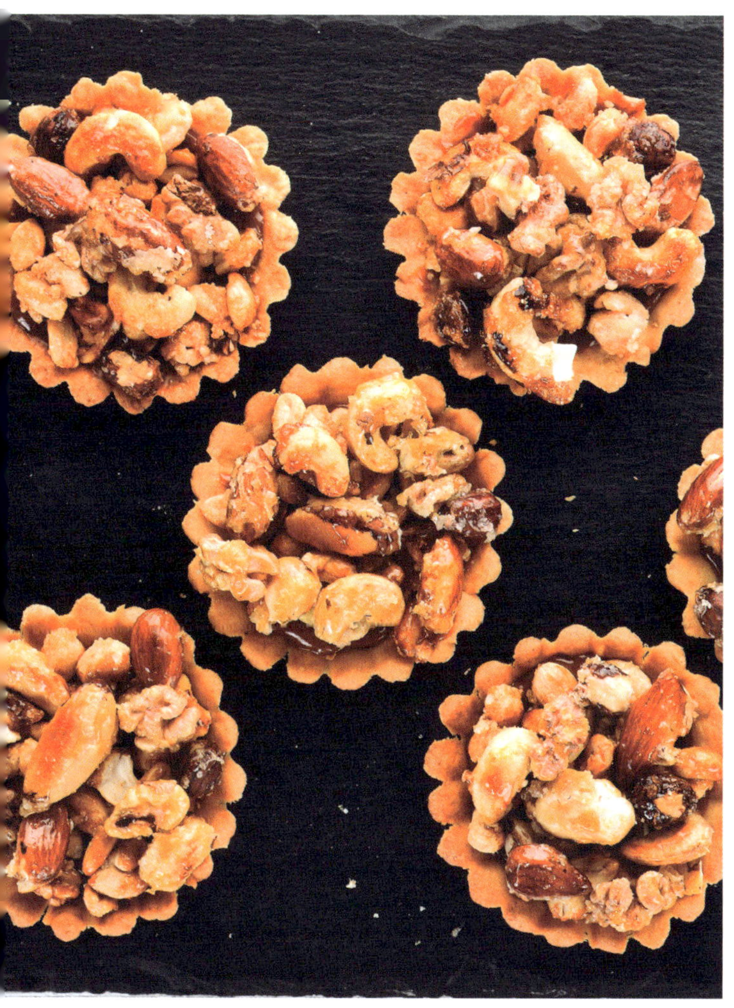

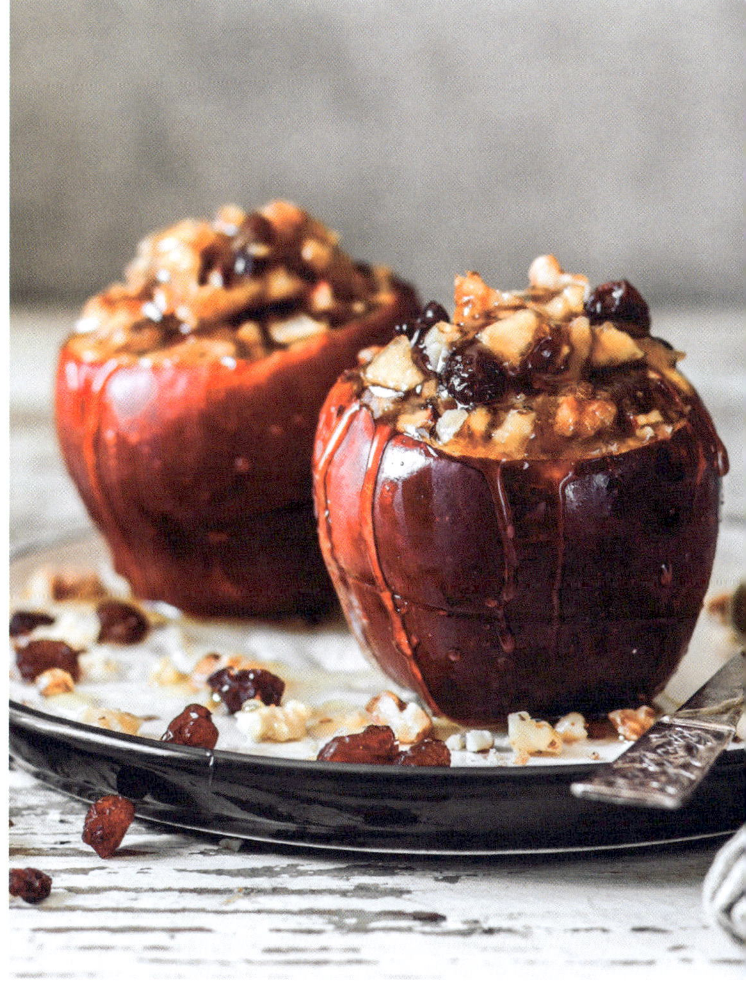

Caramelised Nut Clusters

MAKES 8

PREP + COOK TIME: 45 MINS

VEG

Baked Apples

SERVES 4

PREP + COOK TIME: 30 MINS

VEG • GLUTEN FREE

Pumpkin Pie

SERVES 2

PREP + COOK TIME: 50 MINS + COOLING

VEG

1 sheet frozen shortcrust pastry, thawed

2¼ cups (500g) mashed cooked pumpkin

½ cup (125ml) thickened cream or coconut cream

2 large eggs

½ cup (155g) maple syrup

1 tsp cinnamon

¼ tsp nutmeg

¼ tsp ground cloves

⅛ tsp ground ginger

¼ tsp salt

Zest of 1 orange

Whipped cream and cinnamon to serve

1 large or 2 small pie dishes

Roll out pastry and cut out circles to line pie dishes. You may need to cook one at a time depending on the size of your air fryer.

Prick pastry case with a fork and place in air fryer. Cook at 160°C for 8-10 minutes.

Combine pumpkin, cream, eggs, maple syrup, spices, salt and orange zest in a large bowl. Mix well then pour into prepared cases.

Place in air fryer and cook at 170°C for 25-30 minutes or until set.

Allow pumpkin pies to cool completely.

Top with whipped cream and cinnamon to serve.

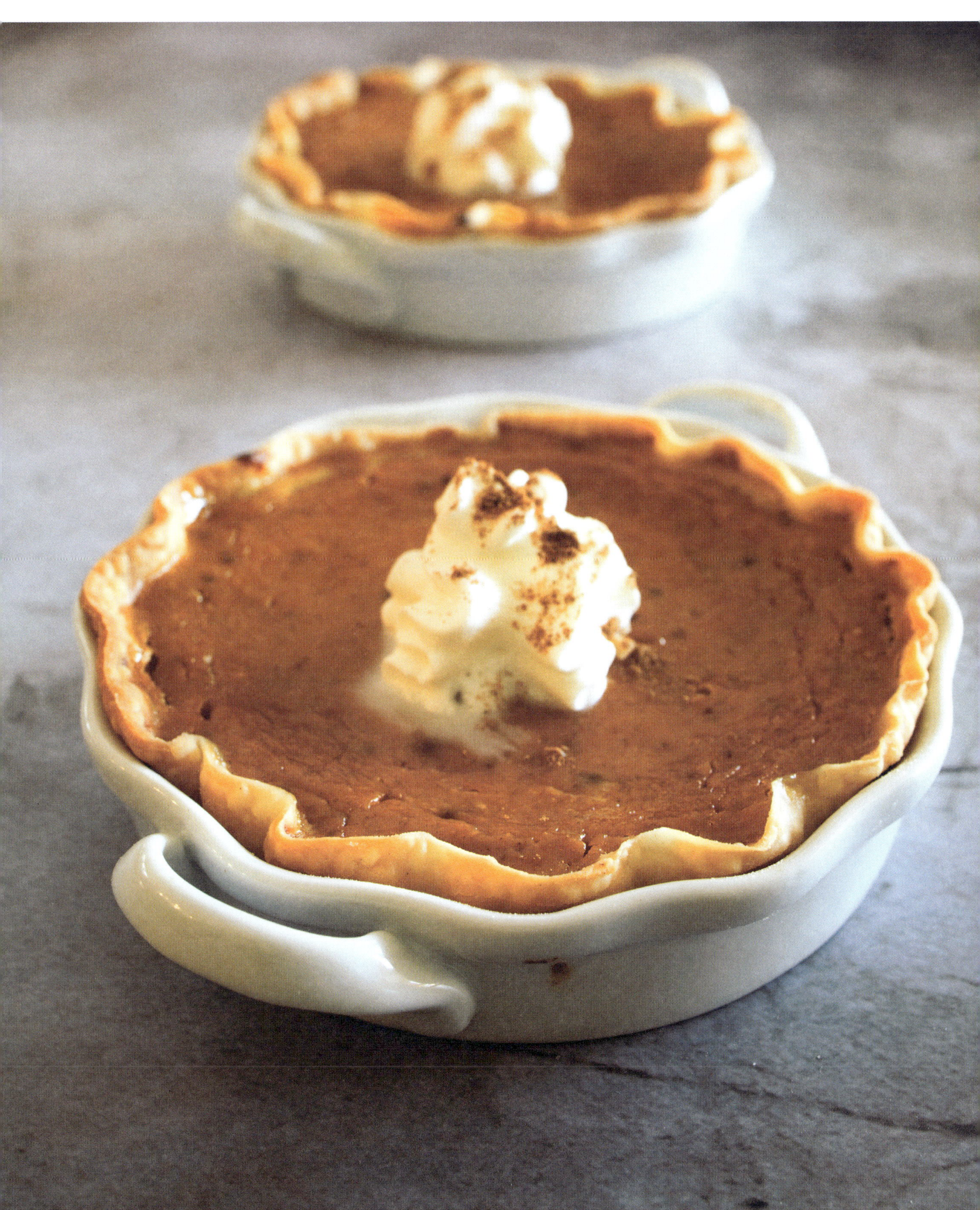

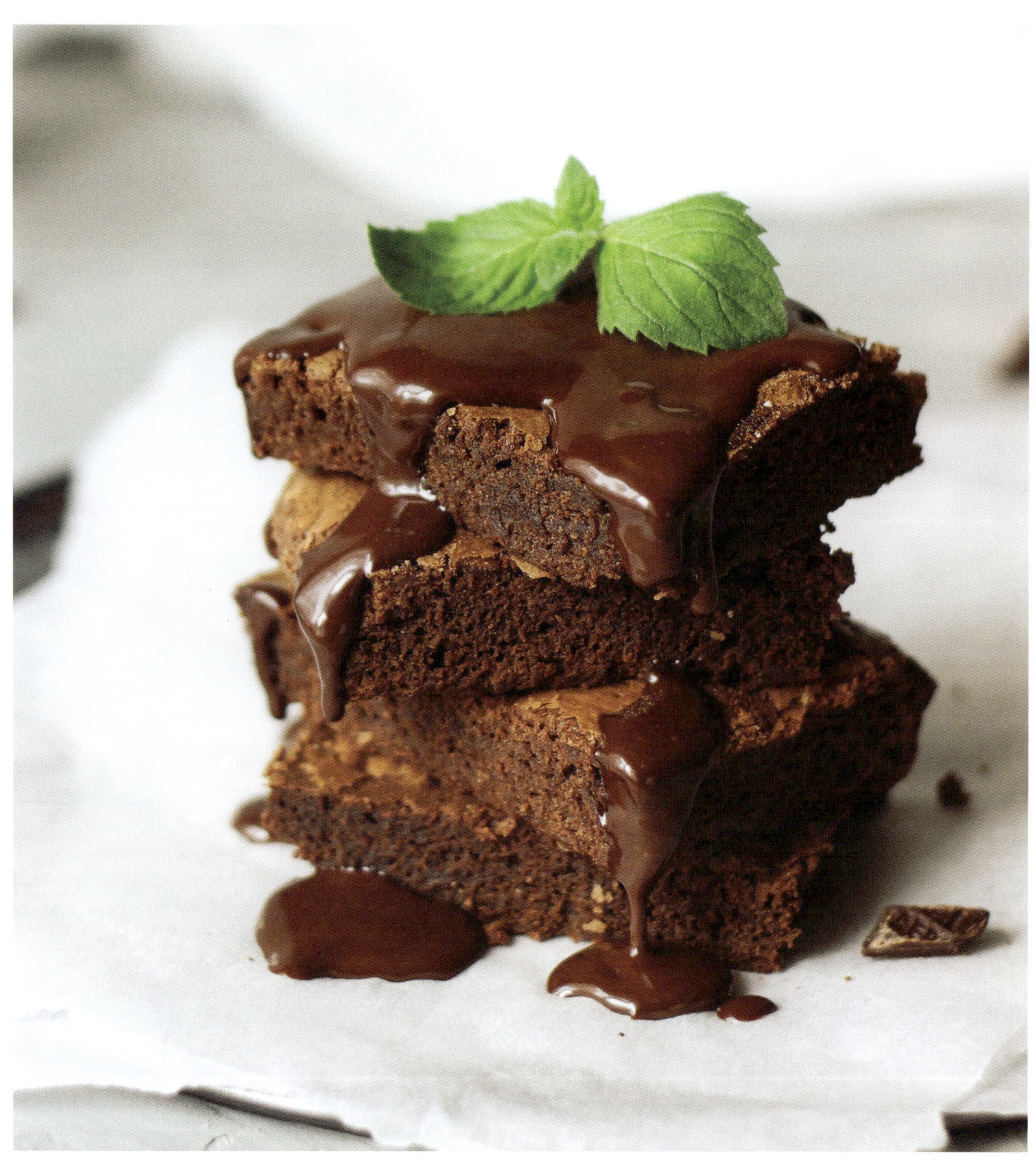

Chocolate Brownies

SERVES 8

PREP + COOK TIME: 35 MINS

VEG

CHOCOLATE BROWNIES

115g butter, melted

1 cup (220g) sugar

2 large eggs

1 tsp vanilla extract

½ cup (60g) plain flour

⅓ cup (35g) cocoa powder

1 tsp baking powder

100g chocolate, melted

Baking pan

Preheat air fryer to 175°C. Grease the baking pan.

In a large bowl, mix together the melted butter and sugar using an electric hand mixer until light and fluffy. Add eggs, vanilla, flour, cocoa and baking powder. Mix well to incorporate.

Pour batter into the prepared baking pan and cook for 20-25 minutes until firm on top but still soft and fudgy inside.

Cut into squares and drizzle with melted chocolate to serve.

BAKLAVA

1⅔ cups (200g) pistachios
1⅔ cups (200g) walnuts
1 tsp ground cinnamon
250g filo pastry
250g unsalted butter, melted
1 cup (200g) caster sugar
¾ cup (200ml) water
½ cup (180g) honey
2 tbsps lemon juice
Baking pan

Place nuts and cinnamon in a food processor. Pulse until finely chopped.

Unroll filo pastry. Cut through the whole stack, trimming the pastry to fit a baking dish that will fit inside your air fryer. Cover the filo sheets with a damp cloth.

Place two sheets of filo in the baking dish. Brush with melted butter, and repeat until you have eight sheets of buttered and layered filo.

Cover pastry with nut mixture then add remaining pastry sheets, brushing each one with butter.

Cut into diamond or square shapes all the way to the bottom of the dish. Transfer to air fryer and cook for 25 minutes at 180°C until golden.

Meanwhile boil sugar and water until sugar is dissolved. Add honey and lemon juice. Simmer for 15-20 minutes. Allow to cool.

Remove the baklava from the air fryer and immediately pour over the cooled syrup. Leave to cool before serving.

PEACH TART

2 sheets frozen shortcrust pastry, thawed
8 peaches, sliced
4 tbsps butter, melted
1 tsp ground cinnamon
4 ramekins or small flan tins

Cut the pastry to fit into four ramekins or small flan tins. Trim the edges and prick with a fork.

Arrange the peaches in the flan tins. Drizzle with melted butter and sprinkle with cinnamon.

Working in batches, cook at 150°C for 15-20 minutes, until peaches are soft and pastry is golden brown.

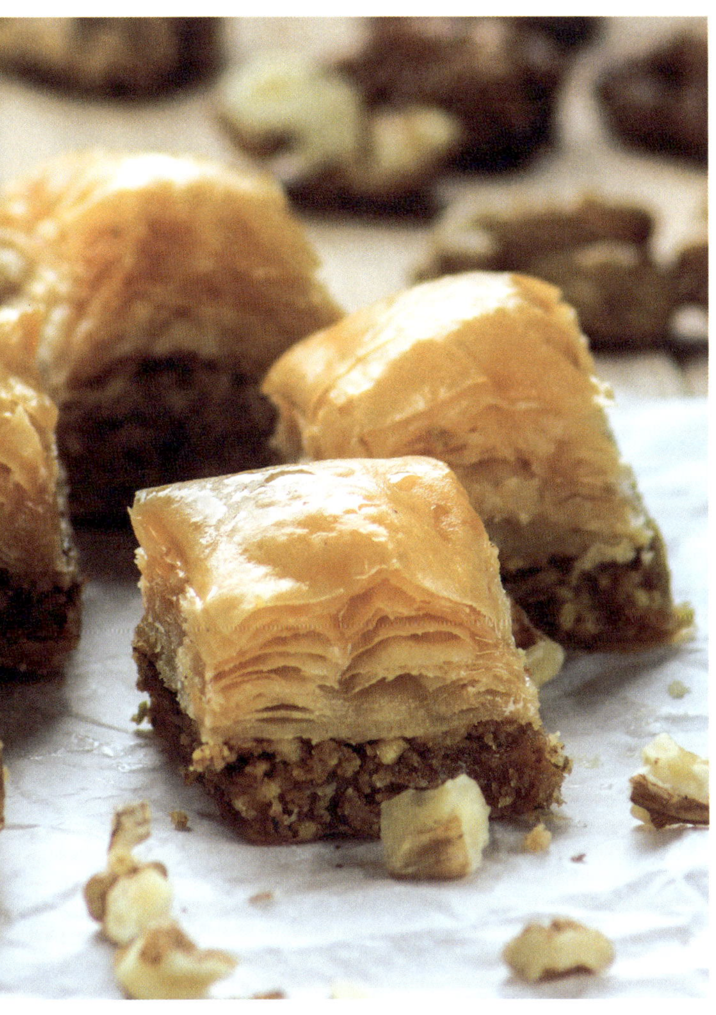

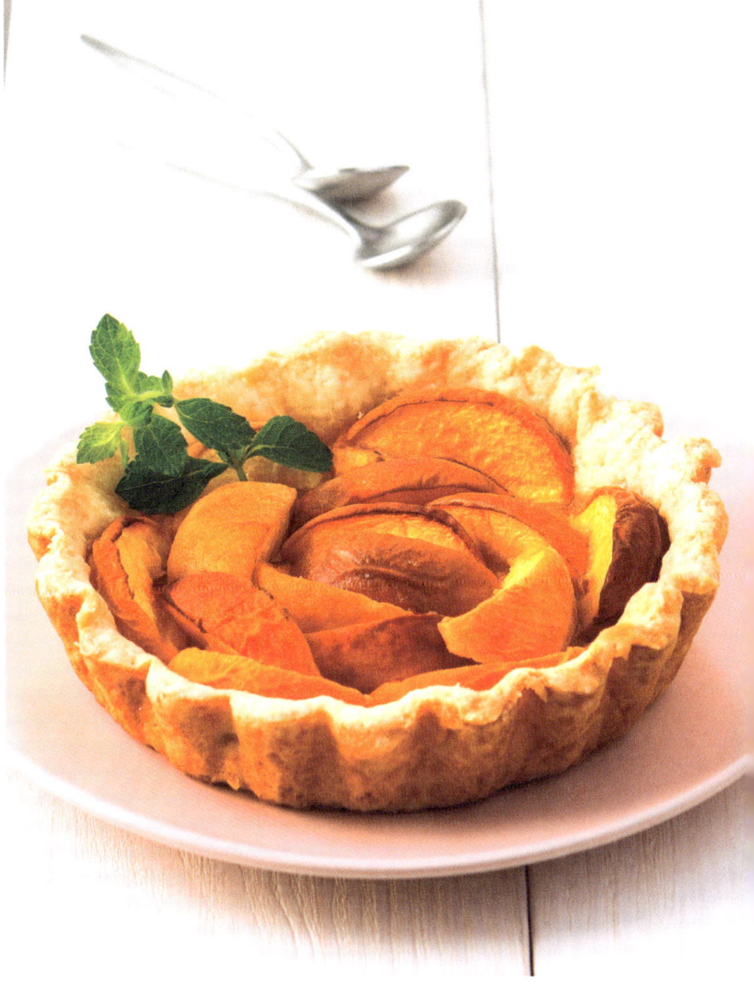

Baklava

SERVES 12

PREP + COOK TIME: 45 MINS

VEG

Peach Tart

SERVES 4

PREP + COOK TIME: 30 MINS

VEG

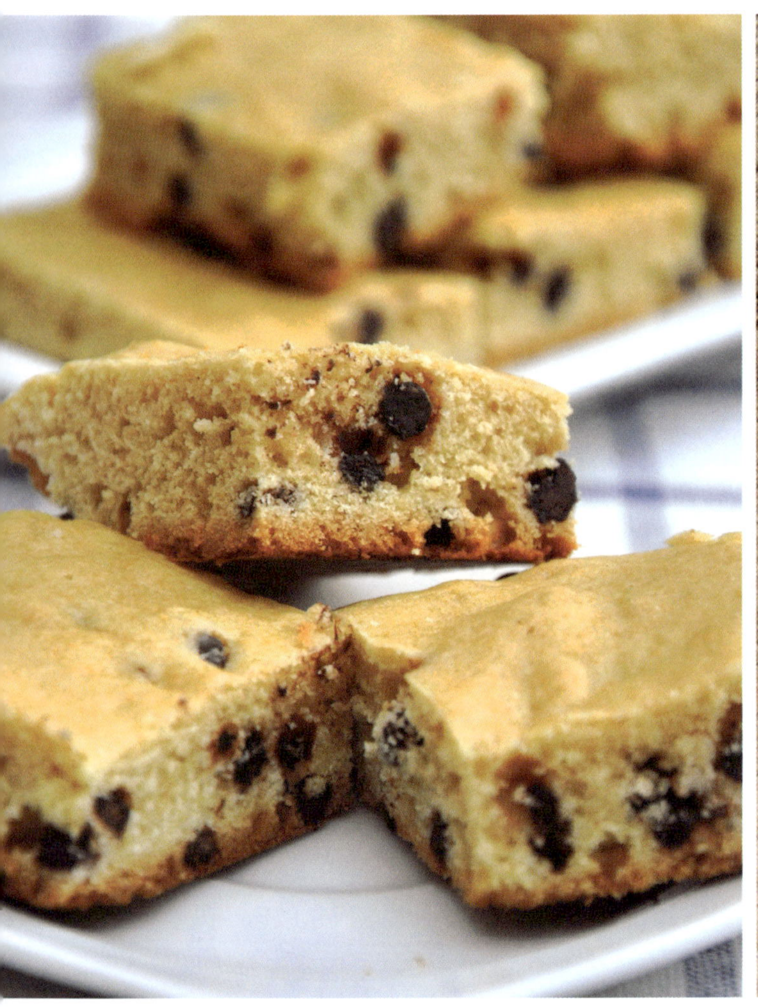

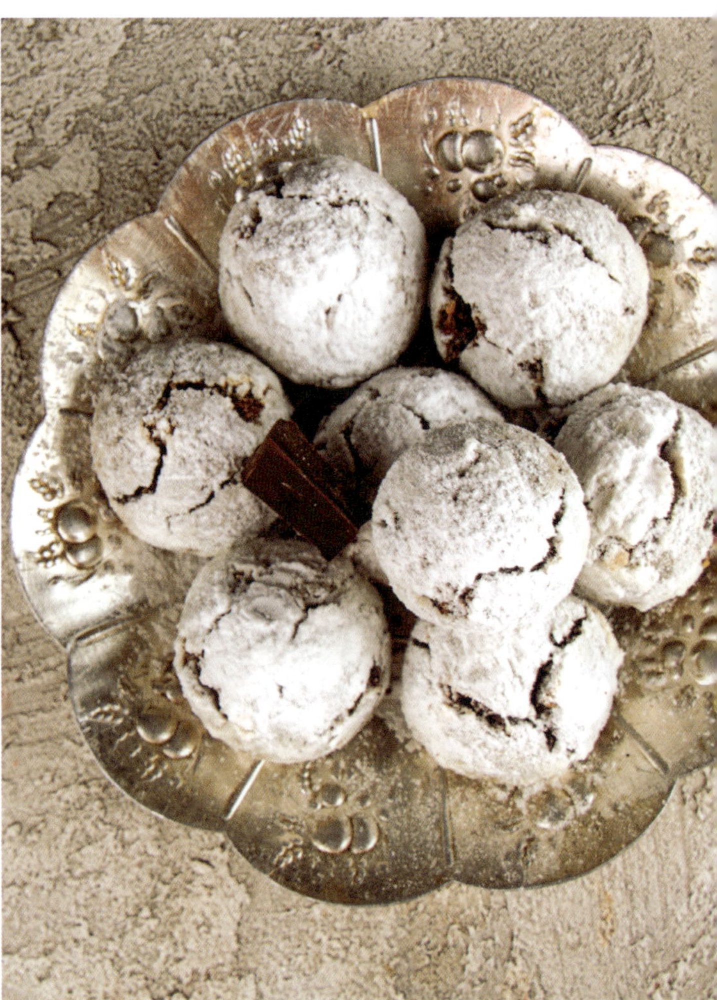

Chocolate Chip Blondies

SERVES 4

PREP + COOK TIME: 20 MINS

VEG

Shortbread Chocolate Balls

MAKES 10

PREP + COOK TIME: 30 MINS

VEG

CHOCOLATE CHIP BLONDIES

6 tbsps unsalted butter, melted
1 cup (155g) dark brown sugar
2 egg yolks
1 tsp pure vanilla extract
1 tsp salt
1 cup (125g) plain flour
1 tsp baking powder
1½ cups (235g) dark chocolate chips
Baking pan

Spray an air fryer baking pan with cooking spray.

In a large bowl mix together the melted butter, brown sugar, egg yolks, vanilla extract and salt.

Fold in the flour, baking powder and chocolate chips.

Pour into the prepared baking pan and place in the air fryer.

Cook at 160°C for 12-15 minutes until golden brown.

Allow to cool before slicing.

SHORTBREAD CHOCOLATE BALLS

¼ cup (25g) plain flour
⅓ cup (75g) caster sugar
2 tbsps cocoa
180g butter, chilled and cut into cubes
½ tsp vanilla extract
10 pieces of good-quality chocolate
Icing sugar, for rolling
Baking pan

Combine the flour, sugar and cocoa in a mixing bowl. Rub in the butter to form a crumble. Continue mixing and then knead to form a smooth dough.

Roll the mixture into 10 balls. Squeeze a piece of chocolate into the centre of each and re-shape the ball around it.

Preheat the air fryer to 180°C.

Place the chocolate shortbread balls onto the baking pan and transfer to the air fryer.

Cook for 12 minutes, turning with tongs halfway through cooking.

Roll in icing sugar while still warm.

Cream Cheese Pie

SERVES 4
PREP + COOK TIME: 30 MINS
VEG

125g cream cheese, softened
1 cup (250g) ricotta
1 cup (250g) cottage cheese
2 tbsps caster sugar
1 tsp ground cinnamon
10 sheets filo pastry
100g unsalted butter, melted
Cake tin

Grease a round cake tin with butter.

Using an electric mixer, beat cream cheese until light and fluffy, then add ricotta, cottage cheese, sugar and cinnamon. Beat well to combine.

Place a sheet of filo in the cake tin and brush lightly with melted butter. Top with another pastry sheet. Continue brushing and layering until there are four layers.

Spoon cheese mixture into cake tin.

Layer the remaining filo sheets on top of the cheese mixture, brushing each one with melted butter.

Take hold of any loose edges and roll and tuck inside the edge of the cake tin. Brush top of pie with melted butter.

Transfer pie to air fryer basket. Cook for 20 minutes at 180°C until golden brown and crisp.

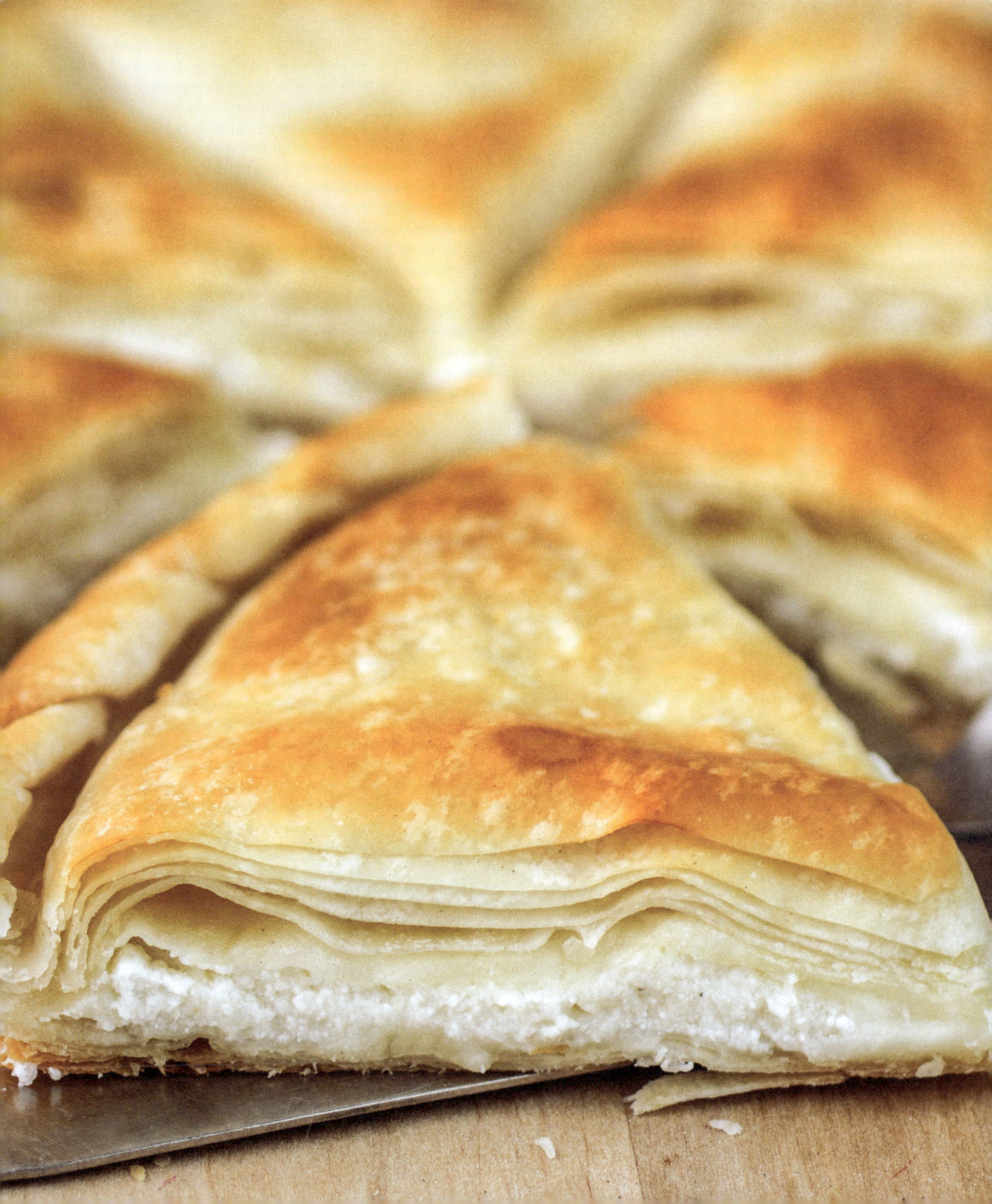

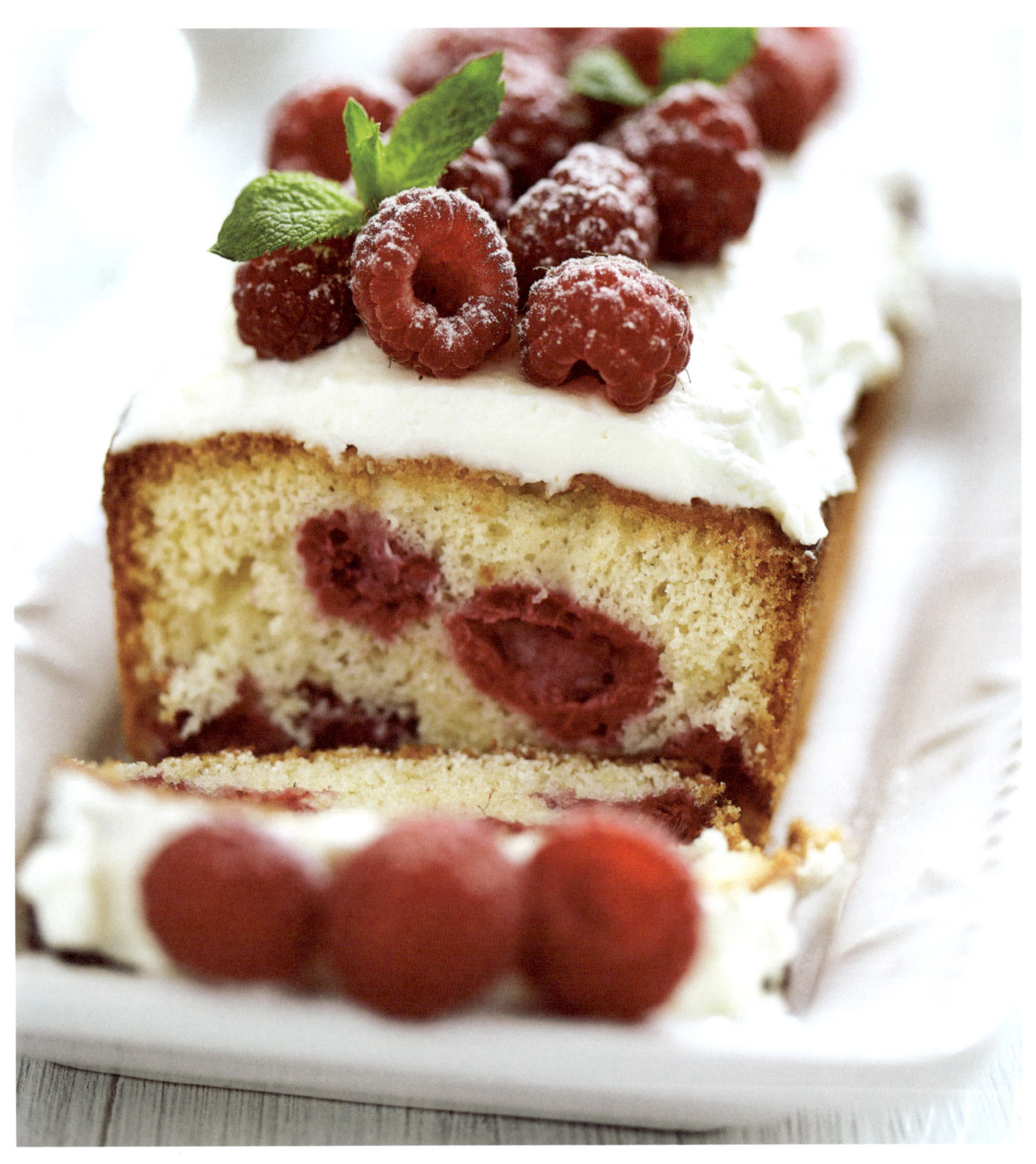

Raspberry Yoghurt Cake

SERVES 6

PREP + COOK TIME: 30 MINS

VEG

RASPBERRY YOGHURT CAKE

½ cup (60g) plain flour

⅛ tsp salt

¼ tsp baking powder

½ cup (125ml) vanilla yogurt

2 tbsps vegetable oil

2 tbsps maple syrup

¾ cup (90g) fresh raspberries + ¼ cup (30g) more to serve

Loaf tin

CREAM CHEESE ICING

120g unsalted butter, softened

225g cream cheese, softened

1 tsp vanilla extract

¼ tsp salt

4 cups (620g) icing sugar

Preheat air fryer to 150°C. Spray a loaf tin that fits into your air fryer with cooking spray.

In a bowl combine flour, salt and baking powder; mix well.

Mix in yogurt, oil and maple syrup, then gently fold in raspberries.

Pour batter into prepared pan and cook for 8-10 minutes. Allow to cool for 10 minutes in the pan, then turn onto a wire rack to cool completely.

Place butter and cream cheese in a large bowl. Mix with an electric mixer until smooth and creamy.

Add vanilla extract and salt and stir well to combine.

With mixer on low, gradually add icing sugar until completely combined.

When the cake is completely cool, spread with cream cheese icing and top with fresh raspberries.

Clafoutis with Blueberries

SERVES 4
PREP + COOK TIME: 35 MINS + CHILLING
VEG • GLUTEN FREE

4 large eggs
1 cup (250ml) milk of choice
¼ cup (90g) honey or maple syrup
1 tsp pure vanilla extract
¼ tsp salt
½ cup (60g) almond meal
¼ cup (30g) tapioca flour
1 cup (125g) mixed berries
4 ramekins

Preheat the oven to 180°C.

Combine eggs, milk, honey, vanilla, salt, almond meal and tapioca flour in a food processor. Blend until smooth.

Pour mixture into the ramekins then add a handful of berries to each one.

Place in air fryer and cook for about 30-32 minutes until set.

Allow to cool, then place in the fridge to chill before serving.

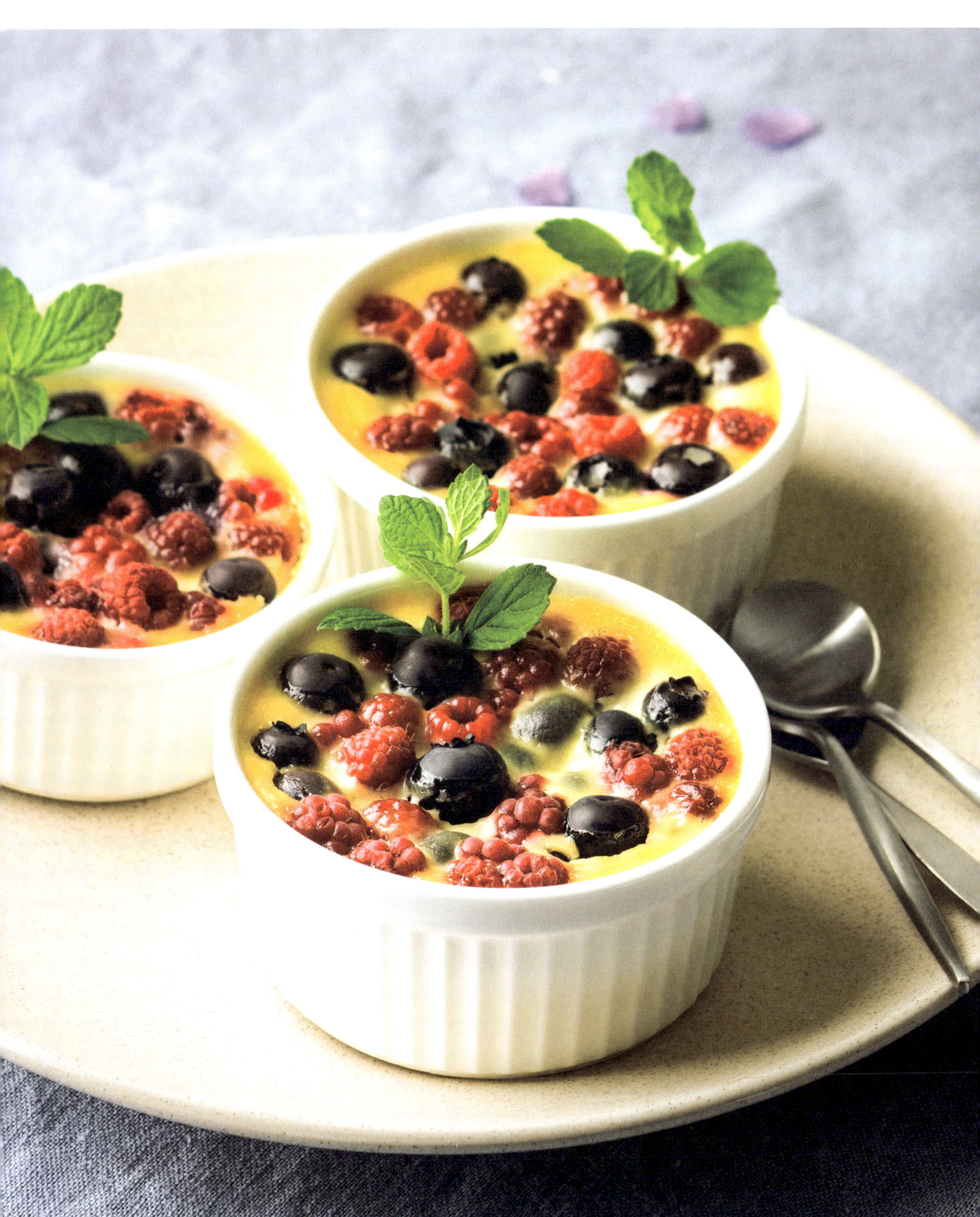

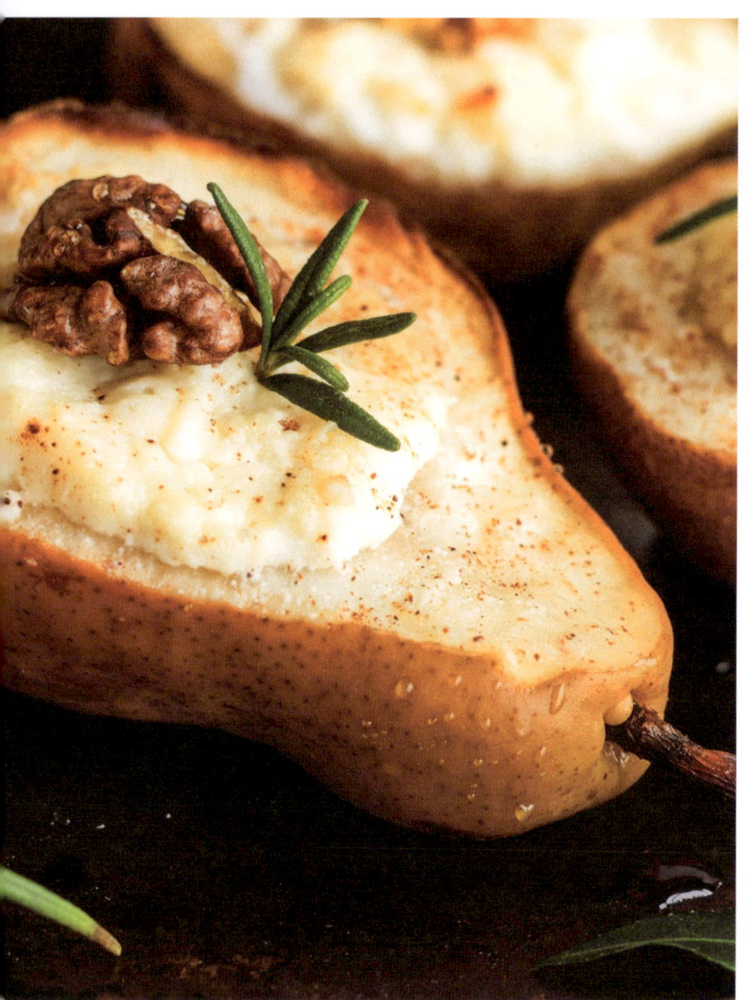

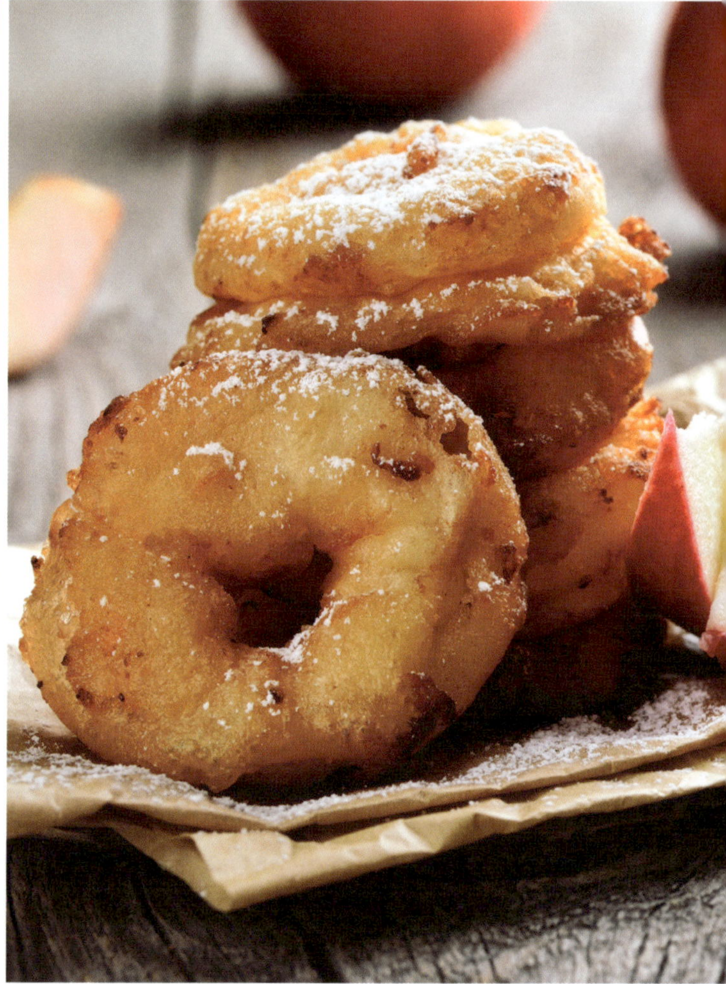

Baked Pears with Ricotta

SERVES 2

PREP + COOK TIME: 20 MINS

VEG • GLUTEN-FREE

Apple Rings

SERVES 8

PREP + COOK TIME: 30 MINS

VEG

BAKED PEARS WITH RICOTTA

2 tbsps butter, melted

1 tsp vanilla powder

½ tsp cinnamon + ½ tsp to serve

2 pears, cut in half and cored

½ cup (125g) ricotta cheese

1 tbsp maple syrup + 2 tsps to serve

4 walnut halves

4 small sprigs rosemary

Preheat air fryer to 175°C.

Combine melted butter, vanilla and cinnamon. Mix well.

Baste pears all over with the butter mixture and place cut-side down in a baking pan that will fit in your air fryer.

Cook for 10 minutes, then baste pears once again and cook for a further 2 minutes.

Transfer pears to a serving plate and baste once more.

Combine ricotta and maple syrup in a bowl. Mix well.

Spoon ricotta on top of the pears. Top each with a walnut half and rosemary sprig. Drizzle with a little more maple syrup and dust with extra cinnamon to serve.

APPLE RINGS

1 cup (125g) plain flour

2 tbsps sugar

2 tsps cinnamon

½ cup (125ml) macadamia oil or other neutral-flavoured oil

4 apples peeled, cored and sliced into 1cm-thick rings

4 tbsps icing sugar

In a bowl mix together flour, sugar and 1 teaspoon cinnamon. Place oil in a small bowl. Dab each sliced apple dry with a paper towel and then dip first into the oil, then into the flour mixture, turning to coat on both sides.

Spray inside of air fryer basket with cooking spray. Lay the apple slices in the basket in a single layer. Work in batches or use a double-layer accessory, if necessary.

Cook at 160°C for 13 minutes. Spray with cooking spray, then cook for a further 2 minutes.

In a bowl mix together icing sugar and remaining 1 teaspoon cinnamon.

Sprinkle the cinnamon sugar over the cooked apples before serving.

PEACH & CHERRY PIES

2 peaches, peeled and thickly sliced
1 cup (200g) fresh cherries, pitted
¼ cup (55g) sugar
2 tsps cornflour
¼ tsp cinnamon
2 sheets frozen puff pastry, thawed

Toss the peaches, cherries, sugar, cornflour and cinnamon together until well combined.

Cut each pastry sheet into four equal squares. Press the pastry squares into silicone cupcake moulds or a greased air fryer cupcake tin. Leave the corners of the squares hanging over the edges of the moulds.

Fill the pastry cups with equal amounts of the fruit mixture. Pinch the corners of the pastry squares together to form parcels.

Place in the air fryer and cook for 10 minutes at 200°C until golden.

BLUEBERRY CRUMBLE

1½ cups (150g) blueberries
¼ cup (30g) plain flour
¼ cup (20g) oats
2 tbsps butter
2 tbsps coconut sugar or rapadura
½ tsp cinnamon
2 ramekins

Preheat air fryer to 180°C.

Place blueberries in ramekins or a small ovenproof dish.

In a large bowl, combine the flour, oats and butter with your fingertips until the mixture resembles breadcrumbs. Add sugar and cinnamon. Mix well.

Spoon the crumble mixture over the fruit. Cook for 15 minutes until golden brown.

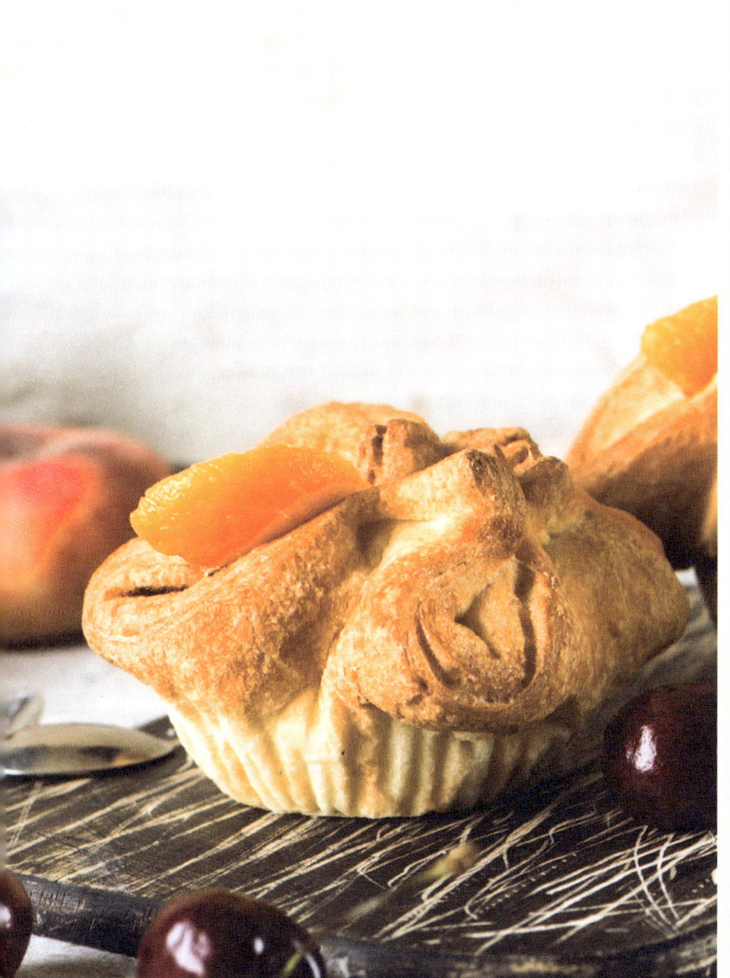

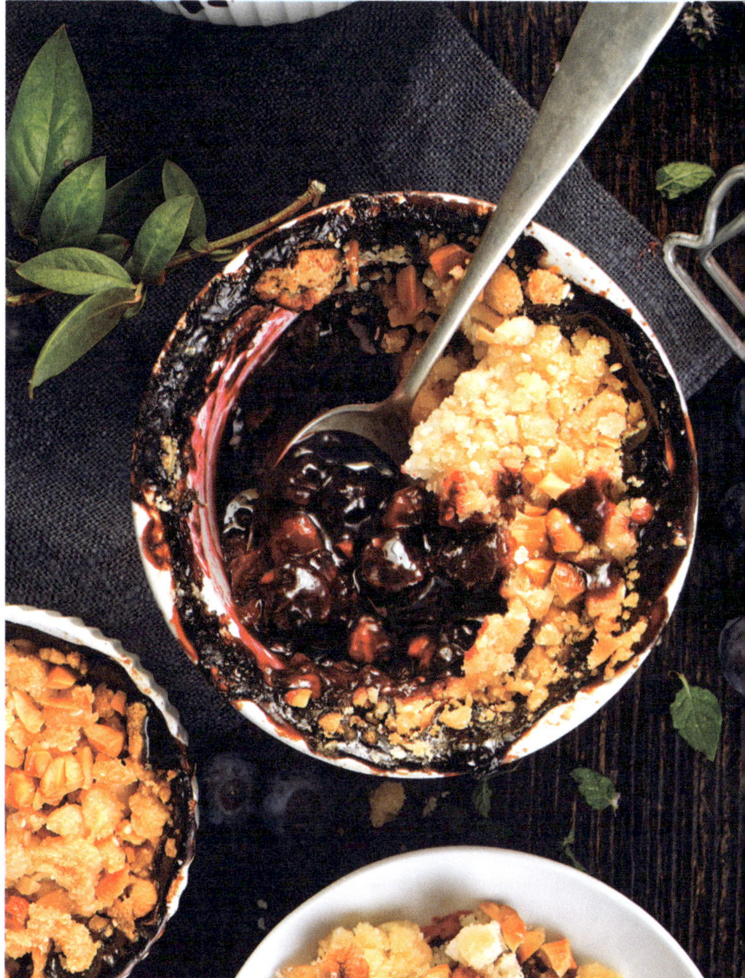

Peach & Cherry Pies

SERVES 8

PREP + COOK TIME: 25 MINS

VEG

Blueberry Crumble

SERVES 2

PREP + COOK TIME: 20 MINS

VEG

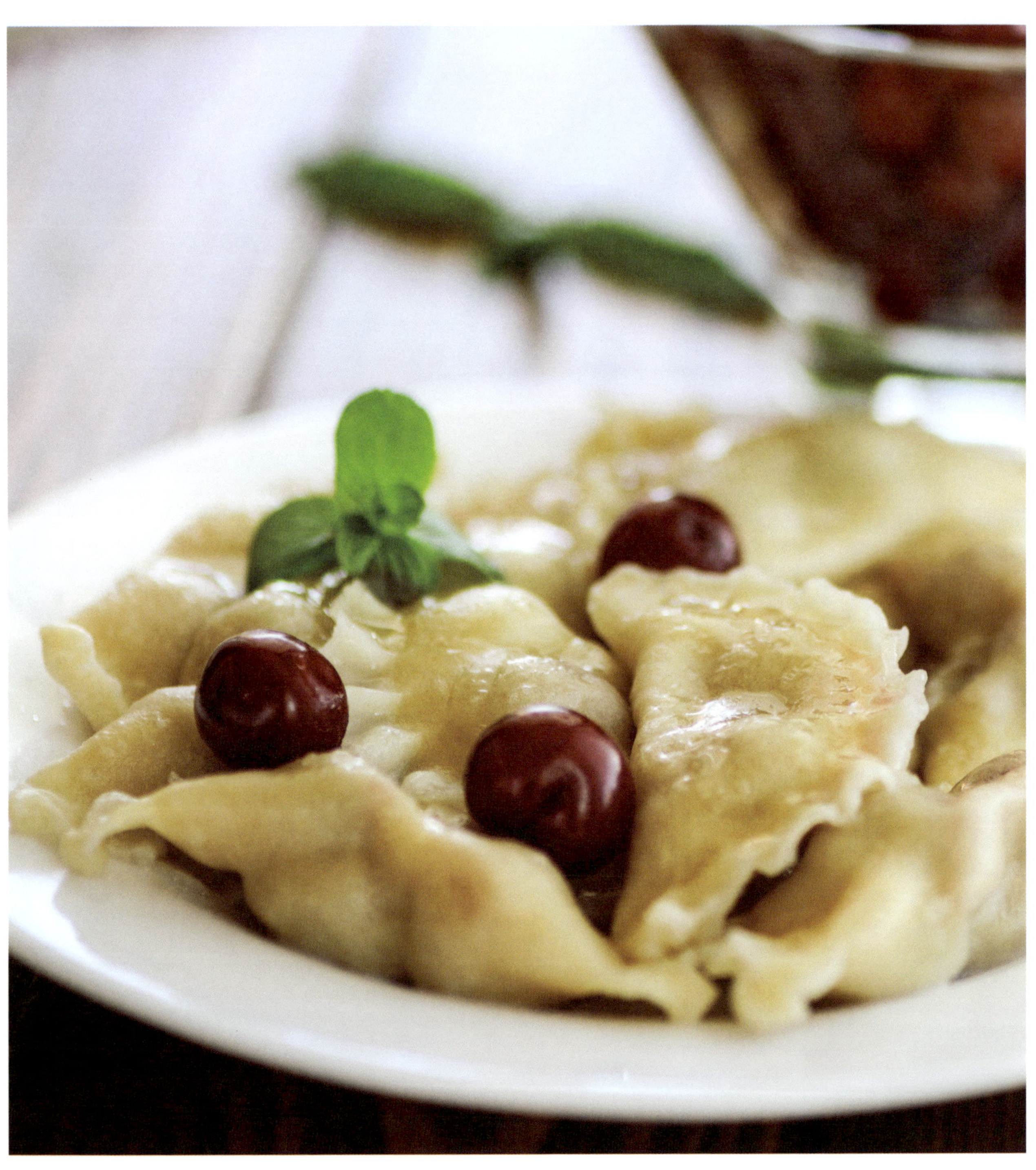

Fruit Dumplings

MAKES 30

PREP + COOK TIME: 45 MINS

VEG

FRUIT DUMPLINGS

DUMPLINGS

2 cups (250g) plain flour

Pinch of salt

1 egg, beaten

2½ tbsps unsalted butter, room temperature, cubed

¾-1 cup (185-250ml) lukewarm water

1½ cups (300g) strawberries, hulled and halved, or pitted cherries

TOPPINGS

2 tbsps unsalted butter, softened

2 tbsps icing sugar

½ cup (125ml) double cream

¼ cup (80g) strawberry or raspberry jam

In the bowl of a large food processor fitted with a dough blade or a large bowl, combine flour and salt. Add egg and butter to the flour mixture. Slowly mix in the water using the food processor or your hands until dough comes together.

Knead on a lightly floured surface until smooth and elastic.

Divide the dough into two pieces. On a lightly floured surface, roll the dough into a thin sheet, about 3mm thick. Use a round cookie cutter or the top of a glass to cut out 7cm-wide circles.

Place a piece of strawberry or cherry in the centre of each circle. Fold the circle in half over the fruit and pinch together the edges to seal. Repeat until remaining dough is used.

Working in batches, transfer to air fryer in one layer. Cook at 175°C for 4-5 minutes, then turn over and cook for a further 4-5 minutes.

Place dabs of softened butter over the dumplings and dust with icing sugar.

Drizzle with double cream and jam to serve.

M&M'S Cookies

MAKES 16
PREP + COOK TIME: 20 MINS
VEG

M&M'S COOKIES

½ cup (80g) brown sugar
60g butter, softened
1 egg
1 tsp vanilla
1 cup (125g) plain flour
¼ tsp bicarbonate of soda
¼ tsp salt
½ cup (80g) M&M'S
½ cup (80g) chopped dark chocolate

In a medium bowl cream together the butter and sugar with an electric hand mixer until light and fluffy. Add the egg and vanilla and mix until smooth and creamy.

In another bowl combine the flour, bicarb and salt and stir to combine. Add dry ingredients to the wet ingredients and mix to incorporate. Fold in the M&M'S and chopped chocolate.

Preheat air fryer to 175°C.

Working in batches form the dough into balls using a cookie scoop or two spoons. Place a sheet of greaseproof paper into the air fryer and place the dough balls, evenly spaced in one layer, in the basket. Flatten slightly with the back of a spoon.

Air fry for 5 minutes but leave the cookies in the air fryer with it closed for another 1-2 minutes. Transfer to a wire rack to cool. Continue with the remaining dough.

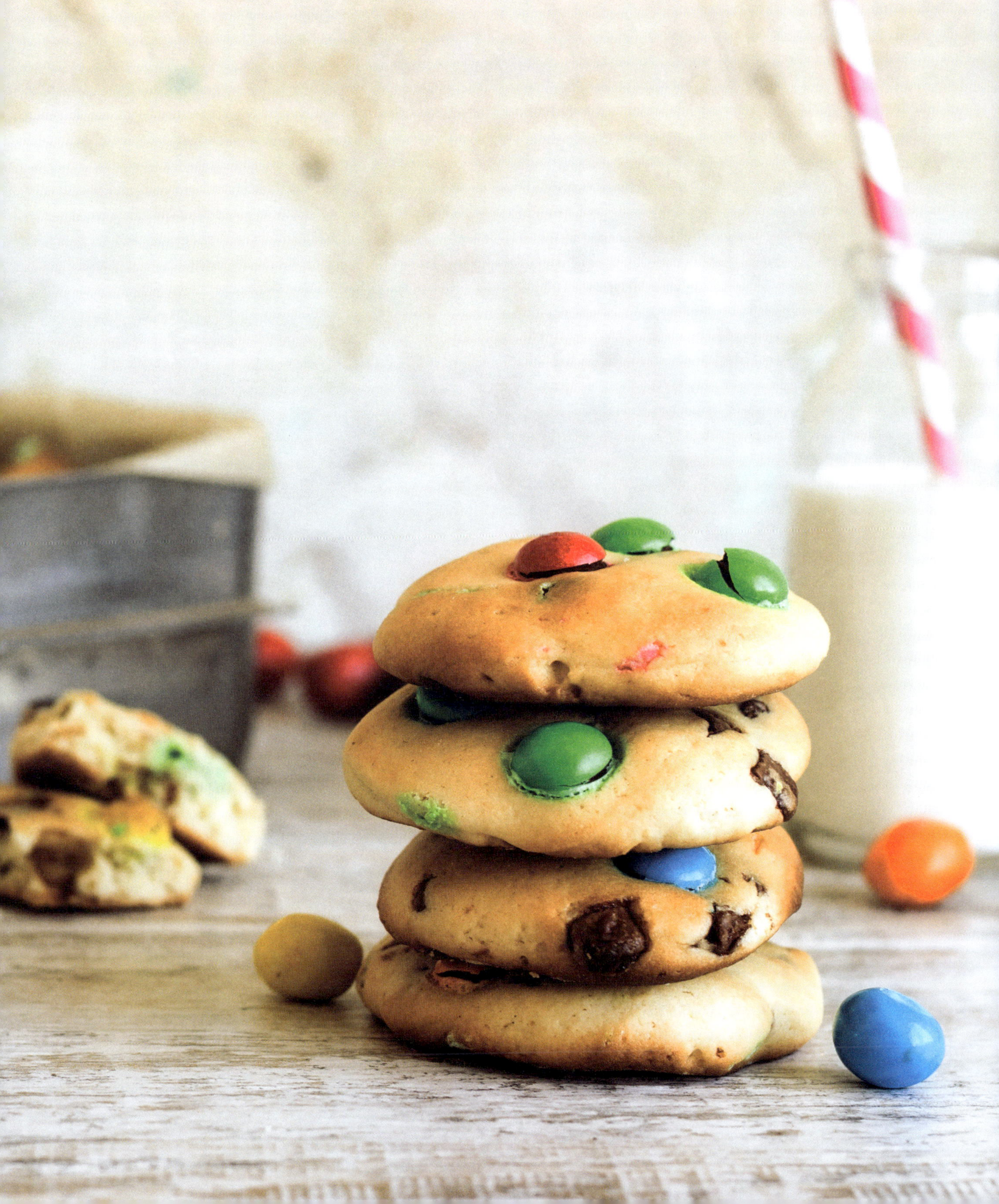

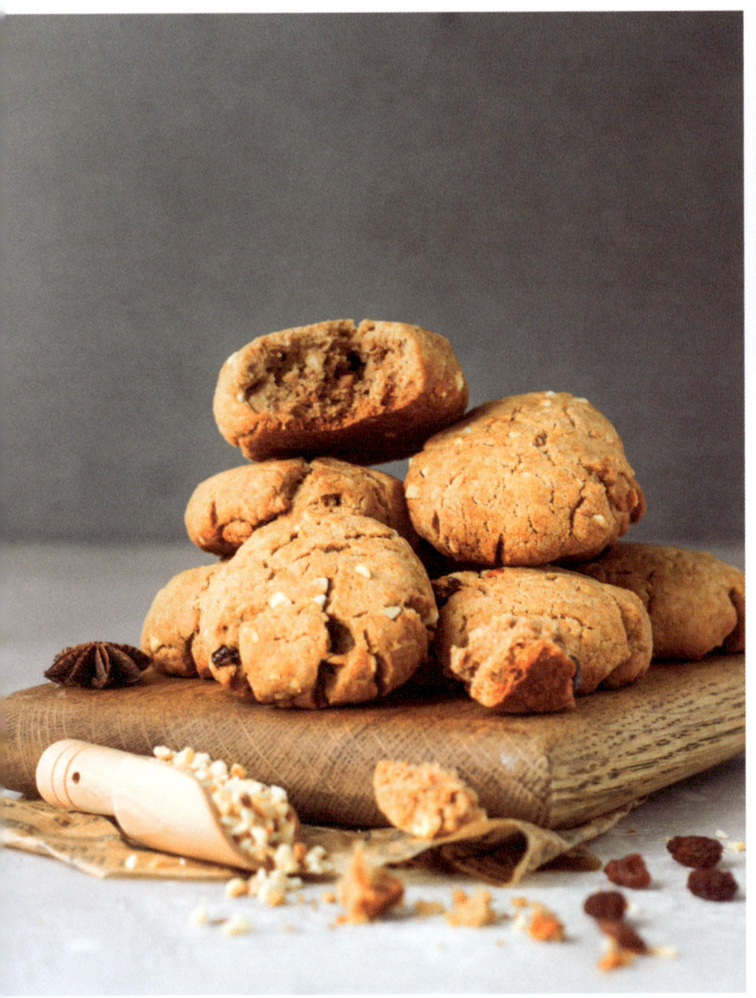

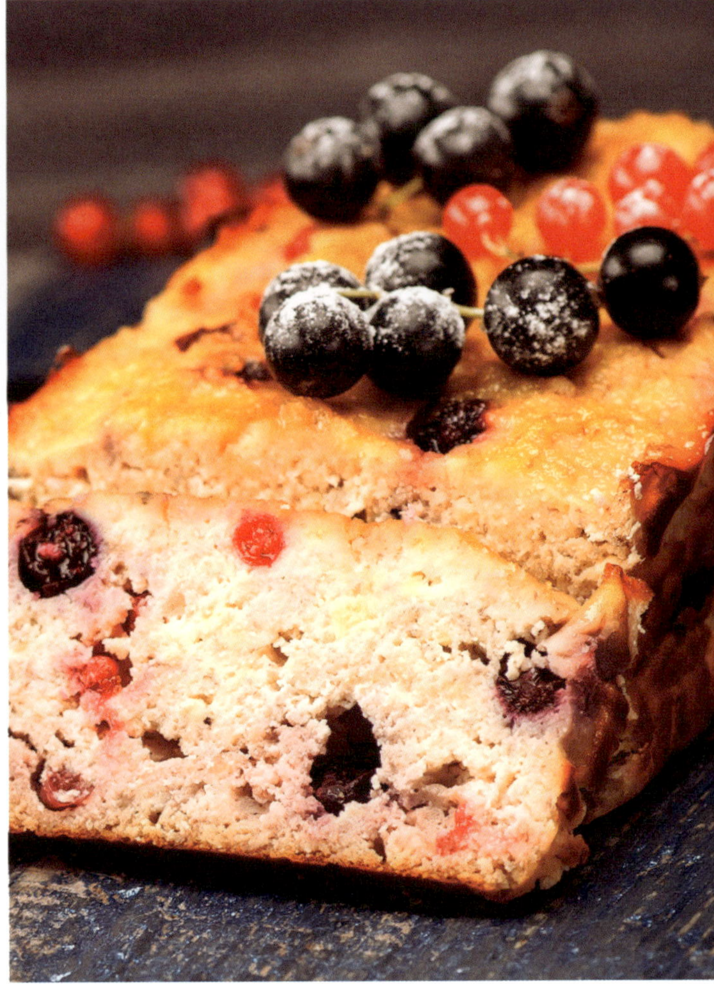

Buckwheat Raisin Biscuits

MAKES 12

PREP + COOK TIME: 20 MINS + 25 MINS CHILLING

VEG • GLUTEN FREE • DAIRY FREE

Easy Berry Cake

SERVES 4

PREP + COOK TIME: 40 MINS

VEG

BUCKWHEAT RAISIN BISCUITS

1 cup (120g) buckwheat flour
½ cup (80g) coconut sugar
⅓ cup (80ml) coconut oil, melted
2 tbsps water
1 tsp vanilla extract
½ tsp salt
½ tsp bicarbonate of soda
1 tsp apple cider vinegar
½ cup (80g) raisins
½ cup (60g) almonds, chopped

In a large bowl, stir together buckwheat flour, coconut sugar, oil, water, vanilla, salt and bicarb. Mix in vinegar.

Fold in raisins and almonds then form dough into a ball. Wrap in plastic wrap and refrigerate for 25 minutes.

Roll dough into 12 balls then press gently to flatten.

Cooking in batches if necessary, arrange biscuits in air fryer basket. Cook for 6-8 minutes at 160°C.

EASY BERRY CAKE

½ cup (155g) rice malt syrup or maple syrup
150g mascarpone cheese
2 eggs
60g butter, melted
Zest of 1 orange
1 tsp vanilla extract
⅔ cup (80g) plain flour
1 tsp baking powder
⅔ cup (80g) mixed berries
Mini loaf tin

Preheat air fryer to 180°C. Line loaf tin with greaseproof paper.

Combine syrup, mascarpone, eggs, butter, orange zest and vanilla in a large bowl. Mix well.

Add flour and baking powder and stir to combine.

Add berries and gently fold through.

Pour cake batter into prepared tin.

Place tin in air fryer and cook for 30-35 minutes or until an inserted skewer comes out clean.

Carrot Cake Cookies

MAKES 24

PREP + COOK TIME: 30 MINS + 1 HOUR CHILLING

VEG • GLUTEN-FREE

½ cup (125ml) coconut oil, room temperature

¾ cup (120g) coconut sugar

1 egg, room temperature

1 tsp vanilla extract

2¼ cups (270g) blanched almond meal

½ tsp bicarbonate of soda

½ tsp salt

1 tsp cinnamon

¼ tsp grated nutmeg

¾ cup (80g) grated carrots, excess moisture squeezed out

½ cup (60g) toasted walnuts, chopped

ICING

125g cream cheese, room temperature

¼ cup (80g) maple syrup

1 tbsp milk of choice

1 tsp vanilla extract

OPTIONAL TOPPINGS

Walnuts, almonds, pumpkin seeds

Grated orange zest

Beat together the coconut oil and coconut sugar. Add the egg and vanilla and mix until smooth. Add the almond meal, bicarb, salt, cinnamon and nutmeg. Mix well to incorporate. Fold in the grated carrots and chopped walnuts. Cover and refrigerate for at least an hour.

Preheat air fryer to 160°C.

Use a scoop to form cookies and then flatten slightly before placing in a single layer in the air fryer. Work in batches, if needed. Cook for 10-12 minutes or until just beginning to turn golden brown around the edges. Set aside to cool.

Beat the cream cheese with an electric hand mixer until softened. Add the maple syrup, milk and vanilla extract and beat until smooth.

Transfer the cream cheese icing to a small piping or bag with a star shaped nozzle. Pipe four or five lines of icing over each cooled cookie. Scatter with almonds, walnuts, pepitas and orange zest, if desired, to serve.

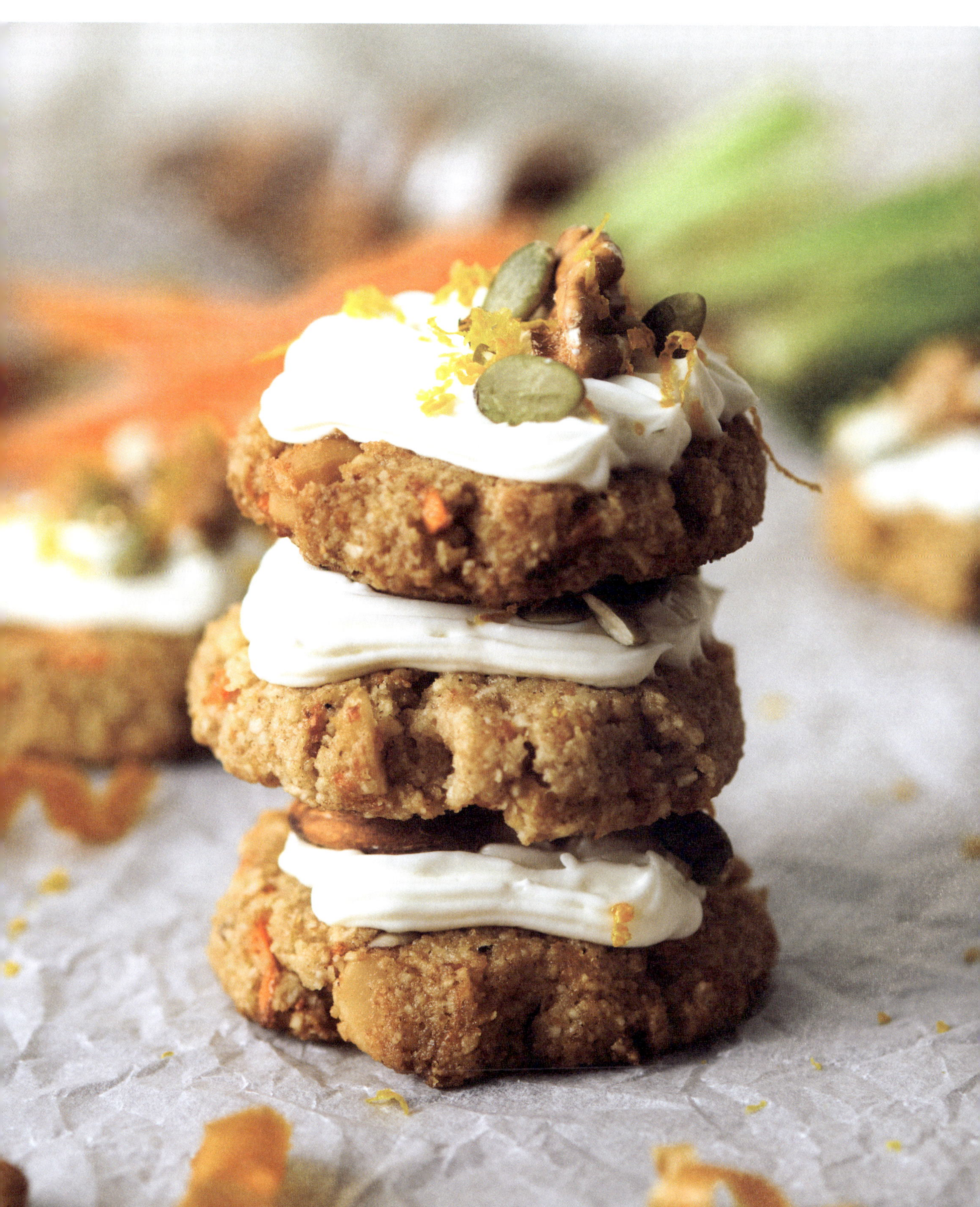

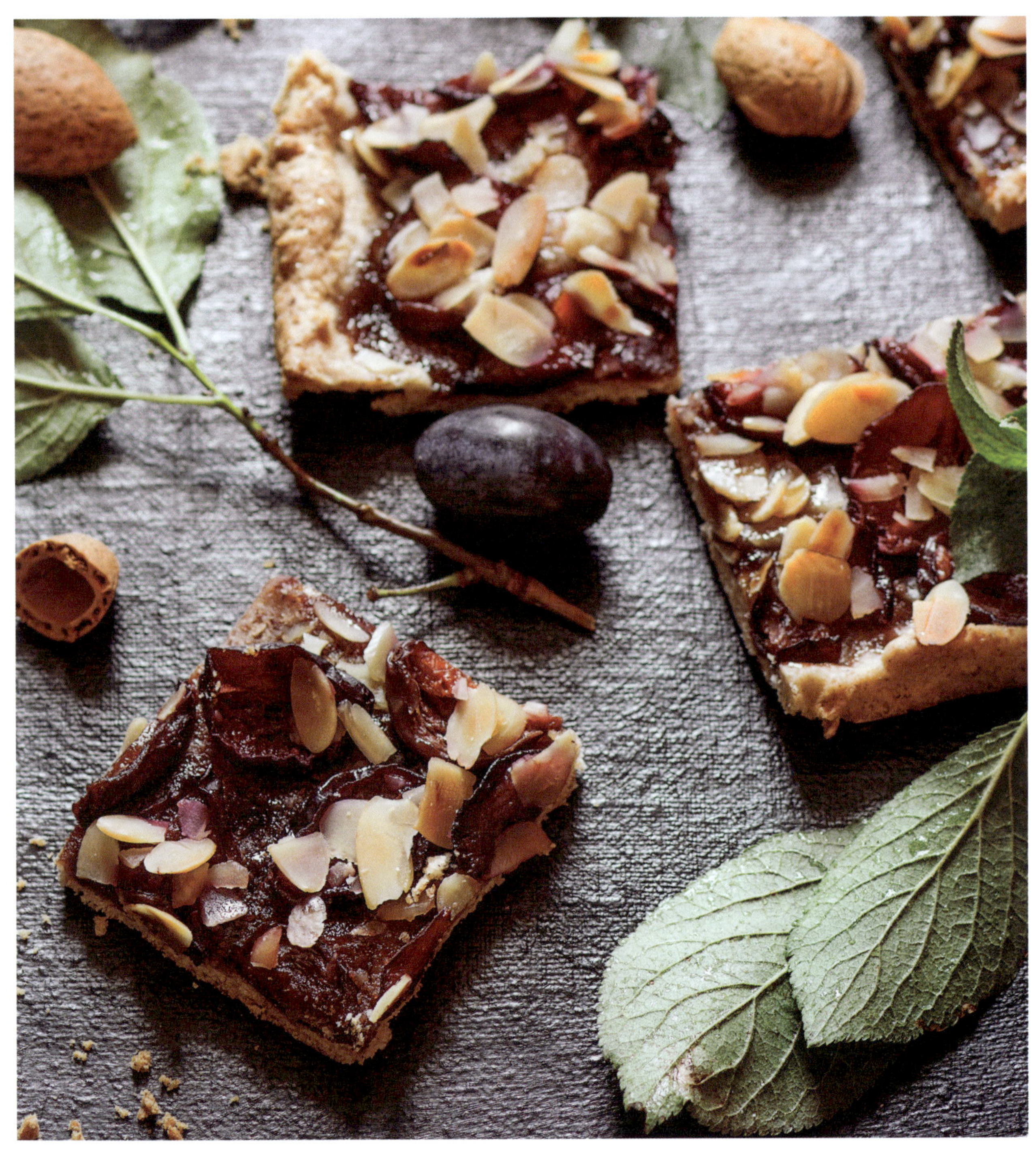

Sliced Plum & Almond Tart

SERVES 6

PREP + COOK TIME: 50 MINS

VEG • GLUTEN FREE

SLICED PLUM & ALMOND TART

ALMOND CRUST

¾ cup (90g) almond meal

¼ cup (30g) tapioca flour

1 tbsp maple syrup

⅛ tsp salt

75g cold butter, diced

1 egg

1 tsp cinnamon

FILLING

6-8 plums, sliced

1 tbsp maple syrup

1 tsp vanilla bean paste

⅓ tsp cinnamon

2-3 star anise

3 tbsps almond meal

2 tbsps milk

¼ cup (30g) flaked almonds, toasted

In a food processor, combine almond crust ingredients and pulse until the dough comes together. Form into a flattened disc, wrap in plastic wrap and place in refrigerator for 30 minutes to chill.

Meanwhile, in a bowl combine the plums, maple syrup, vanilla bean paste, cinnamon and star anise. Stir gently to combine. Set aside to marinate for 10 minutes.

Remove dough from fridge. Place dough between two sheets of greaseproof paper. Roll out to roughly 16cm in diameter. Remove top sheet of paper.

Sprinkle the almond meal into the centre of the pastry leaving a 2cm border. Top with fruit and any juice from the bowl. Brush the crust edges with milk.

Use greaseproof paper to lift tart into air fryer. Cook at 160°C for 25-30 minutes until crust is golden brown and fruit is soft.

Sprinkle with flaked almonds, cut into pieces and serve.

Churros

SERVES 4
PREP + COOK TIME: 30 MINS + 1 HOUR CHILLING
VEG

½ cup (125ml) water
45g butter, cut into cubes
1 tbsp + ¼ cup (55g) sugar
Pinch of salt
½ cup (60g) plain flour
1 egg
½ tsp vanilla extract
½ tsp ground cinnamon

Grease and line a baking tray. Set aside.

Place the water, butter, 1 tablespoon sugar and salt into a large saucepan and bring to the boil over medium heat. Reduce heat to low and gradually add the flour, stirring continuously until the batter is smooth. Remove from the heat and transfer to the mixing bowl of an electric beater or stand mixer. Let cool for a few minutes.

Next add the egg and vanilla and beat well until a sticky dough forms. Transfer to a piping bag (with a star-shaped tip) using a spatula.

Pipe the churros onto the prepared tray. Transfer to the fridge to chill for 1 hour (no more than that or the dough will become too dry).

Preheat the air fryer to 190°C.

Transfer the churros to the air fryer basket being careful not to overcrowd it. (You may need to cook in batches). Lightly spritz with cooking spray. Cook for 10 minutes until golden.

Meanwhile combine the ¼ cup sugar and the cinnamon in a shallow bowl or plate.

When churros are cooked, immediately roll them in the cinnamon sugar to fully coat.

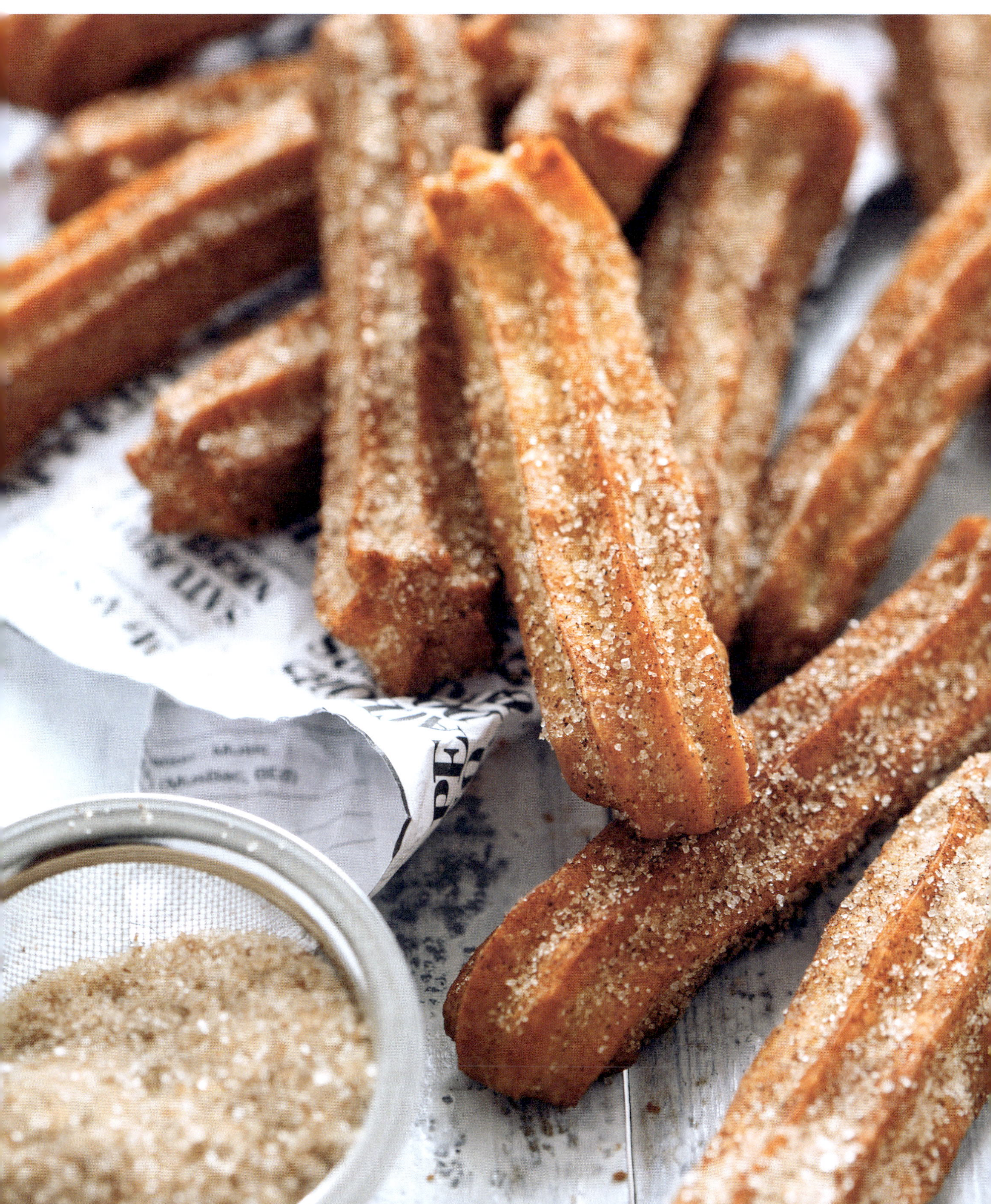

Index

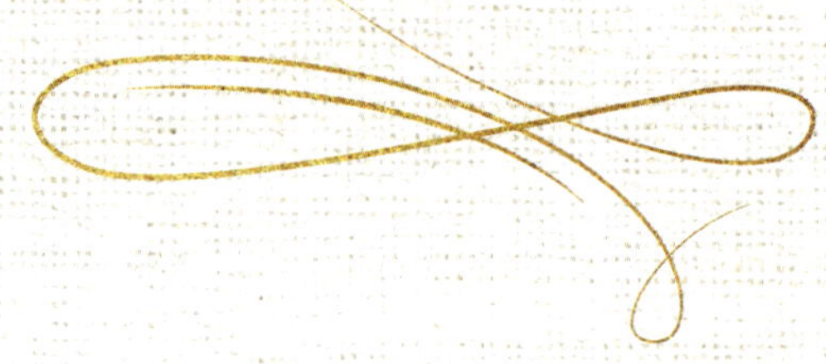

B

C

D

E

F

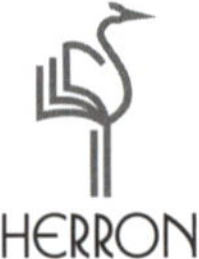

First Published in 2023 by Herron Book Distributors Pty Ltd
14 Manton St
Morningside
QLD 4170
www.herronbooks.com

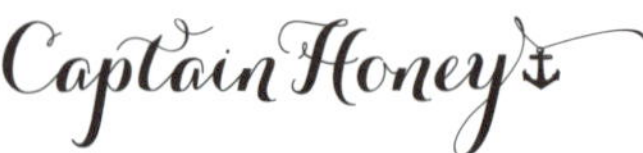

Custom book production by Captain Honey Pty Ltd
12 Station St
Bangalow
NSW 2479
www.captainhoney.com.au

Recipes in this book were previously published in: *Air Fryer* (2020), *Air Fryer Healthy* (2021), *Essential Air Fryer* (2021), *The Best Ever: Air Fryer Cookbook* (2022)

Cataloguing-in-Publication. A catalogue record for this book is available from the National Library of Australia

ISBN 978-1-922944-39-9

All images used under license from Shutterstock.com
except for pg 2 by Monika Grabkowska
Printed and bound in China

5 4 3 2 1   23 24 25 26 27

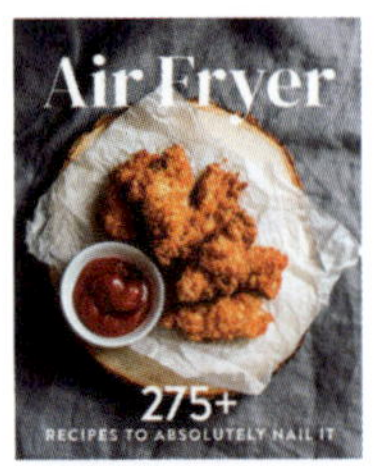

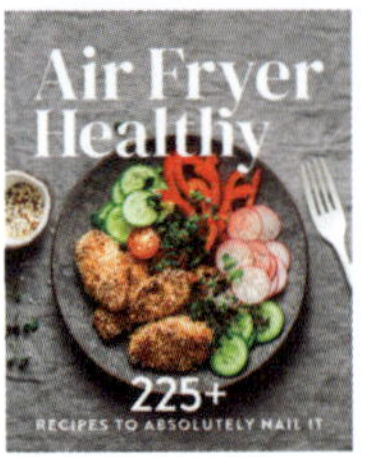

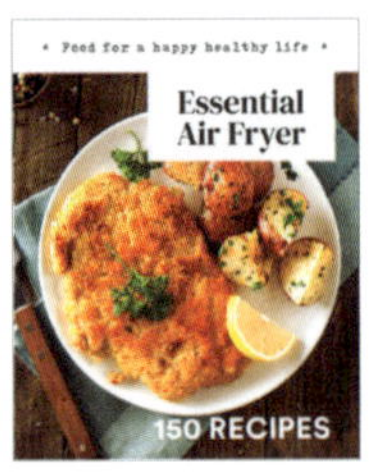

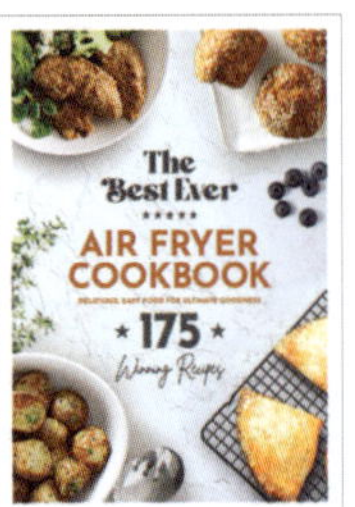

NOTE ABOUT REVIEWS

Thanks to the many customers who sent in complimentary comments about our air fryer cookbooks, or left great reviews on the websites of our key retailers like Kmart.

With thanks, we feature a few of these reviews on the back cover of this book. We appreciate your support and are excited that you loved the recipes.

NOTES FOR THE READER

All reasonable efforts have been made to ensure the accuracy of the content in this book. Information in this book is not intended as a substitute for medical advice. The author and publisher cannot and do not accept any legal duty of care or responsibility in relation to the content in this book, and disclaim any liabilities relating to its use.